P9-BIN-487

Fundamentals of Nutrition

A Series of Books in Animal Science
G. W. Salisbury, Editor

SECOND EDITION

Fundamentals of Nutrition

L. E. Lloyd
MACDONALD COLLEGE
OF MCGILL UNIVERSITY

B. E. McDonald
THE UNIVERSITY OF MANITOBA

E. W. Crampton

W. H. Freeman and Company
SAN FRANCISCO

QP
141
.C77/24,556

CAMROSE LUTHERAN COLLEGE
Library

Library of Congress Cataloging in Publication Data

Lloyd, Lewis E
    Fundamentals of nutrition.

    (A Series of books in animal science)
    Edition of 1960 by these authors, entered under
E. W. Crampton.
    Bibliography: p.
    Includes index.
    1. Nutrition. I. McDonald, Bruce Eugene, 1933–
joint author. II. Crampton, Earle Wilcox, 1895–
joint author. III. Title. [DNLM: 1. Nutrition.
QU145 C892f]
QP141.C77   1978   591.1'3   77-16029
ISBN 0-7167-0566-4

Copyright © 1959 and 1978 by W. H. Freeman and Company

No part of this book may be reproduced by any mechanical,
photographic, or electronic process, or in the form of a phono-
graphic recording, nor may it be stored in a retrieval system,
transmitted, or otherwise copied for public or private use, without written permission from the publisher.

Printed in the United States of America

9 8 7 6 5 4 3 2 1

Contents

Preface to the first edition

The specific object of this book is to integrate the basic facts concerning the nature of nutrients and of their metabolism. Thus we establish a basis for reasoning in the selection of foods and in the compounding of diets and rations adequate for the nourishment of man and animals under specified conditions.

Section I is, in a way, introductory. Its chapters present a brief consideration of the sources of energy in foodstuffs, and of the nutrients required by the animal body for its functioning; a condensed consideration of the scheme of proximate analysis most widely used in food description; an abbreviated description of the general chemical makeup of the animal body and some of its tissues, and of plants and their anatomical parts; and, finally, a few comments on tables of food composition and their use. This section includes a chapter on water and its metabolism, and a chapter on comparative anatomy of the digestive systems of man and of domestic animals as it relates to nutrition.

Section II deals with the description and metabolism of those parts of foods that supply energy to the body, viz, the carbohydrates, fats, and proteins, and ends with a brief consideration of the final common pathway of their degradation. Here we shall see something of the operation of the metabolic machinery of the body with respect to the utilization of energy.

Sections III and IV are concerned, respectively, with the vitamins and the minerals of importance in the nutrition of the body. The nature of these substances as individual nutrients and their roles as components of metabolic catalysts or regulators are discussed on a "functional" basis with a view to further elucidating the way in which the animal body performs its operational functions.

In Section V are introduced some of the quantitative aspects of nutrition. Separate chapters are devoted to consideration of animals as tools in nutrition experimentation; the quantitative description of animals or of their characteristics; the principles of the design of comparative feeding trials and the selection of appropriate criteria by which to describe the results of the imposed experimental treatments; digestibility and balance studies as methods of measuring nutritive values of foods or diets; and the determination of physiological fuel values of foods, their use, and their limitations as measures of useful energy of foods. In this section we begin to see the importance of a knowledge and an assessment of individual variability in interpreting nutritional data, and hence of the indispensable role of statistics in nutrition.

Section VI treats the nutrient needs of animals. The phenomena of growth, pregnancy, and lactation are first discussed as functions influencing nutrient demands. Then the fundamental basis for, and the computation of, the requirements of the animal body for its maintenance, activity, production, and reproduction are dealt with in some detail. Finally, the nature, uses, and limitations of feeding and dietary standards are briefly treated.

In this textbook, which is intended for students beginning their first serious consideration of the discipline of nutrition, the material is not treated exhaustively. Rather, the object has been to introduce an integrated picture of the field of nutrition and to illustrate the type of facts and figures with which the nutritionist must deal.

Wherever possible, diagrams and charts have been used to supplement the text. Such aids, of necessity, oversimplify the events they are intended to depict, and in some cases they may be expressed in terms or symbols that are not universally accepted. However, this is largely immaterial if we remember that the illustrations are intended merely to depict the plan, the scheme, the method, by which some physiological event functions or is regulated, and how or why this is of nutritional significance. Students who eventually go further in this field will not have been misled by the material as presented in this book; and at the same time those whose formal study of nutrition ends with this course may have obtained through some of the illustrations a better understanding of the functioning of the body and of its nutritional needs.

This book is not fully documented. Specific references have been given where data or direct quotation are involved, or where fundamental historical contributions are mentioned. The omission of extensive citations has been deliberate. It is the authors' view that the basic purpose of an undergraduate textbook is primarily to develop an integrated and coherent picture of the subject rather than to serve as a reference to the literature from which it has grown.

There are at least three reasons for this philosophy. First, it seems to the authors impossible to arrange for satisfactory "living" references to the literature of a discipline such as nutrition. The classical papers of course are landmarks to be noted, but the student surely must utilize current research findings in order not to miss turnings in the road of knowledge that inevitably mark the path of progress in this field. Indeed, it is to make easier the following of new developments in nutrition that such publications exist as *Nutrition Abstracts and Reviews,* published by the Commonwealth Bureau of Animal Nutrition, Rowett Research Institute, Bucksburn, Abderdeenshire, Scotland. Here is presented a continuous coverage of the scientific nutrition literature from some 600 recognized world sources that is truly up to date in the sense that most of the references appear before they are a year old.

In a field as rapidly expanding as that of nutrition it seems especially desirable that the student be directed by his instructor to pertinent current scientific literature as one means of compensating for the fact that textbooks are in some respects old before they are printed. Suggested readings appended to most of the chapters herein will enable the interested student to amplify the subject matter of this book.

Second, there may be some doubt that the references in a fully documented textbook can ever serve as a satisfactory basis on which to familiarize the undergraduate student with the work and thinking of the innumerable scientists who contribute through their research to the subject. For example, a single statement or paragraph in a chapter on some phase of the problem of cellulose utilization cannot enable the student to appreciate the position the bacteriologist holds on the nutrition team. And to document the statement would merely shift the responsibility for it from the author of the text to the research worker who originally was led by his research or philosophy to that observation. Thus, documentation of undergraduate textbooks can be carried to the point where the author appears to be more concerned with showing the sources of his specific information than in developing an integrated, informative statement of the subject matter.

Third, there is the overall problem of undergraduate teaching, especially as it applies to the discipline of nutrition. It has been the authors' experience, after many years of developing a collegiate course in this subject, that students require training in the several operations that are part and parcel of the overall utilization of scientific literature, viz: the search of published literature and the use of abstracting journals in this connection; the preparation of bibliographies in acceptable form; the writing of meaningful, precise, and brief abstracts of published scientific papers; and finally the assembly and integration of such abstracts in the preparation of scientific manuscripts for oral presentation or for publication.

This last phase of training has been introduced in the course by the authors as laboratory work which accompanies Sections I-IV, inclusive, of this text. The assignments are made individually to the students, to avoid problems of limited copies of some references, and to encourage independent effort. In this laboratory course the authors have seized the opportunity of using assignments to familiarize the student with the current literature as well as with the classical researches applicable to the subject matter as developed in this book. Such a program has proved a satisfactory solution to the problem of full documentation of the text itself. Not the least of its benefits is the opportunity it offers the instructor of interpretation of researches that warrant special consideration.

E. W. Crampton
L. E. Lloyd

Preface to the second edition

The objective of the second edition of *Fundamentals of Nutrition* remains the same as that of the original edition: to integrate the basic facts concerning the nature of nutrients, their metabolism and physiological function, and all the factors that influence the degree to which they are required by the animal body. It is still our belief that good applied nutrition depends upon fundamental knowledge of this nature.

The book is designed primarily for those students of nutrition who have completed, or are taking concurrently, a course in biochemistry. Some prior knowledge of physiology, microbiology, and genetics would be helpful, but is by no means essential. We believe that, because it covers fundamental concepts, the book can be used by students majoring in either human or animal nutrition. In the second edition, we have made a greater attempt to draw examples from both fields.

The general format of the first edition remains intact: the order of sections and chapters is the same in both editions. The revisions made in the second edition relate primarily to the content. We have completely revised the material of some chapters whereas in others the changes have been chiefly designed to clarify the presentation of the first edition.

Section I maintains its original character, and the revisions made in Chapters 1 through 6 were designed for greater clarity and precision.

Section II again deals with the metabolism of carbohydrates, fats, and proteins, and concludes with a chapter describing their interrelating biochemical pathways. Because of developments in this area of biochemistry since 1957, we have revised extensively this latter chapter, as well as those dealing with soluble carbohydrates, fats, and proteins.

Section III examines all the known vitamins, discussing the sources, physiological functions, and symptoms of deficiency of each one. We have revised the chapter describing the vitamin B complex to clarify the presentation of the material, whereas we have rewritten the chapter on the fat-soluble vitamins to incorporate recent findings in respect to vitamins A and D, and to a lesser extent, in respect to vitamins E and K.

Section IV, dealing with the various minerals and their metabolism, has been subjected to major revision. This is mainly because current evidence indicates that several of the mineral elements considered to be either possibly essential or nonessential in 1957 are in fact truly essential to the body. In particular, the number of trace elements classified as essential has doubled over the past twenty years.

Section V, which is still devoted to the quantitative aspects of nutrition, has undergone relatively minor revisions, with the exception of Chapter 24. The first edition of this chapter was devoted principally to physiological fuel values; the second edition of the chapter deals with the energy value of foods from a broader base by outlining a number of systems of describing this characteristic of foods.

Section VI investigates the nutrient needs of animals. In our revision of Chapter 27, we have deleted details about endocrinologic activity in reproduction and lactation, replacing it with information on how these conditions affect nutrient requirements. We have altered Chapters 28 and 29 primarily to clarify our presentation of energy and protein requirements, whereas we have revised considerably the final chapter on dietary or feeding standards to place greater emphasis on the philosophy, application, and value of such standards.

We would like to point out that our philosophy regarding reference lists, which we outlined in the foreword to the first edition, applies to the second edition as well. We still believe that "viable" references should be provided by the instructor of the course in which this text is used. Notwithstanding this position, we have updated the suggested readings by including new references that we consider to be of key value.

Throughout the second edition, quantitative data are given in metric units, except where reference has been made to actual research data that were expressed originally in avoirdupois units. Because of the stated intention of many countries to convert to the SI system of measurement, we seriously considered using the joule in place of the calorie. However, the complete replacement of the calorie seemed premature and the expression of both units throughout the book seemed cumbersome. For these reasons we retained the calorie system; however, the method of converting calories to joules is described in Chapter 24.

The use of "boxes" throughout the second edition is an innovation we hope will prove useful and interesting to the reader. These boxes are of two types: one describes some application of the fundamental problem being discussed; the other provides a brief biographical description of an individual who contributed in a direct way to the subject matter under consideration. This diversion from the basic instructive material of the book is designed to stimulate the reader to a wider perusal of subjects related to each topic.

L. E. Lloyd
B. E. McDonald
E. W. Crampton

Section I
INTRODUCTION

The subject of nutrition concerns the nature of foods and food nutrients, and the needs of humans and animals for these substances. In order to deal with such matters we must be able to describe foods in such a way that they can be usefully compared for nutritional value. Similarly, we must be able to describe the animal body itself, in particular its operation as a metabolic machine. Plants also are biological machines, built of the same chemical units as animals. Since the foods of animals consist of plants as well as of other animals (or their tissues), we shall find that the same general scheme can be used to describe both animals and their foods.

The physical organization, the anatomy, of an animal affects its nutritional needs, and we must therefore know something of the "architecture" of the body.

Of rather special importance in the subject matter which introduces nutrition proper is an understanding of the fundamental role played by water in the metabolic economy of the animal body. The cells which collectively make up the metabolic machine are, except for the skeleton and the epidermal tissues, watery (lyophilic) gels. Indeed, the body is 50%–90% water, the amount depending partly on its physiological age; and continual maintenance of the normal concentration of water is more critical to the survival of an animal than the provision of an exact supply of most other nutrients. From an entirely different viewpoint, not only is water a diluent of other nutrients in foodstuffs, but its concentration largely determines their stability in storage. Consequently, a whole chapter in this section has been devoted to water and its several roles in nutrition.

Thus, the contents of Section I consist of bits of material which at the outset may seem unrelated in any logical sequence to one another, but which are nevertheless intimately related to nutrition.

Chapter 1
Nutrition defined

Nutrition had its beginning as an art, the foundations of which were a blend of instinct, habit, experience, folklore, and conjecture. By the term *instinct* we refer to "congenital attributes of the mind which are distinct from habit, and which impel an animal under certain circumstances to act in a certain way without previous experience."[*] There is no escape from the premise that instinctive reactions are congenital. Darwin believed that instincts gradually change by the elimination through natural selection of those that discourage the survival of a species, and by the hereditary continuance, with genetic modification, of those that help the species to adapt to a changing environment.[†]

The instinctive reactions to hunger are present at birth in all animals. Young animals seem instinctively to eat almost anything they can get into their mouths, so that an important concern of nutrition at this stage is to make them distinguish food from inedible material. For example, in a modern method of pig raising the youngsters are weaned before two weeks of age; sometimes they are then confined in warm pens bedded with sawdust and fitted with containers of dry meal. In a matter of a few hours they will begin to seek food, but, having no judgment about food, they are as likely to start eating the sawdust as the meal. If this happens, the bedding must be removed so that the only material they can get into their mouths is the meal and they

---

[*]*Cambridge Encyclopedia*, The Cambridge Society Ltd., Montreal (1932).
[†]Darwin, C., *The Origin of Species*, A. L. Burt Co., N.Y. (1859).

form the habit of going to the feeder to satisfy their hunger. In a day or two the bedding can be replaced, since the pigs will have learned where their feed is to be found.

Learning by experience is likely to be slow and perhaps painful, and one of the objectives of the "art" of nutrition is to direct the selection of food and to establish desirable eating habits. Dietitians and animal feeders are continually faced with the problem of dealing with beliefs and prejudices about foods and their use that have arisen as explanations for customary eating habits and feeding practices. For example, science may prove that butter, vegetable shortenings, and lard can be nutritionally equivalent, and food technology may make them physically indistinguishable, but it will be the artfulness of the dietitian (or the force of practical economics) that will persuade the public to make these products really interchangeable in the diet. Traditionally, vegetable oils are for salad dressings, lard is for pie crust and cakes, and butter is for the table. In the minds of the diehards they may be substituted in one direction but not in the other.

Before people moved about the world so widely, and before foods were shipped so easily, it was possible without a knowledge of nutrients to gain enough practical experience in feeding to become a highly successful dietitian or livestock feeder. Such persons were indeed skilled artisans, and within the normal range of their experience they got along very well.

The chemist enters the field of nutrition

Nutrition remained essentially an art until the chemist became interested in the nature of foods. One of the first advances was the description of foods in terms of chemical entities or groups of entities with unique nutritive properties. This paved the way for the discoveries that not all foods contain every necessary nutrient and that in most foods the proportions of the various nutrients are inadequate to the body's needs. Consequently, it was learned that by appropriate combinations of foods the assortment of nutrients in the diet could be made to approximate the body's needs.

This was a period of rapid strides in nutritional knowledge. It was the beginning of the era of scientific feeding. It had its share of growing pains, but fact was steadily being separated from conjecture as nutrients became better characterized and the needs of the body became more fully understood.

The physiologist, endocrinologist, and microbiologist join the team

Increasing knowledge of the needs of the animal was the result of an increasing interest by the physiologist in the workings of the nutritional machinery.

The elucidation of the physiology of such functions as digestion, muscle movement, reproduction, and lactation, especially when it included the pertinent chemistry, began to make it possible to relate diet to health and performance. Some nutritional deficiency states could now be assigned causes, and be corrected by amending the diet.

The important role of the endocrine system in regulating, and of the enzyme systems in catalyzing, the metabolic processes involved in the utilization of the energy and the nutrients of food became apparent when the endocrinologist and the enzymologist joined the nutrition team. The discovery that the enzymes themselves consisted of specific combinations of amino acids, and that their coenzymes and cofactors in the functioning systems were often vitamins and/or mineral elements, made clear why these nutrients had to be present in nutritionally adequate rations.

At this stage nutritionists had a working knowledge of at least

25 carbohydrates

15 fatty acids

20 amino acids

13 mineral elements

20 vitamins

as sources of energy or as essential agents in metabolism.

Still there were embarrassing gaps in nutritional knowledge. The marked difference between carnivora, omnivora, and herbivora in their ability to make use of foods of high cellulose content, and the variability between individuals within these groups, have brought into prominence the nutritional role of intestinal microorganisms. It has been clearly shown that rations offered to the host animal must be adequate for the nourishment of its symbiotic population of microflora, and that some apparent control of harmful species of microorganisms can be accomplished by including antibiotics in the rations. Nutrition thus has expanded into the field of microbiology.

Genetics and mathematics

Finally, we must not forget that both the geneticist and the mathematician (statistician) play important, though sometimes indirect, roles in the field of nutrition: no small fraction of the variation among animals in their response to food is genetic—a fact that must be considered in interpreting nutritional research; and the conduct of efficient research and the analysis and description of the findings have made the statistician an indispensable member of the nutrition fraternity. Only with an adequate appraisal of the inevitable variability between individuals can we interpret our observations and arrive at valid conclusions.

The discipline of nutrition

In dictionary terms, nutrition is "the series of processes by which an organism takes in and assimilates food for promoting growth and replacing worn or injured tissues." If we now attempt to think of a field of knowledge broad enough to embrace the subject matter included in Webster's innocent-sounding definition and try to describe it in terms of the several recognized branches of learning mentioned in the preceding paragraphs, we may envision animal nutrition (as distinct from plant nutrition) as a montage of several biological disciplines grouped around the age-old arts of homemaking and husbandry, as in Figure 1.1. In the case of human nutri-

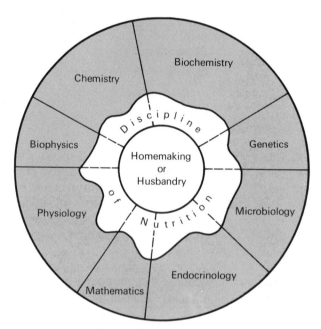

Figure 1.1
The discipline of nutrition.

tion, consideration also must be given to the social sciences. For example, it is generally recognized that the eating habits of population groups may have a cultural origin, that the socioeconomic status of families may influence their choice of foods, and that psychological factors may play a fundamental role in an individual's food consumption pattern.

Such a representation of the subject matter of nutrition gives a clue to the formal training that a qualified nutritionist must anticipate receiving. This is not to say that he must be master of all, or even qualified equally in each of the subjects. Nevertheless, he must have some working understanding of the contributions to be expected from each of these disciplines. Another fact is demonstrated by this diagram: a nutritionist may have started out as a chemist, a physiologist, a geneticist, a husbandman, or a dietitian, so that he may retain a special interest in some particular aspect of the subject. The area covered by nutrition is now so broad that no one can expect to be an authority in all of its branches. Most of the nutrition research of today is done by collaborative effort. The facts are concisely expressed by the comment that nutritionists "no longer hunt alone."

If Figure 1.1 represents a valid concept of the biological and physical components of the discipline of nutrition, it is evident that to understand the nature of the nutrients themselves, to grasp the way in which they perform their roles, to perceive the consequences of their deficiency or of their imbalance in the diet, and to be able to prepare nutritionally adequate diets it is necessary to call upon subject matter ordinarily considered a part of chemistry, biochemistry, physiology, endocrinology, microbiology, or biophysics. Because of genetic variability among animals, statistics frequently is needed to interpret observations in which both genetic and nutritional factors are involved.

Obviously it is impossible in a textbook on nutrition to cover all of these disciplines in depth. However, none of them can be ignored because they are in fact the foundation upon which nutrition rests.

Chapter 2
The nutrients and their proximate analysis

We shall be concerned with those substances that the animal* body utilizes, either as sources of energy or as parts of its metabolic machinery. These substances are called nutrients, and this chapter is devoted to naming and grouping them according to their general chemical nature, which is the basis of the most widely used scheme for the nutritional description of foods.

Nutrient versus energy

The animal is a machine in the sense that it requires for its operation an assortment of "parts," a complement of catalysts, and a supply of substances as sources of energy. Substances used in the body for energy are often referred to as nutrients, but *energy itself is not a nutrient*. Rather it is a property that some nutrients possess. For example, starch is a nutrient only because it is a potential source of energy. It loses its identity almost immediately after being ingested, and eventually is completely degraded to carbon dioxide and water, having yielded its energy little by little in its passage through the metabolic machine. Its path is fascinating to follow, as we shall see. But it is like coal or oil in an internal combustion engine: it is useful only as fuel. There are a number of nutrients of this type.

---

*We shall often refer to the animal, the animal body, or the requirements of the animal. In all cases not otherwise indicated, the term *animal* is used in contrast to *plant*, and not to distinguish between humans and other animals, because the metabolic machinery is essentially the same in the human, in the farm animal, and in the laboratory rodent.

Other nutrients are useful in an entirely different way. They yield no appreciable energy to the body, but can be found in the body or its fluids by chemical analysis. They are destroyed only after their usefulness as chemical entities is past, and even then they can be identified in excretory products. Thus, calcium remains as calcium, or as a recognizable compound of it, from ingestion to excretion; it performs its function by virtue of being calcium. Also in this category are amino acids, vitamins, and mineral elements. Some of these may perform their functions almost independently, but they are usually found combined into complex molecules, such as enzymes or hormones.

Then there are a few nutrients that perform specific roles, but, when present in excess of requirements, the surpluses may be used as sources of energy. Such surpluses when used for energy become impossible to identify as to specific origin. Fats, proteins, and the 5-carbon sugar ribose fall into this third grouping. Some fat is required to supply the essential fatty acids, but most of the fat of the diet is used merely as fuel. On the other hand, proteins, as packages of amino acids, are ordinarily so expensive that they are eaten or fed only in amounts sufficient to ensure adequate supplies of needed amino acids. Surpluses of protein therefore are normally incidental and relatively small, and they contribute only a minor part of the body's energy requirement.

The sugar ribose is part of deoxyribonucleic acid (DNA), which accounts for 10%–15% of the dry weight of cell nuclei. DNA is normally found only in cell nuclei, where it is associated with chromosomes. Indeed, in a given species individual cells contain DNA in proportion to the number of chromosomes in the cell. DNA is made up of coiled chains of nucleotides, each containing one or another of the bases adenine, guanine, cytosine, or thymine, a molecule of deoxyribose, and a phosphate ester.

In addition, all nuclei contain 2%–20% (dry weight) of ribonucleic acid (RNA). The two substances DNA and RNA are essential and major parts of chromosome structure. Nucleoli, found at specific points along the chromosomes, are incased in an elastic membrane of a lipid nature and they also contain high concentrations of ribonucleoprotein. It is obvious then that the sugar ribose, being a part of the reproductive machinery of the animal, is an indispensable structural element of the body.

When used as fuel, nutrients are functionally nonspecific. That is, the amount of energy that such nutrients yield may differ somewhat, but the body uses the energy from one source or from another without preference once the molecule has been digested and absorbed. Thus, once digested, simple and compound sugars, the more complex starches, and the celluloses are practically equivalent sources of energy.

Similarly, while surplus proteins differ from surplus fats in the amount of energy yielded per gram of digested nutrient, the nutrients within each of these categories are about equal in energy value.

The problem of describing nutrients

To understand the basis of dietary requirements and the practical problems of ration formulation, we need some scheme of describing nutrients qualitatively and quantitatively. For entities such as mineral elements or specific amino acids or vitamins—indeed, for all nutrients that are physiologically specific in function—we can and shall use for descriptive purposes the accepted chemical names of the substances. But in the case of nutrients that are of interest only as sources of energy, the separate naming of each is unnecessarily cumbersome and in practice impracticable. We shall resort to considering such materials in groups, each of which can be characterized by some chemical property.

For example, sugars, starches, and cellulose consist chemically of carbon, hydrogen, and oxygen, the last two always in the same proportion as in water. Such materials are called *carbohydrates.* Sometimes there is reason to subdivide this broad group into the structurally course cellulose-like components, called *crude fiber,* and the other carbohydrates, called *nitrogen-free extract.*

Similarly, the amino acids as normally found in most foods are combined into *proteins;* and as a group, proteins are alike in that they all consist of about 16% nitrogen (by weight). It is then feasible and sufficiently accurate for our purpose in considering the first principles of nutrition to estimate the amount of protein in a food by multiplying the chemically determined amount of nitrogen by the factor 6.25. In foods and in the body there may be other nitrogen-containing substances, such as nucleic acids; our method of estimating the amount of protein includes such molecules, and thus we are really expressing the total of all nitrogen-containing molecules in terms of their protein equivalent. But this error is not usually important, especially if we are concerned mainly with the energy value of the protein portion of the food.

The fatty substances that are potential sources of energy for the body are numerous, and to determine them separately would ordinarily not yield enough extra useful information to make the fuller analysis worthwhile in the routine description of foods. When used in the body for their energy, all of the common neutral fats are digested and metabolized in a similar fashion and yield essentially the same quantity of energy per gram. Their molecules are all soluble in ether, and this common property is used to determine their total concentration in foods. They are thus logically described as *ether extract.* There may be small amounts of other ether-soluble materials in some foods, so the amount of ether extract is not a precise measure of neutral fat content, but it is a good enough estimate for a general description of foods.

Another shortcut used in the nutritional description of foods is to lump all the inorganic substances together under the general heading of *ash.* This simplifying device is not employed when the intent is to describe any nutritionally important inorganic nutrients. Rather, its purpose is to make possible, in lieu of any direct chemical determination, the estimation of the amount of carbohydrate by difference.

The Weende food analysis scheme

Henneberg and Stohmann, working at the Weende Experiment Station in Germany, devised in 1865 a scheme for the routine description of animal feedstuffs. It is now commonly referred to as the *Weende analysis* or the *proximate analysis*. At that time the nutritionally important components of protein had not been recognized, all neutral fats were considered to be nonspecific sources of energy, and vitamins were unknown. However, the multiplicity of the carbohydrates and the practical difficulties of their separate chemical determination were clearly recognized. These workers believed that for nutritional description the carbohydrates could be grouped into (1) the starches and the sugars, and (2) a coarse fibrous fraction. The latter they isolated as an insoluble residue after boiling the food sample first with dilute acid and then with dilute alkali. These procedures were intended to simulate the acidic gastric digestion and the subsequent alkaline intestinal digestion of ingested food. The insoluble residue they called *crude fiber*.

With analytical figures for ether extract, ash, nitrogen, and crude fiber of a moisture-free food sample, they needed only to convert the value for nitrogen to its equivalent in terms of protein (i.e., N × 6.25), add to this the other three group values, and subtract the total from the original weight of dry sample, thus *by difference* to arrive at an estimate of the "soluble carbohydrates." This fraction they called *nitrogen-free extract* (NFE).

The majority of foods in human diets, as well as those in the diets of some laboratory animals used in nutrition studies, are so low in crude fiber that this fraction can often be disregarded, and the custom has gradually become general, especially in human nutrition, to omit the crude fiber determination. When this is done it is the *total* carbohydrate that is estimated "by difference."

Other components of nitrogen-free extract   Probably because the chief components of nitrogen-free extract (NFE) are sugars and starches, we are prone to forget that this fraction includes all the nonfibrous, ether-insoluble, water-soluble organic materials of the food (or other material analyzed). Thus all water-soluble vitamins must be included in this fraction. Quantitatively, the vitamins are an insignificant part of the NFE, but in any broad charting of the makeup of foods in terms of the Weende partition these vitamins are part of the NFE in the same way that the fat-soluble vitamins are part of ether extract.

Being determined by difference, the figure for NFE is also subject to an appreciable but variable error that may be as large as the algebraic sum of any analytical and/or sampling errors of each of those fractions determined by direct analysis.

Variability of average Weende analysis values It is appropriate at this point to comment on the errors to be expected in numerical values obtained from the several parts of the Weende analysis. These arise from several sources. Errors in the chemical manipulations—that is, analyst's errors—are usually negligible. Sampling errors, however, are often large because foods and the residues of animal digestion are not usually homogeneous. In addition, different lots of foods called by the same name are seldom identical in "proximate" makeup. Consequently, average composition figures found in tables of food composition are not necessarily applicable to a particular lot of a foodstuff.

Nevertheless, it is often more feasible to estimate the protein, or the fat, or the carbohydrate, of some particular lot of a foodstuff by referring to tables of average composition than to obtain specific values by analysis. When average values are used in this way it should be remembered that the composition figures given for natural foods may be subject to coefficients of variation such as those listed in Table 2.1.

Table 2.1
Coefficients of variation applicable to fractions of the Weende analysis of food

Fractions	*Coefficients of variation (%)*
Crude protein	8
Ether extract	15
Crude fiber	12
Nitrogen-free extract	3

For example, if the average crude protein content of corn meal is given in a table as 10%, it is probable that two samples out of three purchased at random would on analysis give values between 9.2 [10 minus 10 (8%)] and 10.8 [10 plus 10(8%)] percent protein (see Figure 2.1). Similarly, corn meal may average 72% NFE, and hence two samples out of three might be expected to give values between 69.8% and 74.2% (that is, 72 ± 3%).

Importance of the Weende analysis The Weende scheme of food analysis is the basis for the description of foods reported in the usual tables of food composition. With appropriate adjustment for water content of products as purchased or as eaten, it is also a common basis for purchasing food and

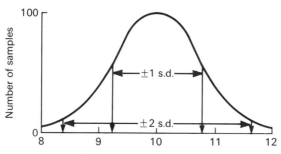

Figure 2.1
Distribution of samples as to protein content of food A, which by analysis shows an average protein content of 10% with a coefficient of variation of ±8% (see Chapter 21). Two samples out of three can be expected to contain 9.2%–10.8% of protein, while ninety-five out of a hundred contain 8.4%–11.6%.

for formulating rations. In addition, the determination of the Weende fractions is frequently the starting point for more detailed analysis for specific nutrients.

Above all, it partitions all biological materials, including foods, feces, urine, and body tissues and fluids, into fractions, or *proximate principles,* that the chemist, the physiologist, the bacteriologist, the dietitian, the husbandman, and the food or feed processor continually refer to in connection with the products and processes having to do with the nourishment of the animal body.

The Weende proximate analysis as a "chemical" procedure is set out in flow sheet form in Figure 2.2. In the first step, the sample of food (or other biological material to be analyzed) is oven dried. The loss in weight during drying measures, of course, the moisture content of the original material. The dried sample is then subsampled to obtain three portions. One is extracted with dry diethyl ether. The extract is then heated to drive off the solvent, and the residue is weighed as ether extract; or the loss in weight of the sample as a result of the ether treatment can be taken as the measure of the ether extract. When this method is followed, the fat-free residue may be ignited. The incombustible material remaining will be the "ash" of the sample.

The second subsample is subjected to Kjeldahl procedure in order to determine its nitrogen content. This value is multiplied by the factor 6.25 to obtain a figure for *crude protein.*

The third subsample is boiled for 30 minutes in dilute sulfuric acid and filtered; the residue is boiled in dilute sodium hydroxide. The still insoluble material is filtered off, dried, and weighed as crude fiber plus ash. Loss on ignition is then crude fiber, and the residue is ash. This ash figure should not be used as a measure of mineral content because variable amounts of inorganic material may be found in both the acid and the alkali filtrate.

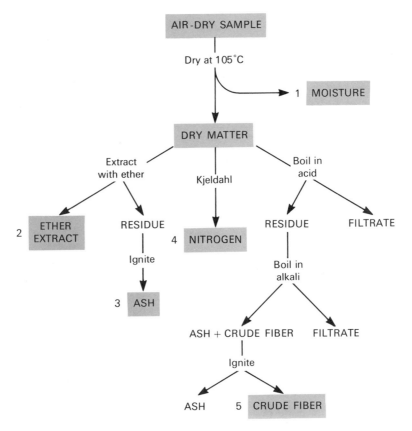

Figure 2.2
The Weende proximate analysis.

Nutrient makeup of proximate principles

Before leaving this subject we should specifically relate to the proximate analysis the several nutrients with which we shall be dealing in this book. We shall thus also delimit the extent to which the Weende scheme can be expected usefully to describe specific nutrients and groups of nutrients found in the animal body and in its food.

Carbohydrates   The total number of edible materials that are carbohydrate by definition is large. There are, for example, a dozen or more that are found in everyday foods, either as one of six or seven "sweet" sugars, or in combinations of them comprising numerous more complex molecules such as the starches, hemicelluloses, or celluloses. The monosaccharide sugars are classified according to the number of carbon atoms in their molecules. Thus there are 5-carbon or pentose sugars, and 6-carbon or hexose sugars. All pentose sugars have the same empirical formula, $C_5H_{10}O_5$; the empirical formula of all hexoses is $C_6H_{12}O_6$. The complex carbohydrates are merely polymers of the simple sugar units, as $(C_5H_8O_4)_n$ or $(C_6H_{10}O_5)_n$. Cellulose, for example, has been estimated to consist of 1000–2000 hexose units polymerized into the long fibrous chains characteristic of the cellulose structure. The distribution of the carbohydrates between the Weende nitrogen-free extract and crude fiber fractions is shown in Table 2.2.

It will be seen that the carbohydrate portion of our foods and feeds consists either of single 5-carbon or 6-carbon units, or of larger molecules formed by combinations of such structures. Before the larger molecules can be useful in nourishing the body they all must be degraded by enzymes in the digestive tract to their simple 5- or 6-carbon units; or, in the case of cellulose and perhaps of some of the hemicelluloses, to either the 2-, 3-, or 4-carbon molecules of acetic, propionic, or butyric acids, respectively. (These three

Table 2.2
Some common carbohydrates of foods and their distribution
between the Weende nitrogen-free extract and crude fiber fractions

Classification	Name	Monosaccharide unit	Reaction to Weende fiber procedure	Fraction of feed in which found by Weende analysis
Monosaccharides (single saccharide unit)	Arabinose Xylose Ribose etc.	$C_5H_{10}O_5$	Completely soluble	Nitrogen-free extract
	Fructose Galactose Glucose Mannose etc.	$C_6H_{12}O_6$		
Oligosaccharides (2–10 saccharide units)*	Lactose Sucrose Raffinose etc.	$(C_6H_{10}O_5)_n$		
Polysaccharides (over 10 saccharide units)	Glycogen Starch	$(C_6H_{10}O_5)_n$		
	Hemicellulose Pectin	$(C_5H_8O_4)_n$ $(C_6H_{10}O_5)_n$, Hexuronic	Partially but variably soluble†	Crude fiber
	Cellulose	$(C_6H_{10}O_5)_n$		

*Only disaccharides are nutritionally important.
†According to van Soest and McQueen [*Proc. Nutr. Soc.* **32**(1973):123], sequential extraction with acid and alkali removes about 80% of the hemicellulose and 20%–50% of the cellulose. Lignin, although not strictly a carbohydrate, frequently is grouped with the crude fiber fraction in the Weende analysis. However the above authors claim that only 10%–50% of the lignin remains in the crude fiber fraction.

acids are products of digestion by microflora inhabiting the digestive system of animals, such as herbivores.)

The nutritional significance of the fact that carbohydrates are all assemblies of 5- or 6-carbon units is that they have potentially about the same energy value, roughly between 3.75 and 4.25 kilocalories per gram of dry substance. Except for small amounts of ribose, carbohydrates can be considered useful primarily as sources of energy. These facts make it clear that even though the carbohydrate portion of a food or a diet is estimated "by difference" in the Weende scheme of analysis, little, if any, useful information is lost by this group treatment.

The digestible or the metabolizable energy the body ultimately obtains from the nitrogen-free extract, from the crude fiber, or from the total carbohydrate (i.e., the nitrogen-free extract plus the crude fiber) of a food, is a somewhat different matter, since the completeness of the digestion of these two groups of carbohydrates is often appreciably different. This matter will be considered later when the question of digestibility is dealt with. For the moment it will suffice to note that celluloses and hemicelluloses yield less useful energy to nonherbivores than do the carbohydrates of the nitrogen-free extract category.

Crude protein   *Crude protein* is also a group name; it refers collectively to the sum of up to 20 nutrients, the amino acids, each of which has one or more specific roles in metabolism. In addition, each of these protein components, if present in excess of that needed for its specific function, may, following absorption, be split into a nitrogen-containing entity NH_3 and a deaminized residue, the latter becoming a nonspecific source of energy.

Most of the amino acid residues that can be metabolized for energy contain 3-carbon atoms. In any case, only that fraction of an amino acid that is equivalent to some intermediate in the metabolism of sugars (or of fats) is so used. However, the potential energy in proteins, as measured by their complete combustion in a bomb calorimeter, is considerably greater than that in carbohydrates. This is true because with protein, oxygen is required not only to oxidize the carbon, but, unlike carbohydrate, is required also to oxidize some of the hydrogen atoms; and the heat of water formation is much higher than that of carbon dioxide. Thus, typical pure proteins yield 5.25–5.75 kilocalories of gross energy per gram.

Nevertheless, the amount of *nutritionally useful* energy of protein is not greatly different from that of carbohydrate. This is so because the amino group that is split off in the deaminization of each "discarded" amino acid forms urea, which is eliminated in the urine. Urea,

$$NH_2—C—NH_2$$
$$\overset{\|}{O}$$

contains combustible carbon and hydrogen, and this part of the potential energy from protein is lost the the body. In humans it amounts to about 1.25 kilocalories per gram of protein, so that the maximum usable energy from typical protein does not exceed 5.50 − 1.25 or 4.25 kilocalories per gram; this is usually reduced further by the incompleteness of digestion to about 4 kilocalories per gram. This can be stated in another way: whereas carbohydrate yields to the body, on the average, about 95% of its potential energy, only some 70% of the potential energy of protein can be used to meet energy needs. Protein is obviously not normally the preferred source of energy in nutrition.

Box 2.1   The van Soest method for fiber determination

The generally unsatisfactory nature of the Weende method for estimating the crude fiber content of foods and feeds has been recognized for many years. Boiling with dilute acid and with dilute alkali, which is taken to simulate gastric and intestinal digestion, frequently bears little relationship to the availability of complex carbohydrate determined by digestibility studies with animals. Although many attempts have been made to modify the crude fiber method or to devise new methods, until recently few approaches have proven satisfactory. Not all of the problems encountered in describing the less-available portion of foods of plant origin are analytical. There are conflicting opinions about what constitutes plant fiber. In addition, hemicellulose, cellulose, and lignin differ in chemical composition and biological availability among different plant species and within different constituents from the same plant. Methods of describing the fiber fraction in plant foods that have received fairly widespread acceptance are those based on the use of neutral and acid detergents to separate the various constituents of the cell wall.

Much of the early work on the use of detergents in the analysis of fiber was carried out by P. J. van Soest and his colleagues at the Animal Husbandry Research Division, United States Department of Agriculture, Beltsville, Maryland. These workers have devised procedures for determining the amount of neutral-detergent residue*, which represents the cell-wall constituents of the plant, and for determining the amount of acid-detergent fiber†, which is comprised primarily of cellulose and lignin, in plant materials. These detergent procedures permit estimation not only of the total amount of cell-wall material in a feedstuff, but of the relative proportions of hemicellulose, cellulose, and lignin contained in the cell walls‡.

*van Soest, P. J., and Wine, R. H. *J. Assoc. Off. Agric. Chem.* **50**(1967):50.
†van Soest, P. J. *J. Assoc. Off. Agric. Chem.* **46**(1963):829.
‡van Soest, P. J., and McQueen, R. W. *Proc. Nutr. Soc.* **32**(1973):123.

Incidentally, crude protein, by itself, describes only the energy of this nitrogenous fraction of foods. Without other information the figure for the amount of crude protein in a food gives no reliable clue to the makeup of its nutrient units, the amino acids. Of these acids we shall learn more later. It is sufficient here to tabulate them as some of the nutrients that we must deal with in nutrition (see Table 2.3).

Table 2.3
The amino acids of foods classified according to their indispensability in the diet of adult humans

Dispensable	Semi-dispensable	Indispensable
Glutamic acid	Arginine	Lysine
Aspartic acid	Glycine	Tryptophan
Alanine	Histidine*	Phenylalanine
Serine	Proline	Methionine
Hydroxyproline	Cystine	Threonine
	Tyrosine	Leucine
		Isoleucine
		Valine

*Histidine is essential for growing infants; according to a recent study [Kopple, J. D., and Swendseid, M. E., *Fed. Proc.* **33**(1973):671A], it may also be essential for adult humans.

Lipids, fats, and ether extract   In a beginning course in nutrition there is a tendency to use almost interchangeably the terms *lipid, fat,* and *ether extract.* In particular, when we record the total of the ether extractives, we often designate it merely as *fat.* This rather loose usage of these terms does not often lead us astray, for reasons that will in due course become obvious. But it may be well at the outset to define these terms in a more specific way, in order to have a clearer conception of what substances are included in that fraction of the Weende analysis called ether extract.

Lipids are naturally occurring substances soluble in organic solvents, such as diethyl ether. A classification of these substances is given in Table 2.4.

Calorie value of ether extract   This classification does not include all of the substances that may be found in the ether extract of foods or of tissue of the animal body. In general, the presence of substances other than triglycerides in ether extract dilutes its useful energy. They are mentioned here chiefly to show what a mixture the ether extract of foods may be. In foods of animal origin, such as meat fats, lard, or butter, it may be composed almost entirely of triglycerides. But in foods of plant origin, as much as half the total ether extract may be composed of sterols, waxes, and various other lipids. Since the nonglyceride lipids yield little utilizable energy to animals, the

Table 2.4
Classification of lipids

Class	Subclass	Description and examples
Neutral lipids	Acylglycerols	Esters of glycerol and fatty acids; e.g., triglycerides. Primary constituents of dietary and tissue lipids.
	Fatty acids	Monocarboxylic acids, chains ranging in length from 3 to 24 carbon atoms. Usually contain even number of carbon atoms.
	Waxes	Long-chain hydrocarbons or long-chain alcohols and their fatty acid esters.
	Sterols	Cholesterol, its fatty acid esters, and compounds derived from it; e.g., sex and adrenal hormones, bile acids, vitamin D. Phytosterols; e.g., β-sitosterol, campesterol, ergosterol.
	Terpenoids	Compounds containing repeating units of the 5-carbon isoprene group. Included in the group are the carotenoids, xanthophylls, tocopherols, vitamin A, squalene, vitamin K.
Phospholipids	Phosphoglycerides	Lecithin, phosphatidyl ethanol amine, phosphatidyl serine, phosphatidyl inositol, plasmalogens.
	Sphingolipids	Ceramide, sphingomyelin, cerebrosides, ganglioside.

caloric value of *ether extract* is characteristic of specific foods: a single energy value, such as 9 kilocalories metabolizable energy per gram, while perhaps satisfactory for the fats of animal origin, the refined vegetable oils, or the shortenings prepared from them, is usually too high for the ether extract of foods of plant origin.

The usefulness of the ether extract of the Weende scheme as a source of energy is dependent almost entirely on its total content of triglycerides. Ether extract values by themselves give no indication of the particular fatty acids in the fraction, nor of the amount of nonglyceride lipid. These values, therefore, are only an indication of the energy of a feed, which in turn is subject to considerable variation from one type of feed to another because of the possible variation in the composition of the lipid fraction.

Ash—the inorganic nutrients   The Weende analysis includes an inorganic fraction—the total of the noncombustible substances of the material. The quantity of *ash* in a feed or in some biological product does not of itself give

Table 2.5 Makeup of the proximate principles of the Weende food analysis

- **Organic**
  - **Nitrogenous**
    - Protein
      - Dispensable amino acids — Glutamic acid, aspartic acid, alanine, serine, hydroxyproline
      - Semidispensable amino acids — Arginine, glycine, histidine, cystine, tyrosine, proline
      - Indispensable amino acids — Lysine, tryptophan, phenylalanine, methionine, threonine, leucine, isoleucine, valine
    - Non-protein — Nucleic acids, amines, etc.
  - **Lipid**
    - Neutral
      - Acylglycerols — Triglycerides
      - Sterols — Cholesterol, vitamin D, etc.
      - Terpenoids — Carotene, vitamin A, xanthophylls, etc.
    - Phospholipids
      - Phosphoglycerides — Lecithin
      - Sphingolipids — Sphingomyelin
  - **Carbohydrate**
    - Water-soluble vitamins — Thiamin, riboflavin, niacin, vitamin B_6, pantothenic acid, biotin, folacin, vitamin B_{12}, ascorbic acid
    - Nitrogen-free extract
      - Monosaccharides — Simple pentose or hexose sugars
      - Oligosaccharides — Compound sugars
      - Polysaccharides ("soluble") — Starches
    - Crude fiber
      - Polysaccharides ("insoluble")
        - Celluloses
        - Hemicelluloses
- **Inorganic — Ash**
  - Essential elements
    - Macro — Ca, Mg, Na, K, P, Cl, S
    - Micro — Mn, Fe, Cu, I, Zn, Co, Mo, Se, Cr, Sn, F, Ni, V, Si
  - Possibly essential elements — As, Ba, Br, Cd, Sr
  - Potentially toxic elements — Cu, Mo, Se, As, Cd, F, Pb, Hg, Si
  - Nonessential elements — Al, Sb, Bi, B, Ge, Au, Pb, Hg, Rb, Ag, Ti

information about any specific nutrient, and frequently the figure is used only to calculate the amount of carbohydrate by difference. The combination of mineral elements found in foods of plant origin is so variable that the ash figure of our analysis is useless as an index of the quantity of any particular element, or even of the total of the nutritionally essential ones. In the case of certain animal products, such as bone, milk, or cheese, whose composition is relatively constant, the approximate quantities of calcium and phosphorus can be predicted from the total ash figure.

Thus, so far as useful information about the inorganic nutrients of foods is concerned, the ash figure is merely a starting point for specific analysis for one or another of some 21 to 26 mineral elements required by the body, and for a few about which information may be needed because of their toxic nature.

Classification of the nutrients

To summarize this chapter, Table 2.5 identifies the principal nutrients by name and indicates the fractions of the Weende analysis into which they fall.

The table makes it clear that the Weende analysis does not describe nutrients individually; when this is necessary, some other scheme of description must be used. But, in spite of limitations that will be more apparent later, *the Weende analysis is the basis for the everyday chemical description of foods, body tissues, and excreta that are of concern in such calculations as the estimation of digestibility and utilization of foods and the establishment of feeding standards for all animal species.*

Suggested readings

A. O. A. C. *Official Methods of Analysis* (11th ed.). Edited by William Horowitz. Published by the Association of Official Analytical Chemists, Washington, D.C. (1970).

Crampton, E. W., and Harris, L. E. *Applied Animal Nutrition,* Chap. 2. W. H. Freeman and Company, San Francisco (1969).

Davenport, J. B., and Johnson, A. R. *Biochemistry and Methodology of Lipids,* Chap. 1. Wiley Interscience, New York (1971).

Munro, H. N. "An Introduction to Nutritional Aspects of Protein Metabolism." In *Mammalian Protein Metabolism,* Vol. 2. Edited by H. N. Munro and J. B. Allison. Academic Press, New York and London (1971):3–39.

Van Soest, P. J., and McQueen, R. W. "The Chemistry and Estimation of Fibre," *Proceedings of the Nutrition Society* **32**(1973):123.

Waksman, S. A., and Stevens, K. R. "The System of Proximate Chemical Analysis of Plant Materials," *Industrial and Engineering Chemistry, Analytical Edition* **2**(1930):167.

Chapter 3
Water and its metabolism

In the discussion of the Weende analysis in Chapter 2, and in the review of the nutrients that must be considered in nutrition, no specific reference was made to water. The omission was intentional because this component of foods and of all living biological substances is so important that it warrants separate and specific consideration. Strangely enough, the dietitian and husbandman often do not consider water a nutrient, perhaps because they are more often concerned with its physical rather than with its chemical properties. Indeed, one dictionary* devotes nearly a quarter of a page to the definition of water and the different senses in which the word is used without once suggesting it is a food or a nutrient. Yet a nutrient, according to this source, is a substance "furnishing nourishment."

Water makes up about 75% of the weight of the adult animal body and as much as 95% of the weight of the newborn. Water is an integral part of the structure of the soft tissues of the body in that the cell contents are lyophilic gels. Thus they readily take up and release water as a part of the biophysics of metabolism.

---

*Webster's New Collegiate Dictionary, G. & C. Merriam Co., Springfield, Mass. (1975).

Functions of water in the body

Water's unique physical properties are, of course, very important in nutrition. One of these is a high specific heat, the highest of any substance known. It is this physical property that makes water so indispensable for dispersing the heat produced by some of the chemical reactions in metabolism. For example, enough heat is generated in the body by the oxidations resulting from a few minutes of exercise to coagulate the proteins in the participating muscle cells. This is prevented only by prompt dissipation of the heat by the body water.

Water is also important in the adjustment of body temperature to environmental temperature. The ingestion of large amounts of cold water may so cool the body that increased oxidation is necessary to maintain body temperature. To avoid this chilling, animals and people may voluntarily restrict their water intake during cold weather to below optimum. On the other hand, in hot weather the intentional ingestion of large amounts of water to cool the body may upset osmotic relations sufficiently to cause what is called *water intoxication*. This is an occupational hazard in some industries where men work under high temperatures. Water intoxication is due actually to an excessive loss of body salts through sweating. This loss may be avoided by ingesting extra salts, either in saline drinking water or as salt tablets.

The ingestion of hot fluids may cause internal body temperatures to rise. This of course induces sweating, which cools the body. Hot drinks are sometimes used in medical practice when it is desired either to temporarily increase body temperature or to induce sweating.

The movement of nutrients to the cells of body tissues and the removal of metabolic end products from the cells is accomplished by virtue of the solvent properties of water. Most of the end products of metabolism that must be removed from the body are filtered out of the blood by the Bowman capsules of the kidney. The filtrate is then concentrated by reabsorption of water and certain threshold substances. However, there is a limit to the degree to which the body can concentrate the filtrate from the kidneys; therefore, the quantities of end products (usually urea and salts) that must be eliminated through the urine determine the minimum amount of water required for this purpose. The amounts of water required for the excretion of chlorides and of carbonates are practically identical and appear to be additive, but the requirement for the elimination of urea is somewhat less than that for the salts, and the requirement for elimination of urea and that for salts are not additive.

It is evident therefore that the quantity of minerals consumed in the diet or otherwise ingested has a direct bearing on the amount of water that must be ingested. In addition, the amount of protein in the diet is important—high-protein foods increase the quantity of urea that must be eliminated.

Water is also present in living plant tissues, though often there is much less of it than in the animal body. Here too it plays a vital role in the transfer of nutrients in the living organism.

Water a diluent of nutrients in foods

Thus water is a component of virtually all natural products used for food. The water content of different foods is highly variable and its diluent effect on other nutrients is often large, as is evident from the examples in Table 3.1.

Table 3.1
Diluent effect of water on the concentrations of protein and energy in foods

Food	Approx. % protein in		kcal per 100 g in	
	Food as eaten	Dry matter of food	Food as eaten	Dry matter of food
Bread (white)	8	13	275	425
Apple	trace	2	58	360
Potato	2	9	83	380
Turnip	1	10	40	362
Lettuce	1	23	17	340
Egg	13	49	162	622
Beef	20	63	182	585
Milk, whole	3	27	65	500
Cheese	25	40	398	635

Consequently, it must be accounted for in any chemical description of the concentration of nutrients in the dry substance of a food.

We can see from Table 3.1 that while the energy contributed to the diet by different foods as eaten is highly variable, the caloric value of their dry matter differs greatly from about 375 only when the foods contain large amounts of fat, like cheese, whole milk, or egg, or are of especially high protein content, like beef. For example, the differences in metabolizable energy food value between lettuce, potato, apple, and turnip, as eaten, are almost entirely due to different dilutions by water. Similarly, one egg of average size (2 ounces) furnishes about 70 kilocalories, 2 ounces of cheese about 225 kilocalories; this difference is due entirely to the fact that the egg calories are diluted with more than twice as much water as the cheese calories are.

The dilution of protein by water results in values for some foods that may lead to assigning the food to the wrong protein category. For example, we might, erroneously, think of milk and lettuce as low-protein foods, whereas they are both actually high-protein supplements. Similarly, the very high protein content of cheese, egg, and beef is masked by the values expressed on an "as purchased" basis. Indeed, fruits are about the only natural foods whose dry substance is very low in protein. Most natural foods that are primarily sources of carbohydrate carry 1 gram of protein for every 35–40 kilocalories of metabolizable energy; that is, roughly 10% of their energy is provided by protein. This is a rule of thumb sometimes applied to adult diets in comparing their protein level with dietary standard requirements. This proportion can be applied to foods regardless of their water content. Products in which appreciably more than 10% of the energy is derived from protein are considered high-protein foods or protein supplements. The use made of this information will be described later, but here we are interested only in a way of categorizing foods, irrespective of their water content.

Finally, the differing water content of foods affects the quantities that must be eaten to meet some specific energy or nutrient demand. Thus, we must eat some 500 grams of lettuce but only about 20 grams of cheese to obtain the same amount of energy we would from 100 grams of potatoes.

Water and food storage

The livestock feeder, too, must face the problem of water in feed, and in addition to considering equivalent energy and nutrient values, he must often consider the fact that feeds containing over 14% or 15% moisture will not store satisfactorily. Unlike human foods, livestock feeds cannot be refrigerated for storage.

Because in the process of making dry hay there are important losses in feeding value from the shattering of leaves or from leaching during adverse curing weather, many farmers attempt to preserve the original feeding value of the fresh grass by cutting and ensiling while it is still immature. If, by careful curing, excessive loss in feeding value has been avoided, then the chief difference in feeding value between the grass as pasturage, as grass silage, and as dry hay is in the quantity that must be eaten daily in order to supply the same amount of energy. Except for minor differences in digestibility, which usually do not exceed 5%, this difference in necessary intake is due to the differing water content of the three forms of forage.

Table 3.2 compares the water content of certain forages with the quantities required to be eaten daily by cattle in order to meet energy requirements.

Table 3.2
Effect of water content of forage on the amount of feed
required daily by a 450-kg cow producing 15 kg of milk

Feed	Water content (%)	Daily requirement (kg)	Normal daily capacity for the feedstuff (kg)
Dry hay	10	16.5	18.0
Grass silage	70	40.0	45.5
Pasture grass	75	54.5	63.5

Chemical role of water

Water plays a chemical role in the changes undergone by energy-yielding nutrients in the body. Most of the digestive changes in dietary carbohydrates, fats, and proteins are hydrolytic; that is, they entail the addition of water to the substrate. Indeed, practically all enzyme-catalyzed reactions in the body entail (1) addition or subtraction of water, (2) addition of oxygen or removal of hydrogen, (3) addition or removal of phosphoric acid, or (4) splitting or formation of a carbon–carbon linkage.

It is evident then that we must count water among the nutrients required by the body, and also *account for it* in the description of foods.

The turnover of water in the body

A very common rule of thumb calls for the drinking of about 1 liter of water for every 1000 kcal of food consumed by an adult human. But from this figure it is easy to get an erroneous impression of the total amount of water that is involved daily in the operation of the body. The total water turnover in the body may be exceedingly large. A part of the water that is secreted from various tissues in the body is not lost but is reabsorbed at other points and reused. Nevertheless, there is a considerable loss of water from the body. It is this loss that must be replaced by ingested fluid or by metabolic water from the diet.

Table 3.3 gives the approximate minimum and maximum 24-hour water turnover for adult humans and indicates the wide range there may be between individuals.

The amount of water turnover depends in part on what and how much the individual eats, and on his activities. For example, when very dry foods are ingested, salivary and intestinal secretions increase in order to maintain the necessary consistency of the ingesta during their passage through the digestive system. If insufficient fluid is available, dysfunctions such as constipation are likely to result. Under certain conditions, the secretion of fluid from the gall bladder may increase to as much as four times the normal amount. Such increases may result from ingestion of large quantities of fats that require bile for their emulsification. Elimination of urine by the kidneys is, of course, highly variable, and depends on a number of factors, among which the amount of water ingested for cooling purposes is important. Insensible perspiration does not vary as markedly as some other losses, but exercise increases the secretion of sweat. As we have already noted, it does not necessarily follow that the body sweats only because of exercise. Loss of water in the form of milk applies, of course, only to females, and it may be appreciable.

Table 3.3
Water turnover each 24 hours in adult humans

Category	Secreted from	Minimum (ml)	Maximum (ml)
Recovered by the body	Salivary glands	500	1500
	Stomach	1000	2400
	Intestinal wall	700	3000
	Pancreas	700	1000
	Gall bladder	100	400
	Lymph glands	700	1500
Total recovered		3700	9800
Lost from the body	Kidney (urine)	600	2000
	Colon (feces)	50	200
	Skin (insensible)	350	700
	Sweat glands	50	4000
	Mammary glands	0	900
Total lost		1050	7800
Total turnover		4750	17600

SOURCE: Adolph, E. F., *Physiol. Rev.* **13**(1933), no. 3.

An adult human metabolizes daily a minimum total of almost 5 liters of water, and a maximum that may be more than three times this amount, depending on circumstances. The minimum necessary daily ingestion of water—that is, the new water that must come into the body to replace daily losses—is normally about 1 liter. Some of this will be a part of the foods eaten, and some will be taken as beverage. The necessary daily intake may run as high as 7 or 8 liters if large amounts of water are being lost, either in the urine or in the sweat.

Absorption of water

Most of the water ingested by an animal is absorbed by organs of the digestive tract; the extent to which absorption actually occurs is determined by a number of factors. One of these is the osmotic relations inside the small intestine. If food solutions are more concentrated than the blood or tissue fluids in this part of the digestive tract, water is drawn into the lumen of the gut from these two body fluid sources. This is one way the body maintains the optimum consistency of the ingesta during their passage through the small intestine. On the other hand, if food solutions in the small intestine are less concentrated in water than the body fluids in the walls of the tract, absorption from the ingesta begins almost at once. It is believed that the rate of absorption from the small intestine depends in large measure on the nature and proportions of the solutes in the lumen of the intestine. Water is most readily absorbed when it is taken alone as beverage, or when taken with food that, after gastric digestion, forms a solution with osmotic pressure lower than that of blood plasma.

Another factor that affects the absorption of water in both the small and the large intestine is the nature of the carbohydrate component of the foods eaten. Certain food materials (specifically, polysaccharides, such as pectin) form gels in the digestive system that tend to hold water, and hence reduce its absorption from the intestine. Since this increases the water content of the feces, such foods are generally laxative. Food components other than carbohydrates are usually much less important to the water-holding capacity of foods.

Metabolic water

Metabolic water is water formed during metabolism by the oxidation of hydrogen-containing foods. Oxidation produces water nearly in proportion to the caloric value of the food or food component, yielding 10 to 15 grams of water per 100 kcal of metabolizable energy in the diet. Table 3.4 gives the yield of metabolic water from the carbohydrate, the protein, and the fat content of foods.

The calculation of the yield of metabolic water can be illustrated for a monosaccharide $C_6H_{12}O_6$. The molecular weight of this nutrient is 180, of which 108 weight units are accounted for by hydrogen and oxygen in the proportion of water. Thus, glucose yields 60% of its molecular weight as

Table 3.4
Yield of metabolic water from each 100 grams of typical dietary carbohydrate, protein, and fat

Nutrient	Metabolic H_2O formed by oxidation (g)	Average caloric value (kcal)	Metabolic H_2O per 100 kcal metabolizable energy
Carbohydrate	60	400	15.0
Protein	42	400	10.5
Fat	100	900	11.1

water. More complex carbohydrates, such as sucrose and starch, yield slightly less water per unit molecular weight—57.9% and 55.5%, respectively.

Similar calculations can be made for a typical protein and a typical fat. Although the results are only average values, they are satisfactory for use with a mixed diet.

An example will illustrate. Consider a diet that has been analyzed to contain 10% protein, 20% ether extract, and 55% carbohydrate (for simplicity, considered to be glucose). The other components of the diet can be disregarded since they yield neither metabolizable energy nor metabolic water. Using the conventional Atwater figures of 4, 9, and 4 kcal per gram of protein, fat, and carbohydrate, respectively (see Chapter 24), and the values given in the last column of Table 3.4, we may calculate the metabolic water from 100 grams of this diet as follows:

10 g protein	$\times 4 =$ 40	kcal yields	40 $\times$ .105 =	4	g metabolic water
20 g fat	$\times 9 =$ 180	kcal yields	180 $\times$ .111 =	20	g metabolic water
55 g carbohydrate	$\times 4 =$ 220	kcal yields	220 $\times$ .150 =	33	g metabolic water
Total	440	kcal yields		57	g metabolic water

To put it another way, for every 100 kcal of metabolizable energy in this diet 12.9 grams of metabolic water are formed. Of course, the figures we have used are not completely accurate for all types of diet, but we shall not go far wrong in estimating 13 grams of metabolic water formed for every 100 kcal of metabolizable energy in a typical mixed human diet. The significance of the metabolic water is that it represents a part of the water intake, and consequently its total can be deducted from the estimated daily water requirement.

Daily water intake requirements

The quantity of water to be ingested in a 24-hour period is considerable when compared to the weight of dry food metabolized. As a *very rough rule,* the water needed by an average man for sedentary living is about 1 milliliter for each kilocalorie of metabolizable energy of his diet. This rule can also be applied, *again very roughly,* to most species that are on a maintenance diet. Taking approximately 4 kcal per gram of dry substance as the metabolizable energy of a typical mixed diet, we see that, by weight, four times more water than dry food must be ingested to meet this requirement. Appreciable exercise, lactation, or environmental temperatures high enough to cause sweating will increase further the quantity of water needed.

Not all of the water required must be in the form of beverage, because, as we have already seen, practically all foods contain free water in addition to that which will be formed by metabolism. Furthermore, many foods, such as soups, are actually consumed in a watery state.

The human 24-hour water requirement is sometimes calculated by determining the amounts lost from the body through different channels. These losses differ from time to time with respect to storage in tissues, and to the needs for temperature regulation. When these two are zero, as would be the case with idle adults in comfortable environmental temperatures, the maintenance requirement may be calculated from body surface and caloric intake, as shown in Table 3.5.

Table 3.5
Minimum daily water losses
for an adult human

Mode of loss	Water (ml)
Urinary	$400A$
Fecal	$30A$
Basal extrarenal	$250A$
Exercise	$1.73 \times 0.4E$

SOURCE: Adolph, E. F., *Physiol. Rev.* **13**(1933), no. 3.

In this table, A is the surface area of the body in square meters, and E the kilocalories consumed in excess of the basal energy requirement. For purposes of calculating the daily water needs, the approximate surface area of a man in square meters may be calculated from his weight according to the equation

$$\text{Surface area (meter}^2) = 0.12 \times W_{kg}^{0.66}$$

and his daily basal energy requirement (E) according to the equation

$$E \text{ (kcal)} = 70 \times W_{kg}^{0.75}$$

The surface area formula is a slight modification of one originally proposed by Meeh, while the formula for basal energy requirement is Brody's. Both will be discussed in detail in Chapter 28. They are useful at this point merely for calculating water requirements according to the figures in Table 3.5.

For example, consider an adult male weighing 70 kg and consuming daily 2500 kcal of metabolizable energy. The sum of his daily urinary, fecal, and basal extrarenal water losses would be calculated as

$$\text{Water}_{ml} = (400 + 30 + 250) \times 0.12 \times 70^{0.66}$$
$$= 1346 \text{ ml}$$

To this we must add for exercise

$$\text{Water}_{ml} = 1.73 \times 0.4[2500 - 70(70^{0.75})]$$
$$= 559 \text{ ml}$$

Thus, total necessary daily water intake for this example is $1346 + 559 =$ 1905 ml. Of this we can estimate $(13 \text{ ml} \times 2500 \text{ kcal})/100 = 325 \text{ ml}$ will be provided from metabolic water, and approximately another 500 ml will come from free water in foods as eaten, leaving about 1 liter to be taken as beverage.

Drinking water for laboratory animals

It is traditional to supply water to farm animals, of course, but in "small animal" husbandry giving drinking water is a relatively modern improvement in practice. It is a curious fact that, traditionally, drinking water was given only to rats in the laboratory. It was a common supposition that rabbits and guinea pigs "did not drink" and that, in any case, the provision of drinking water to these animals was the cause of outbreaks of diarrhea. It was assumed that the green food that always formed a part of their daily rations would satisfy their needs for water, and even today some professional breeders hold this view. Mice were given a wet mash or bread soaked in milk or water, often with a little green food; no water was given apart from that used to prepare the wet mash. It is now well recognized that the provision of drinking water has a beneficial effect on the health of all laboratory animals.

Amounts of water normally consumed by several species of laboratory animals are given in Table 3.6. These figures do not necessarily represent minimum requirements, but they are the quantities consumed voluntarily by animals seeking to quench their thirst.

Table 3.6
Grams of drinking water consumed by various species of laboratory animals

Species	Approx. adult wt.	Av. daily water intake	Intake per kg wt.
Mouse	25	6	240
Hamster	90	8	89
Albino rat	300	24	80
Guinea pig	800	84	105
Rabbit	2400	328	137

Influence of type of diet on water requirements

In practical terms, the need of the body for water is chiefly to replace that which has been evaporated as sweat plus that lost in the urine. The metabolic water furnished to the body from hydrogen-containing foods just about replaces the fecal water loss. In general, the water loss easiest to reduce is that required for the formation of extra urine. This loss can be decreased by selecting foods containing moderate to small amounts of protein, with no more than the necessary amounts of minerals, and by including foods with high contents of preformed water.

Table 3.7 indicates the water needed for the complete metabolism of 100 kcal furnished by various foods. If we assume that the net deficit of water per

Table 3.7
Grams of water needed for metabolism of each 100 kilocalories furnished by various foods

Food	Preformed water	Met. water formed	Water lost in dissipation of heat	Water lost in excreting end products	Net deficit of water
Protein	0	10.3	60	300	350
Starch (CH_2O)	0	13.9	60	0	46
Fat	0	11.9	60	0	48
Beef	25	11.3	60	119	143
Eggs	47	11.1	60	154	156
Milk	127	12.5	60	123	43
Bread	14	13.2	60	69	102
Apples	150	13.9	60	56	−48

100 kcal furnished by food represents the amount of water that must be restored to the body, it is evident that the protein, carbohydrate, and fat contents of foods greatly affect the amount of water that should be ingested. Special attention should be called to the position in Table 3.7 of milk, a product that is itself almost 90% water, but which because of its high protein, and especially its high mineral content, actually leaves the body water-deficient. This, of course, has important implications for the feeding of young animals whose natural diet includes milk. It has often been erroneously assumed that animals being given unlimited quantities of milk do not require water, but it is now well known to pediatricians, and is becoming better understood by livestock feeders, that in addition to the milk a young mammal may be given, additional fluid in the form of water is also required. In fact, in experimental tests, calves given liberal allowances of skim milk

voluntarily drink about an equal amount of water; and when water is made available to water-deprived animals, their consumption of feed increases and their weight gains markedly improve.

It should be evident from Table 3.7 that excessive intake of protein and the ingestion of unnecessary minerals should be avoided whenever water is limited in supply.

Thirst

Many persons give little thought to the water requirement of individuals on the assumption that thirst is a satisfactory guide to the quantity of fluid the body needs. When animals are sweating rapidly, however, thirst sensations are not strong enough to demand intake of enough water to balance the water losses from the body. It has been shown that under intense activity a man will voluntarily drink only about half as much water as what is needed to replace his losses from sweating plus those from the excretion of urine. Only after food and rest does a person crave the water needed to wipe out the accrued deficit. This means that persons suffering from water privation, as in heat exhaustion, may have to be compelled to drink.

Effects of water restriction

Persons who do not replace heavy sweat losses suffer a series of changes, which may be summarized as follows:

  1. Increase in pulse rate and in rectal temperature.

  2. Increase in respiration.

  3. Tingling and numbness of fingers and feet.

  4. Increase in concentration of blood.

  5. Diminution of blood volume and more difficult circulation.

The difficulty and inadequacy of the circulation of blood under these conditions leads to difficult breathing, to gastro-intestinal upsets accompanied by nausea and appetite failure, and eventually to difficulty in muscular movements and to emotional instability.

Most of the difficulties noted above are basically the result of inadequate circulation, particularly peripheral circulation; when this occurs a person is said to be suffering from exhaustion. Exhaustion of this type, which is the most characteristic disability brought on by dehydration, has no permanent effects if it is relieved promptly.

Table 3.8
Effect of water restriction on the food intake, weight gain, and food efficiency of growing rats

Test no.	No. of rat pairs	Av. initial wt.		Av. water intake			Av. food intake			Av. weight gain			Av. gain/food		
		Water ad libitum (g)	Water restr. (g)	Water ad libitum (ml)	Water restr. (ml)	Extent of restr. (%)	Water ad libitum (g)	Water restr. (g)	Extent of red. (%)	Water ad libitum (g)	Water restr. (g)	Extent of red. (%)	Water ad libitum (g/100g)	Water restr. (g/100g)	Extent of red. (%)
1	12	88	83	286	140	51	225	171	24	68	35	49	30	21	30
2	10	103	97	275	133	52	212	169	20	50	28	44	24	17	29
3	30	52	51	297	139	53	183	118	36	72	32	56	39	27	31
4	30	86	84	325	159	51	205	145	29	58	26	55	28	18	36
Mean						52			27			51			31

Coefficient of variability: food intake = 12%, gain = 23% of the means.
Percent reductions necessary for significance at $P = 0.05$ and $n = 82$: food intake = 4%, gain = 7% of the means.

However, it has been found in experiments with animals that dehydration to the extent of a weight loss of 10%–12% results in a rise of body temperature. This is the characteristic condition of heat stroke, and it usually comes on suddenly. It is the result of the overheating of certain tissues, and unless promptly relieved it is fatal.

The more immediate effects of regular water restriction are a reduction in voluntary food intake and a decreased metabolism of the food eaten. These effects are especially marked in young growing animals. The extent of these changes in food consumption and in the use made of the food in terms of body gains is indicated by the results of a series of tests carried out in the Department of Nutrition at Macdonald College; these are shown in Table 3.8.

It will be noted that when water is restricted to 50% of that which was voluntarily consumed by those animals on *ad libitum* allowances there was a reduction of some 27% in voluntary food intake, a 50% reduction in weight gain, and almost one-third reduction in the efficiency of the metabolism of the food that they did consume. It may also be significant that all of the animals on restricted water rations were highly irritable and in some cases bad tempered. This seems to indicate that unnecessary restriction of the supply of water to animals of any age or any species is to be avoided as much as possible.

Suggested readings

Adolph, E. F. *Physiology of Man in the Desert*. Interscience, New York (1947).

Drury, D. R. "Metabolic Activities of the Kidney," *Annual Review of Physiology* **17**(1955):215.

Lee, D. H. K. "Terrestrial Animals in Dry Heat: Man in the Desert." In *Handbook of Physiology, Section 4: Adaptation to the Environment*. Edited by D. B. Hill, E. F. Adolph, and C. G. Wilber. American Physiological Society, Washington, D.C. (1964):551–585.

Leitch, I., and Thompson, J. S. "The Water Economy of Farm Animals," *Nutrition Abstracts and Reviews* **14**(1944):197.

MacFarlane, W. V. "Terrestrial Animals in Dry Heat: Ungulates." In *Handbook of Physiology, Section 4: Adaptation to the Environment*. Edited by D. B. Hill, E. F. Adolph, and C. G. Wilber. American Physiological Society, Washington, D.C. (1964):509–539.

McCance, R. A. "Man's Need for Water," *Proceedings of the Nutrition Society* **16**(1957):103.

National Academy of Sciences–National Research Council. *Recommended Dietary Allowances*. (8th ed.). National Academy of Sciences, Washington, D.C. (1974):21–24.

Chapter 4
General composition of
the animal body and its tissues

In chapter 2 we named the nutrients that we shall be considering in some detail in later chapters. We also described the Weende analysis, the most common method of quantitatively describing groups of some of these nutrients (protein, ether extract, crude fiber, nitrogen-free extract, and ash). We shall now consider in a general way why some of these nutrients or groups of nutrients are needed by an animal. This can be done for most of them by examining the makeup of the body, its tissues and its fluids. If we learn, for example, that some particular vitamin is a necessary part of an enzyme system without which blood sugar cannot yield its energy to the body, the reason for the inclusion of the vitamin in a diet becomes obvious.

The physiological functions of specific nutrients will be dealt with in later chapters; here we shall describe the animal body in terms of its nutrient, or proximate, composition.

Plant versus animal tissue

At the outset we should note that, unlike plant tissues, many animal tissues have almost the same composition in many different species. The calcium and phosphorus content of the skeleton, for example, is essentially the same for all animals. Thus, while the amount of ash in a food of plant origin may give almost no indication of the amount of either of these elements, the ash figure for bone is a useful indirect measure of both. Further, the amino acid makeup of muscle protein of different species of animals appears to be almost identical. Thus, the nutritional value of lean meat from all sources is about the same—which is not the case for proteins of plant origin.

Data for the proximate composition of the animal body are not numerous, perhaps because of the difficulty of satisfactory sampling. It is a major undertaking to prepare a steer for chemical examination! How, for example, would we go about obtaining the 1-gram samples, dry weight, for a chemical analysis from which we might estimate the average protein content of the whole body? Each fluid, each tissue, and, to some extent, each individual animal shows variations with respect to nitrogen content. Even sampling each separate tissue still raises the question of how these should be weighted to take account of their differing proportions in the body. It is not at all surprising therefore that data are meager for the chemical makeup of the animal body as a whole.

Typical proximate composition of the adult body

From the data available it appears that the typical composition of an entire adult mammalian animal is approximately

Water	60%
Protein	16%
Fat	20%
Ash	4%

The composition of different species of animals varies somewhat, but the differences between species are fairly small. The largest of these variations are in fat and in water. Those animals that are characteristically fat carry less water in the body than those that are less fat. Thus, the steer and the hog carry nearly 25% fat and correspondingly only about 55% water. On the other hand, the mouse and the horse (both relatively active species) carry less fat and more water. Man is apparently more variable than other large animals in this respect, and incidentally, there are less data for the composition of the human body than for other species.

One might conclude from the above figures that there is no carbohydrate in the body. This is not true, but for the most part the carbohydrate which is present is not a structural part of the body, and in amount it changes rapidly from hour to hour. To be strictly accurate we should list about 1% of the body weight as carbohydrate. This is chiefly in the form of liver glycogen, together with smaller amounts of muscle glycogen and blood sugar.

High variability of water and fat   Figures for the average composition of
the adult animal body as a whole, which include water and fat, are not of
much use in predicting the makeup of individuals because the water and fat
content are subject to fairly wide variation. Age, for example, markedly affects the water content of the body, since aging is accompanied by dehydration. This can be illustrated by typical figures for the bovine and human
species:

Bovine	*% Water*	*Human*	*% Water*
Embryo	90	Embryo	93
Newborn calf	80	Newborn infant	72
6- to 12-month calf	65	2-month infant	70
Mature steer	55	Adult	65

The ether extract content of the animal body is almost entirely triglyceride,
with small amounts of phospholipids also present. The kind of triglyceride,
however, differs with the species, with the diet, and with the age of the
animal. Variations with age are usually more a reflection of the type of food
that animals of different ages normally consume than of age *per se*.

In general, as the fat content of the body increases, its water content decreases. This change may occur quite quickly in response to changes in feed,
and it may be marked. For example, the carcass of a thin steer may contain
about 18% fat and 57% water, whereas that of a fat steer may contain as much
as 41% fat and as little as 41% water.

Average fat-free composition of the body   To avoid the complication of
fatness, the composition of the body is usually expressed on a fat-free basis.
The average figures then become

Water	75%
Protein	20%
Mineral	5%

On this basis the protein content of the body appears relatively constant.
Once maturity has been reached, the quantity of protein is not affected appreciably either by age or by diet; and the fraction of the total body weight
that is protein appears to be a hereditary characteristic of the individual.
Skeletal muscle usually accounts for most of the body protein. This should
not be taken to imply that skeletal muscle is primarily a structural element,
like the skeleton itself. It is true that the shape and size of the musculature

affect the external shape of an individual; however, from the physiological standpoint this is incidental to the fact that skeletal muscle functions as a "contractile machine," as we shall see shortly.

Significance of ash value   The percentage of ash in a body is an indication of the size of its skeleton. The major components of the ash are fairly constant, irrespective of species. Calcium makes up about 1.5% of the total body weight, phosphorus about 1.0%, and together they account for over 70% of the total ash of the body. Other mineral elements, which appear to be required only in trace amounts, are now known to be essential because they are components of certain enzymes or enzyme systems. The mineral components of the body will be dealt with individually in some detail in Section IV of this book.

Makeup of muscle

One of the basic characteristics of living animals is movement. Not only does the whole animal have the ability to move from place to place, but its separate parts may perform independent movements. Body or tissue movements are accomplished through cycles of contraction and relaxation of muscles of various sorts: some muscles are under voluntary control, whereas others perform their movements involuntarily. Muscle activity requires energy, the ultimate origin of which is the food ingested. We might almost say that the object of food intake is directly or indirectly to permit muscle activity. There are, of course, other functions of the body that require energy, but under normal conditions energy for muscle activity accounts for most of the dietary energy requirement.

The general makeup of muscle, particularly of skeletal muscle, is of some interest to nutritionists because it is an important part of the diets of most species of carnivora and omnivora, and may also constitute a part of the diet of herbivora. Depending on the species and plane of nutrition, 45%–60% of the weight of an adult animal's body is accounted for by skeletal muscle; of this, 75% is water. The dry matter of muscle has been partitioned as shown in Table 4.1.

The proteins of muscles serve not only as "contractile machinery," but also as an expendable reserve of amino acids. Adenosine triphosphate (ATP) acts as the immediate source of energy for muscle contraction. ATP also is important for its "plasticizing effect," that is, its ability to inhibit or reverse the interaction of actin and myosin. Creatine phosphate serves as a readily available source of energy for maintaining ATP levels. Glycogen and triglycerides are "fuel" reserves.

Table 4.1
Composition of mammalian skeletal muscle

Fresh skeletal muscle			
Water, 75%			
Dry matter, 25%	Protein, 70%–75%*	Myofibrillar, 55%†	Myosin Actin Tropomysin Troponin α-Actinin β-Actinin
		Sarcoplasmic, 33% ("Myogen")	Soluble enzymes Myoglobin Hemoglobin Globulin
		Stromal and particulate, 12%	Reticulin Collagen Elastin Mitochondrial and other particulate proteins
	Fat, 10%–12%		Triglyceride‡ Phospholipid Cholesterol
	Other substances, 12%–14%	Nitrogenous, 45%§	Creatine phosphate Creatine Amino acids ATP, ADP Anserine, carnosine Nucleic acids
		Carbohydrate, 45%	Glycogen Phosphorylated sugars
		Ash, 10%	Phosphorus Potassium Sodium Magnesium Calcium Zinc Chloride

*Percent of dry matter.
†Percent of protein.
‡Primary constituent of Fat, although the proportion varies with age, species, etc.
§Percent of other substances.

Muscle—the contractile protein   Movement requires a source of energy and a mechanism for converting it to physical action. The outstanding feature of muscle is the high efficiency with which it converts chemical energy to physical action. Muscle fibers are composed of many parallel *myofibrils*. The functional unit of a myofibril is the *sarcomere*, a bundle of thick and thin protein filaments that interdigitate with each other in a hexagonal array: each thick filament is surrounded by six thin ones, and each thin filament by three thick ones. During contraction the thin filaments slide along the thick filaments. The overall result is a shortening of each sarcomere, without any change in the length of the filaments themselves (see Figure 4.1). The con-

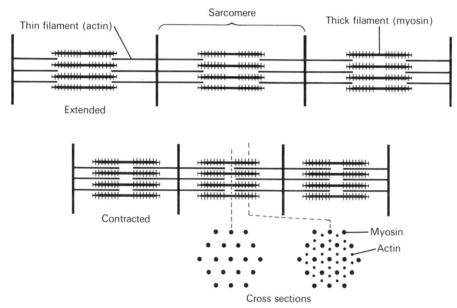

Figure 4.1
The structure of muscle. (From Linus Pauling and Peter Pauling, *Chemistry*, W. H. Freeman and Company, San Francisco, 1975.)

tractile protein operates with extremely high thermodynamic efficiency. Muscle is capable of converting about two-thirds of the energy of ATP to external work, and when allowance is made for the ATP consumed in activating the contractile machinery, work efficiency increases to more than 95%. This efficiency explains why exercise must be repeated and strenuous to bring about any significant loss in body weight.

The myofibrillar proteins   Myosin and actin are the principal proteins of the contractile apparatus, constituting approximately 55% and 20% of the total, respectively. Apparently actin and myosin interact directly during con-

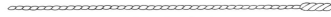

A myosin molecule

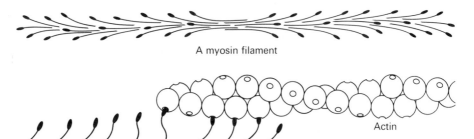

A myosin filament

Actin

Myosin

Figure 4.2
A myosin molecule and a myosin filament. At the bottom of the figure, a myosin filament is shown creeping along an actin filament by the interaction of the combining groups in the myosin heads with the complementary regions of the actin molecules. (From Linus Pauling and Peter Pauling, *Chemistry*, W. H. Freeman and Company, San Francisco, 1975.)

traction, although several minor proteins, such as troponin, are intimately involved in the regulation of this interaction.

The thick filaments of skeletal muscle are made up of aggregates of myosin molecules. The globular heads of the myosin molecules stick out from the filament to form the so-called cross-bridges, which are the portions of the myosin molecules that interact with ATP and with actin (see Figure 4.2). The thin filaments are made up primarily of actin but they also contain troponin, tropomyosin, α-actinin, and β-actinin. Actin in muscle consists of polymers of the globular G-actin molecule. The polymerized form, referred to as F-actin, contains the divalent cation Mg^{++} and the nucleotide ADP tightly bound to it in the ratio of one mole of each per mole of G-actin monomer. Troponin, a globular protein, is of utmost physiological importance because it is a calcium receptor; together with tropomyosin, it is responsible for the calcium sensitivity of actin: the presence of Ca^{++} causes a change in the troponin molecule, which in turn renders the active sites of actin available for interaction with myosin. Removal of Ca^{++} from troponin-tropomyosin, which is an energy(ATP)-requiring process, reverses the sequence, thereby bringing about disengagement of the filaments and relaxation of the muscle.

Because of its relationship to the post-mortem changes of rigor mortis, the interaction of Ca^{++}, ATP, and the myofibrillar proteins is of interest not only to the physiologist but to the meat scientist.

Sarcoplasmic and stromal proteins   The *sarcoplasm* is the intracellar fluid of muscle. Sarcoplasmic protein is made up primarily of glycolytic and associated enzymes. In fact, glyceraldehyde phosphate dehydrogenase, which makes up 20% of the sarcoplasmic protein in rabbit muscle, and four or five other major enzymes account for about 50% of the sarcoplasmic protein. Nevertheless, there are in the sarcoplasm a great variety of enzymes, such as those that participate in the metabolism of fat and protein. The sarcoplasm contains myoglobin in addition to the soluble enzymes; although myoglobin is not a major constituent of muscle, its quantity and color greatly influence the appearance of the meats we eat. In general, high levels of myoglobin are found in red muscle and in large species, especially sea mammals, where it functions as an oxygen store during deep dives. By contrast, the pectoral muscles of chickens contain virtually no myoglobin.

The *stroma* is defined as the fraction of muscle that is insoluble in neutral aqueous solvents. Collagen, elastin, and reticulin are the primary proteins of the stromal fraction, which constitutes 10%–15% of the total muscle protein. The connective-tissue proteins are also important constituents of skin, bone, tendon, cornea, and blood vessels. These proteins resist digestion, and because of their structure they contribute a "background" toughness to meat.

Collagen is characterized by high levels of the amino acid glycine and the imino acid proline. It also contains two unique hydroxy amino acids, hydroxyproline and hydroxylysine. Since they have been found only in collagen, analysis of the content of hydroxyproline in a tissue is used as a measure of the amount of collagen present. The formation of hydroxyproline is of particular interest to the nutritionist because vitamin C is needed for the conversion of some of the proline residues in collagen to hydroxyproline. This conversion occurs after proline has been incorporated into the polypeptide chains that will eventually make up the collagen molecule. Thus, the rate of excretion of hydroxyproline in the urine has been used as an index of collagen turnover in the body.

Elastin is also rich in glycine and proline but, unlike collagen, it contains very little hydroxyproline and no hydroxylysine. It forms a major part of the aorta and of elastic ligaments such as those in the necks of grazing animals. Elastin has been of particular interest to the nutritionist and biochemist during the past few years because copper has been shown to be a cofactor in an amino oxidase enzyme that plays an important role in the formation of crosslinks within and between the elastin molecules.

Appreciable quantities of the proteins of two abattoir byproducts used in animal feeds, dry or wet rendered animal carcass residue with a maximum of 5% blood (meat meal) and a similar product with 6%–30% blood (tankage), are from these connective tissues.

Amino acid composition of muscle   The composition and activity of muscles are of interest to the nutritionist for several reasons. Motility in animals is the direct result of the ability of muscles to convert chemical energy to physical work. A substantial portion of the energy derived from food goes into work, including work associated with such vital processes as the circulation of the blood, breathing, and peristalsis of the alimentary tract. The fact that muscle makes up an appreciable portion of the weight of the body is also of nutritional significance. Growth is largely the accumulation of protein; if this process is to occur, amino acids must be supplied, either directly or indirectly, by the diet. Muscle also serves as an important source of amino acids in the diets of many animals, including man. Muscle meats supply an excellent array of the essential amino acids. Table 4.2 shows that there is little difference in the amino acid composition of muscle from widely differing species.

Table 4.2
Amino acid composition of the muscle of different species,
in grams of amino acid per 16 grams of nitrogen

Amino acid	Steer	Pig	Chicken	Fish
Alanine	5.97	5.95	3.41	5.98
Arginine	6.50	6.64	5.57	6.11
Aspartic acid	8.86	9.60	9.17	9.70
Cystine	1.28	1.26	1.31	1.01
Glutamic acid	14.77	15.58	15.00	13.52
Glycine	5.76	5.31	5.30	5.04
Histidine	3.07	3.00	2.62	3.31
Isoleucine	5.12	5.41	5.34	5.04
Leucine	8.19	8.16	7.36	7.71
Lysine	8.64	9.04	8.00	7.82
Methionine	2.56	2.84	2.53	2.91
Phenylalanine	4.21	4.34	4.00	3.84
Proline	4.64	4.53	4.16	3.71
Serine	4.00	4.29	3.90	4.67
Threonine	4.40	4.99	3.97	4.54
Tryptophan	1.12	1.36	1.02	1.12
Tyrosine	3.45	3.76	3.34	3.84
Valine	5.36	5.70	5.09	5.81

Makeup of epithelial tissue

Epithelial tissues, such as hair, wool, feathers, nails, horns, and hooves, are largely protein in nature. The characteristic substances present in these tissues are the insoluble proteins known as keratins. Keratins are characterized by their high sulfur content, most of which is contributed by the amino acid cystine. Hair, for example, contains approximately 15% cystine by weight, feathers 9%. The high cystine content of keratins is of structural importance because of its formation of disulfide linkages between units making up the keratin molecule. Raw keratins are poorly digested by vertebrates, but steam heating under pressure and fine grinding render the raw products susceptible to attack by digestive enzymes. Properly hydrolyzed feathers contain about 85% protein, of which 80% is digestible. This product, known in the feed trade as *hydrolyzed feather meal,* can be successfully substituted for limited quantities of other protein sources in livestock rations.

Other components of the animal body

The foregoing paragraphs have given a very general picture of the makeup of the principal tissues of the animal body. However, we must not assume that the body does not contain many other substances of interest to the nutritionist. For example, the composition of muscle was considered almost entirely from the standpoint of its protein and amino acid makeup. This is an aid to understanding the physiology of muscle action and the relation it bears to the dietary amino acid requirements. Enzyme systems, on the other hand, not only are composed of protein and amino acids but also frequently include one or more of the vitamins and the inorganic elements. Thus, if we consider the animal body as food, these other components must be taken into account. Table 4.3 illustrates the partial nutrient composition of certain parts of the animal body that are used for food.

Muscle, liver, and kidney, as well as bone, may comprise appreciable parts of the diet of various animals, including humans. Muscle, liver, and kidney carry about 70% water. Their protein content is about 20%, and the fat content of the three ranges from 3% to 11%. It should be noted, however, that muscle and kidney contain very small amounts of carbohydrate. Liver is commonly listed as carrying about 6% carbohydrate, on the average, and this is in the form of glycogen. The quantity of carbohydrate in the liver fluctuates, depending on how recently the animal has consumed food or been physically active, both of which cause the mobilization of glycogen into blood sugar.

Table 4.3
**Partial composition of certain tissues
of a typical animal body, per 100 grams**

Component	Muscle	Liver	Kidney
Moisture (g)	68	70	75
Protein (g)	20	20	15
Fat (g)	11	3	8
Carbohydrate (g)	1	6	0.9
Calcium (mg)	10	7	9
Phosphorus (mg)	180	358	221
Iron (mg)	3.8	6.6	7.9
Vitamin C (mg)	0	31	13
Riboflavin (mg)	0.17	3.33	2.55
Niacin (mg)	4.7	13.7	6.4
Thiamin (μg)	80	260	370
Vitamin A (mg)	0	1.32	0.34

The soft tissues contain almost no calcium but do contain appreciable amounts of phosphorus; and the glandular organs, represented in Table 4.3 by liver and kidney, are rich sources of iron. In general, the thiamin content of muscle is low compared to the level in glandular organs. A notable exception is pork, in which the thiamin level is 4 to 5 times that in beef. Niacin and riboflavin levels also are low in muscle compared to the levels in the glandular organs. Vitamin A is present in fairly large quantities in liver, but is essentially absent in muscle. Vitamin C also is found in some of the glandular organs, but in amounts quite small compared to the human requirement for this vitamin.

Suggested readings

Briskey, E. J., Cassens, R. G., and Trautman, J. C. *The Physiology and Biochemistry of Muscle as a Food 1*. The University of Wisconsin Press, Madison, Milwaukee, and London (1966).

Briskey, E. J., Cassens, R. G., and March, B. B. *The Physiology and Biochemistry of Muscle as a Food 2*. The University of Wisconsin Press, Madison, Milwaukee, and London (1970).

Forrest, J. C., Aberle, E. D., Hedrick, N. B., Judge, M. D., and Merkel, R. A. *Principles of Meat Science*. W. H. Freeman and Company, San Francisco (1975).

Lawrie, R. A. *Meat Science*. Pergamon Press, Oxford and New York (1966).

Price, J. F., and Schweigert, B. S., (eds.). *The Science of Meat and Meat Products* (2nd ed.). W. H. Freeman and Company, San Francisco (1971).

Williams, R. J. *Biochemical Individuality*. John Wiley & Sons, New York (1956).

Chapter 5
General composition of the foods of man and his domestic animals

No detailed consideration of the composition and nutritional properties of specific foods will be included in this book. It will be helpful, however, in understanding some of the fundamental problems of nutrition, to consider the broad characteristics of typical foods, and particularly how it is that food can have markedly different nutritive values.

Foods of animal origin

We have already noted a few of the characteristics of those parts of the animal body that, in the form of meats or by-products of animal carcasses, are used for foods. The composition of meat as we purchase it, for example, is similar to the composition of muscle. The trimmings of carcass cuts, together with some tissues not desired in the human diet, are processed into foods for many classes of farm animals, particularly those species whose diets must contain certain amino acids not abundant in foods of plant origin. We have already noted that the amino acid makeup of muscle tissue is virtually the same for most species; hence meats cut from skeletal muscle are not widely different in food value except that there may be some variation in the amounts of fat and water.

Glandular tissues, on the other hand, consist not only of protein but, in varying amounts, of quantities of vitamins and mineral elements in sufficient concentration to give such tissues nutritional properties different from those of meats cut from muscle. Furthermore, the concentrations of "stored" nutrients in each type of gland are subject to wide variation, depending on the nature of the food eaten by the animal during the weeks prior to slaughter. Variations in the nutrient content of glandular tissues make no difference in the appearance of the material as purchased; consequently, the consumer can do little more than assume that liver, for example, in addition to having a certain protein value, is probably a rich source of vitamin A, niacin, riboflavin, iron, phosphorus, and other nutrients.

Table 5.1 compares the general composition of muscle cuts of beef, glandular tissues (represented by beef liver), and cow's milk. The figures show

Table 5.1
The general composition of the dry matter of three animal "tissues" (figures are parts per million; divide by 10,000 to obtain percentages)

Component	Beef round	Beef liver	Cow's milk
Protein	565,000	650,000	268,000
Ether extract	320,000	107,000	276,000
Crude fiber	0	0	0
Nitrogen-free extract	0	20,000	394,000
Calcium	320	2,300	9,850
Phosphorus	5,200	12,000	7,550
Iron	84	220	6
Thiamin	3	10	3
Riboflavin	6	110	15
Niacin	135	460	7
Carotene	0	263	15

the wide differences there can be and normally are between different foods of animal origin. Generally speaking, foods of marine or of avian origin are considered dietary substitutes for others of animal origin. Table 5.2 shows the differences between some of these products and allows their nutritive properties to be compared with those of the animal tissues listed in Table 5.1.

Table 5.2
General composition of the dry matter of typical foods of marine and of avian origin
(figures are parts per million; divide by 10,000 to obtain percentages)

Component	Halibut	Oyster	Lobster	Chicken	Hen's egg
Protein	745,000	490,000	810,000	595,000	512,000
Ether extract	208,000	105,000	95,000	371,000	460,000
Crude fiber	0	0	0	0	0
Nitrogen-free extract	0	280,000	25,000	0	28,000
Calcium	520	4,700	3,050	4	2,164
Phosphorus	8,400	8,400	9,200	5,900	8,400
Iron	28	280	30	44	108
Thiamin	2.8	7.5	6.5	2.4	4.0
Riboflavin	2.4	10.0	3.0	4.7	11.6
Niacin	368	60	95	235	4
Carotene	10.5	9.6	0	0	27.3

Foods of plant origin

The composition of foods of plant origin varies greatly according to the type of plant from which the food is derived, the age of the plant, the conditions under which it was grown, the part of the plant actually eaten, and modifications that may result from commercial processing or home preparation for serving.

Table 5.3 compares the general composition of a few food products obtained from wheat. Because wheat flour is so important a food, the comparison between it and the wheat germ is of more than passing interest. The latter is a far richer source of important nutrients, but because its lipid deteriorates in storage the germ is usually removed in the manufacture of flour. This practice is not confined to the preparation of wheat by-products but is general in the preparation of cereals for human use. Thus, it is well to remember that foods based on seed endosperm are likely to be deficient in nutrients other than starch.

Cereal grass is the young leaf blade, which is cut when about four inches high and artificially dried. It is a component of some special human diets, and is also a common ingredient in rations for poultry. Its special value lies in its rich store of protein, minerals, and vitamins. It is sometimes referred to as one of the protective foods. It corresponds to such leafy foods of the human dietary as lettuce and spinach.

A comparison of the makeup of cereal grass with the makeup of wheat hay,

Table 5.3
General composition of the dry matter of some foods obtained from wheat
(figures are parts per million; divide by 10,000 to obtain percentages)

Component	Cereal grass	Hay	Whole grain	Bran	Germ	Flour
Protein	376,000	65,000	110,000	175,000	282,000	120,000
Ether extract	61,000	19,000	22,100	35,000	112,000	12,000
Crude fiber	132,000	290,000	22,100	103,000	22,200	0
Nitrogen-free extract	310,000	540,000	825,000	655,000	535,000	710,000
Calcium	20,000	1,600	400	965	940	170
Phosphorus	2,200	750	3,800	13,400	12,300	102
Iron	400	300	35	105	91	8
Thiamin	8		4	2	24	1
Riboflavin	17		1	4	9	0
Niacin	42		45	196	52	8
Carotene	100	100	0	0	0	0

prepared from the almost mature plant and including the nearly ripe seed, illustrates the change that takes place in some of the nutritionally important components of these foods with the aging of the plant. The reduction in concentration of some of the nutrients is due to dilution by the increased amount of crude fiber. Except for herbivora, who can digest crude fiber, this change is comparable to diluting the effective nutrient content with water. However, as we shall see later, crude fiber presents problems of digestibility and palatability that are quite unlike those resulting from the high water content of some foods.

Foods from animals versus foods from plants

In comparing foods of animal with those of plant origin, the absence of carbohydrate in the animal, marine, and avian products (other than milk) is striking. The nitrogen-free extract, chiefly starches and sugars, is less than 3% of most animal tissues used for food. Milk, a product of animal synthesis and intended to be the total diet of the very young animal, is the only exception: it contains almost 40% nitrogen-free extract, by virtue of its high sugar (lactose) content.

Box 5.1 Genetic manipulation of plant proteins

The discovery in the early 1960's that the Opaque-2 mutant of maize contained nearly twice as much lysine as ordinary maize aroused a great enthusiasm among plant breeders around the world for the improvement of the nutritional quality of cereal proteins by genetic manipulation. The subsequent discovery of high-lysine mutants of barley, referred to as *Hiproly,* and of sorghum further heightened the hope that the protein quality of all cereals of economic importance might be improved by genetic selection. The tremendous optimism these discoveries engendered among plant breeders and nutritionists is understandable when one considers that cereals supply 50 percent of the total protein consumed by humans and that another 20 percent comes from plants other than cereals. There is little doubt that, with the possible exception of protein produced by the culturing of single-celled organisms, most of the additional protein required to feed the rapidly increasing world population will be provided by plants.

The development of "man-made" cereals such as *triticale,* an intergeneric cross between wheat (genus *Triticum*) and rye (genus *Secale*), is another exciting and promising area of plant breeding. The development of a new cereal crop such as triticale could not have happened without the intervention of man because the natural offspring (F_1) of intergeneric crosses are almost always infertile. (The classic example of an intergeneric cross is the mule, the offspring of a male ass and a mare.) However, the plant breeder has been able to overcome the problem of infertility through the use of the alkaloid colchicine, which brings about a doubling of the number of chromosomes in the hybrid offspring. These amphiploid offspring are sufficiently fertile that the plant breeder can select for desired traits. Many of the triticale lines have been found to have not only a higher total protein content than either of the parents but an appreciably higher proportion of lysine in the protein.

In addition to genetic manipulation of cereals, plant breeders have made appreciable improvements in plant protein sources such as rapeseed and cottonseed. Plant breeders in Canada have been very successful in developing rapeseed lines that are nearly free of glucosinolates, the antithyroid precursors that had previously limited the use of this high-quality protein even for the feeding of livestock. At the same time, plant breeders in the United States have been equally successful in improving cottonseed by removing the gossypol glands by genetic means.

Although many of the genetic lines currently being developed are inferior in many agronomic characteristics to lines presently being used, plant breeders are confident that nutritionally superior lines can be developed with yields equal to those now in use.

In contrast to meats, the nitrogen-free extract of plant seeds and their milling fractions is normally high, except for plants whose seeds store reserve energy as fats instead of as starch. Peanuts, for example, contain only half the nitrogen-free extract, but twice the ether extract, of wheat grain.

Foods of animal origin contain a consistently high quantity of protein. In general, this protein is of high biological value—that is, the concentration and proportion of indispensable amino acids coincides with the body's needs for growth, reproduction, and so on. In contrast, foods of plant origin vary considerably in protein content. In addition, many plant proteins are deficient in one or more of the indispensable amino acids, and those present may be poorly balanced with respect to the body's requirements.

The figures in Table 5.3 make it obvious that different parts of the same plant can be different enough in proximate composition and in mineral and vitamin components that these variations must be taken into account when considering plant products as foods and feeds. In general, these differences are greater than those between comparable products from different kinds of plants. Thus, cereal grass from oats, wheat, or barley is of quite similar makeup, and the cereal seeds and their milling by-products are also of about the same general composition.

With but few exceptions, single foodstuffs are incomplete nutritionally, and variety in kind of foods is necessary for fully adequate diets for all animal species.

Suggested readings

Dawbarn, M. C. "The Effects of Milling upon the Nutritive Value of Wheaten Flour and Bread," *Nutrition Abstracts and Reviews* **18**(1949):691.

Food and Agriculture Organization. *Amino Acid Content of Foods and Biological Data on Protein.* FAO Nutrition Studies No. 24. Food and Agriculture Organization of the United Nations, Rome (1970).

National Academy of Sciences–National Research Council. *United States–Canadian Tables of Feed Composition.* Publication 1684. National Academy of Sciences, Washington, D.C. (1969).

National Academy of Sciences–National Research Council. *Atlas of Nutritional Data on United States and Canadian Feeds.* Publication 1919. National Academy of Sciences, Washington, D.C. (1972).

Watt, B. K., and Merrill, A. L. *Composition of Foods.* Agriculture Handbook No. 8. United States Department of Agriculture, Washington, D.C. (1963).

Chapter 6
The nutritional significance
of an animal's digestive system

The physiology of digestion in the larger non-herbivores, including man, is essentially the same. Under the influence of a series of digestive enzymes secreted at successive points from the stomach to the large intestine, consumed foods are broken down into their component nutrients so that they can be absorbed. The unabsorbed food residues together with those from any partially digested microorganisms and sloughed epithelial cells of the digestive tract are eventually voided as fecal material.

No attempt will be made in this book to describe the details of digestion in the various animal species with which we are concerned. This information can be obtained, in as much detail as is required, from physiology texts. Rather, our treatment of digestive systems is merely to show how an animal's digestive process has a bearing on the kind and quantity of food or feed the animal can consume and utilize to meet its nutritional requirements.

Digestion and absorption

It is generally assumed that once nutrients are digested from various diet components, they are absorbed. Absorption takes place chiefly from the small intestine; but some nutrients are absorbed directly from the stomach, or from the caecum. Short-chain fatty acids fall into the latter category, being absorbed at the sites of their formation. Sugars, amino acids, mineral elements, and vitamins enter the body through the villi that line the small intestine. Water may be excreted into or absorbed from any part of the large or small intestine.

Rate of digestion

In carnivora and omnivora, both the digestive and absorptive processes following the ingestion of food are normally completed, and residues are voided, within 24 hours. Actually, digestion and absorption are probably practically completed by 4 hours after food ingestion, but dehydration of the residues in the large bowel to the normal fecal moisture content is not completed until several more hours have elapsed.

Capacity of the digestive system

The total capacity of the whole digestive system in an adult man is only about 6 liters, of which the stomach and large intestine account for 1.2 liters each. This means that the adult human stomach can hold a volume of material equal to about 5 cupfuls. Even allowing for the relatively prompt passage into the intestine of the first portions of a meal swallowed, it is obvious that there is a physical limit to the quantity of food a digestive tract of this size can "process." To supply the 3600 calories a working man may need daily would require him to consume some 30 cupfuls of cereal grass—an impossibility from the standpoint of its bulk—though, nutritionally, cereal grass is a reasonably well-balanced food and can serve as the entire diet of animals with digestive systems of sufficient capacity to deal with it.

The herbivorous animals are equipped with a more capacious digestive apparatus. In proportion to her weight, a cow has a digestive tract capacity about nine times that of a man. Not only is every part that has its counterpart in man three to four times more capacious, but in addition the cow has a multiple stomach system whose total capacity per unit of body weight exceeds that of the simple human stomach by more than thirty times.

This system provides space for processing the enormous quantities of foods of low usable energy (such as the roughages) that must be consumed to obtain the energy and nutrients needed for normal maintenance and production. The capacities of various digestive systems are compared in Tables 6.1 and 6.2.

Table 6.1
Capacities of the digestive systems of various species of animals (in liters)

Part of system	Cow	Horse	Pig	Dog	Man
Total gastric system	252	18	8	4	1
Rumen	202				
Reticulum	8				
Omasum	19				
Abomasum	23				
Small intestine	66	64	9	2	4
Caecum	10	34	2	<1	——
Large intestine	28	96	9	1	1
Total	356	212	28	7	6

SOURCE: Adapted from H. H. Dukes, *Physiology of Domestic Animals* (8th ed.), ed. Melvin J. Swensen, Comstock Publ. Assoc., Ithaca and London (1970).

Table 6.2
Relative capacities of the parts of the digestive systems of various species of animals (percent)

Part of system	Cow	Horse	Pig	Dog	Man
Total gastric system	70	8	29	62	17
Rumen	57				
Reticulum	2				
Omasum	5				
Abomasum	6				
Small intenstine	19	30	33	24	66
Caecum	3	16	6	1	——
Large intestine	8	46	32	13	17
Total	100	100	100	100	100

Digestion in herbivora

In herbivorous animals, special digestive or predigestive processes take place in the extra stomach compartments (rumen, reticulum, and omasum) and/or in the functional caecum. (The cow has a multiple stomach; the sheep has both a caecum and a multiple stomach; and the horse has a large functional caecum, but only one stomach.) These structures harbor microflora that attack the cellulose and hemicellulose, producing acetic, propionic, and butyric acids. These fatty acids are absorbed at the sites of their formation and metabolized through the fat pathways, which will be discussed in Chapter 9.

By breaking down the cellulose walls of the cells of food, the bacterial attack exposes the cell contents, including fats, starch, and protein, to "normal" digestive action in the appropriate areas along the tract posterior to the rumen-reticulum-omasum stomach compartments. As though in payment for their living quarters and subsistence, the digestive tract microflora synthesize all members of the vitamin B complex and all of the essential amino acids. The latter can be synthesized from such nitrogen compounds as urea or di-ammonium phosphate, or from food proteins that lack one or more of the indispensable amino acids. Thus, herbivorous animals are indifferent to ration deficiences of specific amino acids and of the members of the vitamin B complex.

Type of food and type of digestive system

We can see now that man and his pigs and chickens must eat foods low in cellulose, whereas his cattle and sheep can subsist largely and often entirely on the bulky, high-fiber forages that, because of their relatively low yield of useful energy per unit of weight of dry matter, must be eaten in large quantities to supply the needed nutrients.

It should be noted, however, that the portion of the digestive tract beginning with the true stomach (abomasum) and including the small and large intestine, but excluding the functional caecum, performs the same function in all species. Thus, before the development of their extra structures young herbivorous animals can be satisfactorily nourished on the same rations that are suitable for omnivorous and carnivorous species. Indeed, "baby foods" are generally suitable for the "babies" of any mammalian species and also for young chickens. For animals of comparable physiological age, specific functions, and activities (lactation, rate of growth, work, etc.), the nutrient and energy needs per unit of metabolic body size ($W_{kg}{}^{.75}$) are remarkably similar. Their rations must differ principally according to the *kind of foodstuff* the animals can process through their digestive tracts.

Suggested readings

Code, C. F., and Heidel, W., (eds.). *Handbook of Physiology, Section 6: Alimentary Canal, Volume 5: Bile; Digestion; Ruminal Physiology.* American Physiological Society, Washington, D.C. (1968).

Morton, J. *Guts: The Form and Function of the Digestive System.* Edmond Arnold Publishers, London (1967).

Williams, R. J. *Biochemical Individuality.* John Wiley & Sons, New York (1956).

Section II
METABOLIC PROCESSES OF THE BODY AND THE ROLES OF THE ENERGY-YIELDING NUTRIENTS

In the preceding chapters we have considered briefly a number of matters that are related in one way or another to nutrition. These must necessarily be understood in any consideration of nutrition, but they are not the core of the subject itself. We have tabulated the nutrients, seen something of how they are grouped for purposes of ordinary description, had a brief look at the makeup of the animal body and of some of its tissues, noted the general nature of the feeds consumed by animals, and considered in some detail water as one of the operating necessities of the animal body.

We are now ready to examine the metabolic pathways—the overall scheme by which the body's cells perform their functions of producing the substances they require and obtaining the energy to carry out this work.

To understand these processes is, indeed, to understand the dietary requirements of the animal body. Every essential component of an adequate diet plays a definable role in the operation of the body. Imbalance between dietary supplies of these operating essentials results in stresses ranging in their expression from slightly reduced efficiency to the inability to survive. The nutritionist must have a working knowledge of the operation of the metabolic pathways in order to prescribe a normal, adequate diet. He likewise depends on such knowledge for the diagnosis of dietary deficiencies.

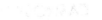

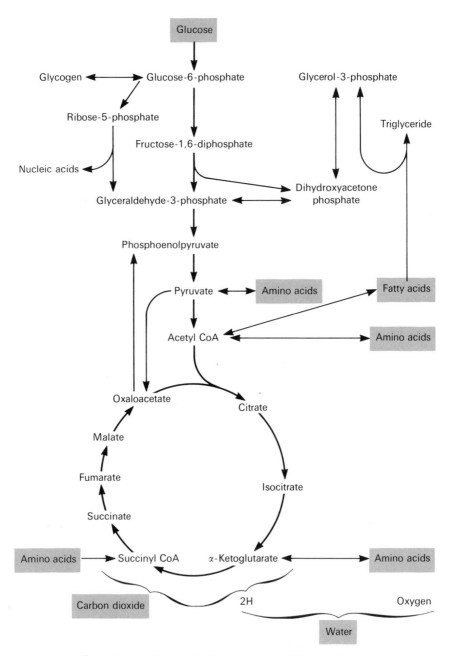

General plan of the metabolism of energy-yielding nutrients in the animal body.

CAMROSE LUTHERAN COLLEGE

In discussing the metabolism of the energy-yielding nutrients we shall omit the detail of chemical formulae and of quantitative thermodynamics. Instead, we shall trace these nutrients from their ingestion to the excretion of their end products, pointing out the paths they follow and the specific roles they play en route in the nutritive economy of the body. Then we shall fit into the overall plan the amino acids, the vitamins, and the minerals. It is out of these that the cells not only manufacture their structural elements, but also synthesize the metabolic regulators of the processes.

Metabolism is the name given to the sum of the chemical and physical processes continuously going on in living organisms and cells. The processes comprise those by which nutrients are synthesized into protoplasm, those by which the protoplasm is broken down, and those by which the energy of the molecules is "captured" in forms that can be used to do the work of making these anabolic and catabolic changes. At the heart of all these activities is a sequence of reactions that begins with the energy-yielding nutrients and ends with the two products of their complete breakdown, carbon dioxide and water. At certain points along this sequence are molecules that perform special functions as they enter into reactions that occur off the main pathway. These "side reactions" usually are involved in the formation of some cell (or tissue) substance; in most cases the ultimate breakdown products of these substances eventually return to the main energy pathway for final disintegration and elimination.

A general plan of this flow is given in the diagram opposite. It shows only a few of the important intermediate products between the energy-yielding nutrients and CO_2 and H_2O. Only a depiction of the general plan is intended. We see that, in the course of its disintegration, blood glucose nourishes the body by providing a number of different substances that are intermediates in the formation of some essential cell component—such as ribose-5-phosphate for the ultimate structure of nucleic acid, or glycerol-3-phosphate for the formation of triglycerides. As the molecules of the main path are, at successive steps, degraded further and further, the energy released from the valence bonds is captured for reuse by the formation of such products as adenosine triphosphate. Thus does our metabolic machine operate. We shall, in the next few chapters, deal with some of the separate phases of this scheme to show where and, to some extent, how the nutrients of the adequate diet are involved in this operation.

Chapter 7
The carbohydrates and their metabolism

Weende nitrogen-free extract
and its component carbohydrates

It is appropriate to begin our consideration of the role of nutrients in animal metabolism with carbohydrates. Well over half the calories of the human diet normally are derived from carbohydrates; and in rations for farm animals, where fat seldom exceeds 5%, carbohydrate makes up at least 75% of the weight. It is to be noted, however, that the carbohydrate of the human dietary is almost all nitrogen-free extract, while in some livestock rations, notably those of ruminants, perhaps no more than one-fourth of the carbohydrate is nitrogen-free extract. Crude fiber represents the principal carbohydrate in rations for ruminants.

For many feedstuffs the term *nitrogen-free extract* is almost synonymous with starches and sugars. As we have seen, nitrogen-free extract does not contain any cellulose. Depending on the source of the material, this proximate analysis fraction may contain some hemicellulose and some lignin. We shall not deal further with the problem of lignin at this point. It is sufficient to say that in feeds where lignin is present in measurable amounts it tends to hamper bacterial attack on cellulose and hemicellulose. It furnishes the animal with no useful nutrient, and to the extent that it is a part of nitrogen-free extract it merely dilutes the potential energy of this fraction. Any hemicellulose in the nitrogen-free extract will be broken down by microorganisms in the digestive tract, as was discussed in connection with crude fiber and its components (Chapter 2).

In most cases, only foods consisting of the leafy parts of plants yield a nitrogen-free extract with appreciable amounts of substances other than starches and sugars. Furthermore, starches and sugars are the only components of the nitrogen-free extract that follow a straightforward course of digestion and metabolism in yielding their energy to animals. Thus, while the percentage figure indicating the amount of nitrogen-free extract in a food will include whatever hemicellulose and lignin may have been made soluble by the crude fiber procedure, the nutritionally effective energy from nitrogen-free extract is likely to be mostly from the starch and sugar components. The steps by which these two types of carbohydrate are reduced to the end products carbon dioxide and water are of particular interest, since eventually the breakdown products of crude fiber and ether extract, and of protein components that yield energy, enter the same "terminal" paths followed by the starches and sugars.

Digestion of nitrogen-free extract

Digestion of starches and sugars of the nitrogen-free extract is accomplished by a group of enzymes produced by the salivary glands, the pancreas, and the epithelial lining of the small intestine. Under normal conditions these enzymes, the α-amylases and disaccharidases, degrade dietary carbohydrate to monosaccharides. Salivary and pancreatic amylases hydrolyze starch to maltose and, in the case of amylopectin, some isomaltose. The disaccharides resulting from starch digestion, together with those of dietary origin, such as sucrose and lactose, are taken up intact and hydrolyzed in the brush border of the mucosal cell by the disaccharidases—maltase, isomaltase, sucrase, and lactase. These enzymes are characterized as being particulate bound, so that any disaccharidase activity in the digesta arises from cells sloughed during the continual regeneration of the mucosal lining.

In close proximity to the disaccharidases in the brush border is the Na^+-dependent monosaccharide transport mechanism, or "pump," which transports glucose and its analogues across cell membranes. This system, which is analogous to other biological-membrane transport systems, is closely associated with the absorption of water and electrolytes. Understanding of this association has been directly applied to the treatment of cholera, where oral administration of glucose and saline solution greatly ameliorates the lethal effects of severe dehydration. The absorption of glucose against a concentration gradient requires energy from ATP, which presumably participates in the Na^+ pump, since a Na^+ gradient is considered the primary driving force in the active transport of sugar through the intestinal wall.

Not all monosaccharides are absorbed at the same rate. Glucose and galactose are rapidly absorbed, whereas fructose is more slowly absorbed by a nonconcentrating mechanism. Active transport of sugars depends on the specific configuration of the sugar molecule: D-glucose has the ability to combine with the "carrier," whereas L-glucose does not; presence of the C-2 hydroxyl and the C-6 carbon greatly increase the affinity of the sugar molecule for the carrier.

Starches and sugars of dietary origin are not usually found in the feces. In fact, their presence in any appreciable quantitites in feces probably reflects a diseased condition in the animal. For example, an animal's deficiency in a specific disaccharidase results in a severe intolerance to that disaccharide. Lactase deficiency, both congenital and acquired, is fairly common in man. Acquired lactase deficiency, which is characterized by the lack of any intolerance to milk during infancy, is particularly prevalent among certain populations.

The metabolism of carbohydrates

Once digested and absorbed, the monosaccharides are transported by the blood to the liver and other tissues where they are metabolized. All of the reactions of intermediary metabolism are catalyzed by enzymes, and theoretically all are reversible. There are several types of reactions in carbohydrate metabolism; those involving the addition or subtraction of phosphorus are of special interest to us here because they usually result in the transfer of a large amount of energy. Accordingly, we shall consider them in some detail in order to clarify the general mechanism of the transfer of energy from one molecule to another.

Primary function of metabolism   The nutrients that are finally absorbed by a living cell supply it with the energy it needs to carry out its many functions, and with the chemical compounds from which it can build its structural and functional components. The resulting chemical reactions, which are referred to collectively as metabolism, also permit the interconversion of the various products of the breakdown of carbohydrate, fat, and protein. This latter aspect of metabolism is important in understanding the conversion of carbohydrate to fat in the fattening animal and the effect of dietary protein/calorie ratios on the efficient utilization of protein by the growing animal; this will be discussed in more detail in Chapter 11.

Because protoplasm is in a dynamic state, part of the work of the cell is the constant replacement of its substance. There is also the work of muscular activity in the vital functions of heartbeat, respiration, digestive tract peristalsis, and the general body movements incidental to maintenance living. If the energy wasted as heat is also included, these cell activities taken together

Box 7.1   Lactose intolerance

Lactose is a disaccharide synthesized by the mammary gland. During digestion this sugar is hydrolyzed into its component monosaccharides, glucose and galactose, by the enzyme lactase. This enzyme reaches maximum activity immediately after birth. Activity remains high throughout infancy, but by late childhood decreases to a very low level in all but the Caucasian race. Lactase activity appears to be confined to the outer cell layer of the intestinal epithelium, possibly in the brush border.

Lactose, which constitutes 7.0% to 7.5% of human milk and 4.5% of cow's milk, seems to have certain beneficial nutritional effects. For example, it stimulates the absorption of calcium and possibly other cations, such as magnesium, manganese, strontium, and barium. Lactose also has been claimed to promote the multiplication of microorganisms that are capable of synthesizing vitamins such as biotin, riboflavin, folacin, and pyridoxine. It has also been suggested that lactose improves the body's utilization of protein.

On the other hand, because of low intestinal lactase activity in a high proportion of non-Caucasian adults, their consumption of lactose in any appreciable quantity can create considerable problems. In such cases, only a portion of the lactose is hydrolyzed—the excess passes down into the lower regions of the gastrointestinal tract, where it undergoes bacterial fermentation. As a consequence, large quantities of fluids are drawn into the intestinal lumen due to the hyperosmotic effect of the unhydrolyzed lactose and its fermented by-products. Lactose intolerance (actually lactose malabsorption) is characterized by abdominal bloating, gaseousness, cramps, flatulence, and watery diarrhea. Initial symptoms are usually observed 30 to 90 minutes after the administration of the disaccharide; diarrhea usually occurs within two hours, and the symptoms disappear by 2 to 6 hours after the intake of lactose.

This situation is of practical concern in developing countries, as well as in school lunch programs in developed countries, where milk has been commonly used in attempts to correct or avoid serious nutritional problems. The argument as to whether lactose intolerance is actually synonymous with milk intolerance has arisen from these practices. There are those who claim that the intake of lactose required to bring about the symptoms of lactose intolerance is greater than what would be consumed with a moderate daily intake of milk, while others have shown that as little as one glass of milk, or its lactose equivalent, will produce gaseousness or cramps in 60% of lactose-intolerant humans.

Hence, caution in the general use of milk and its unfermented by-products is recommended for population groups that are prone to lactose intolerance. It should be kept in mind that the consumption of fermented dairy products, such as cheese and yogurt, will not create any problems in such groups.

See also *Dairy Council Digest* **42**(1971), No. 6, and **45**(1974), No. 5.

represent the energy cost of "maintenance." We shall see later that this amounts to some 93 kcals (389 kilojoules) daily per unit of metabolic size, which is expressed as the three-quarter power of the animal's body weight in kilograms (that is, $W_{kg}^{.75}$).

In addition, energy is needed for the cells' work of synthesizing such products as milk or eggs, or new body tissue, as must be done in growth or fattening. Finally, the cells of skeletal muscles require a certain amount of energy for any activity beyond that of maintenance living.

It is evident that body cells have a constant need for energy, and that the quantity of energy needed varies with the degree and nature of the cells' activity.

Within the cell, metabolism is organized into a series of reactions that permit the orderly transfer of energy from food sources, such as glucose, to processes requiring energy. The transfer of chemical energy from one reaction to another requires that there be a common reactant. The common reactant in most biological systems is the energy-rich compound adenosine triphosphate (ATP). In general, catabolism produces ATP or compounds easily converted to it, while anabolism, which requires energy, consumes ATP.

ATP—the driving force of biochemical processes

ATP, a polyanhydride of phosphoric acid, is characterized by a large negative free energy of hydrolysis under physiological conditions ($-\Delta G^{\circ\prime}$), and is referred to by the biochemist as an energy-rich or high-energy compound. It belongs to a group of phosphorus compounds that are the most prominent high-energy compounds in biological systems. It is important for students of nutrition to distinguish between high-energy compounds, such as ATP, and those of relatively low energy content, such as the phosphate esters (for example, glucose-6-phosphate).

ATP is supplied to the cell principally by biological oxidations. This entails the transfer of electrons from specific substrates to oxygen; free energy produced during this transfer is captured as chemical energy in the form of the energy-rich intermediary ATP. This transfer of electrons to oxygen and the accompanying phosphorylation of ADP (adenosine diphosphate) to ATP is referred to as *oxidative phosphorylation*. The two processes are inseparable; thus, oxygen deprivation is almost immediately lethal to most cells, because they have a constant need for ATP to carry out vital functions. Within limits, the rate of oxidation will vary with the demand for energy.

ATP provides the principal driving force for many biochemical processes, such as muscle contraction, biosynthesis of proteins, fats, nucleic acids, and complex carbohydrates, and absorption of nutrients against a concentration gradient. Reactions that are ATP-dependent fall into two broad categories: (1) reactions in which ATP provides the energy or driving force for an otherwise unfavored reaction and (2) reactions in which part of the ATP molecule is transferred to a suitable acceptor. Reactions in which ATP acts as an energy source are catalyzed by enzymes known as *ligases* or *synthetases*. An example is the conversion of acetate or fatty acids to their coenzyme A derivatives:

$$\text{Acetate} + \text{CoASH} + \text{ATP} \longrightarrow \text{Acetyl SCoA} + \text{AMP} + \text{PP}_i$$

Typical of reactions of the second category are those catalyzed by the phosphotransferases, such as glucokinase:

$$\text{Glucose} + \text{ATP} \xrightarrow{\text{Glucokinase}} \text{Glucose-6-PO}_4 + \text{ADP}$$

Another example is the activation of methionine to *S*-adenosyl methionine, which serves as a methyl donor in many reactions in the body:

$$\text{L-Methionine} + \text{ATP} \longrightarrow S\text{-Adenosyl methionine} + \text{PP} + \text{P}_i$$

Energy pathways—glycolysis and the pentose shunt

Having taken a brief overview of the important features of energy metabolism, we shall now consider in some detail the individual steps involved in carbohydrate metabolism. Our discussion will be restricted to *glycolysis*, or the metabolism of glucose, the principal end product of starch and sugar digestion. We should remember that an enzyme or enzyme complex is required for each step and that free energy $(-\Delta G°)$ is released in many of the reactions. The main route of glucose metabolism in most tissues begins with the phosphorylation of glucose to glucose-6-phosphate. This compound represents one of the major crossroads in the pathway of glucose metabolism, in that there are several alternative metabolic paths into which this product may be diverted. The details in the next few paragraphs may be followed with the aid of Figure 7.1.

Glucose-6-phosphate may undergo molecular rearrangement to form glucose-1-phosphate, which in turn may polymerize to form glycogen. In mammals, glycogen is the form in which glucose is temporarily stored (i.e., between feedings) in liver and skeletal muscle. Glycogen plays an important role in maintaining blood glucose levels and is an important store of readily available energy.

A small amount of glucose-6-phosphate continually enters another route, known as the *pentose shunt* or *hexosemonophosphate* (HMP) *pathway*. In this pathway glucose-6-phosphate undergoes two oxidations by the coenzyme

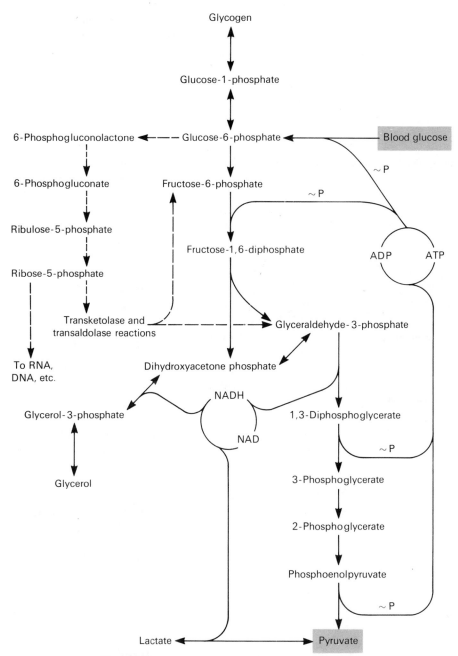

Figure 7.1
General scheme of glucose metabolism in the pentose shunt and glycolytic pathways.

NADP, the final oxidation being accompanied by a decarboxylation to the 5-carbon sugar ribulose-5-phosphate. This pentose in turn undergoes rearrangement to form ribose-5-phosphate and xylulose-5-phosphate. Thus, this pathway is of primary importance as a source of ribose and deoxyribose for nucleic acids (i.e., DNA and RNA) and nucleotide coenzymes (e.g., ATP, GTP). The remaining reactions in this pathway bring about the transformation of the pentose phosphates into hexose and triose phosphates. One of the enzymes catalyzing this transformation is a transketolase that contains thiamin pyrophosphate as a coenzyme. This is a fairly active pathway in red blood cells, which are readily available for analysis, and assay of transketolase activity in erythrocytes is used to estimate the level of thiamin in the body.

The main route of glucose-6-phosphate metabolism in most cells, however, is by the *glycolytic* or *Embden–Meyerhof pathway*. The primary features of this pathway are (1) the transformation of glucose-6-phosphate into a form that can be split into two triose units and (2) the conversion of these triose phosphates to pyruvate. Glucose-6-phosphate is rearranged to fructose-6-phosphate, which is phosphorylated by ATP to fructose-1,6-diphosphate. The next step is the cleavage of fructose-1,6-diphosphate to glyceraldehyde-3-phosphate and dihydroxyacetone phosphate. There is a minor metabolic branch at this point leading from dihydroxyacetone to glycerol. It is by this path that glycerol-3-phosphate is produced as needed for triglyceride synthesis. This path, in reverse, also accepts glycerol from the triglycerides when they are mobilized for energy.

Metabolism of glyceraldehyde-3-phosphate begins with oxidation by NAD and the resulting formation of 1,3-diphosphoglycerate. After several rearrangements, 1,3-diphosphoglycerate yields pyruvate, which stands at the second major crossroad in glycolysis. Two moles of ATP are produced for each mole of glyceraldehyde-3-phosphate converted to pyruvate. The NADH produced by the conversion of glyceraldehyde-3-phosphate to 1,3-diphosphoglycerate can transfer electrons to a number of compounds, including glycerol-3-phosphate. This compound can diffuse into the mitochondria, where it is oxidized: the electrons are first transferred to FAD and then via the oxidative phosphorylation pathway to oxygen. The net result is the formation of 2 moles of ATP for each mole of NADH formed in glycolysis. By contrast, 3 moles of ATP are formed for each mole of NADH formed within the mitochondria. Details of the oxidative phosphorylation pathway (electron transport) will be discussed in Chapter 11.

Pyruvate—an important crossroad in energy metabolism

Pyruvate stands at an important crossroad in glucose metabolism, because it can either enter the mitochondria and be converted to acetyl CoA or remain in the cytoplasm and be reduced to lactate by the oxidation of NADH. The

Box 7.2   The mitochondrion—the powerhouse of the cell

The mitochondrion is a highly structured cellular organelle that is intimately involved in energy conversions, particularly in cells whose metabolism is largely aerobic. In general, the number and distribution of mitochondria within a cell depend on the energy requirements of the cell: cells requiring large amounts of energy normally contain large numbers of mitochondria. Not only does the mitochondrion contain all of the enzymes and cofactors required for oxidation of the various breakdown products of carbohydrates, fats, and proteins, but the enzymes and cofactors of electron transport and oxidative phosphorylation are so arranged in the inner membrane of the mitochondrion as to provide for the most efficient production of ATP—the ultimate energy source for all the processes of life. Three molecules of ATP are produced for each pair of electrons released through oxidation in the mitochondrion, compared to only two molecules of ATP per pair of electrons released in glycolysis.

Inner
Outer   membrane   Intermembrane
membrane   space

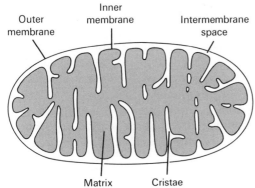

Matrix   Cristae

Diagram of the longitudinal cross-section of a mitochondrion.

The shape and size of the mitochondrion vary with the type of cell. In general, it is watermelon-shaped and ranges from 0.5 to 3.0 μ in length and from 0.1 to 0.6 μ in diameter. It is surrounded by a double membrane: the outer membrane is smooth and is the limiting membrane of the mitochondrion; the inner membrane is folded in a series of invaginations that protrude into the inner space, or lumen, of the mitochondrion. These invaginations, which have the appearance of a series of baffles, are called *cristae*.

The number of cristae in a mitochondrion varies from one tissue to another depending on the requirement for energy. The number of cristae in the mitochondria of heart muscle, for example, is very high compared to the number in the mitochondria of bronchial cells. Close inspection of the inner membrane shows that the inner surface is covered with knob-like structures, which are thought to be the functional units for the production of ATP. The lumen of the mitochondrion contains a viscous medium called the *matrix*, in which are found the enzymes of the citric acid cycle.

Although mitochondria are associated primarily with energy production in the cell, they are also the site of many other transformations, such as the production of acetyl CoA for fatty acid synthesis, the elongation of fatty acids, and the production of oxaloacetate for gluconeogenesis.

formation of lactate is the final, "dead-end" step in glycolysis. During strenuous work, lactate may accumulate in muscle, owing to a marked acceleration in glucose metabolism to pyruvate in order to meet the high demand for ATP.

In the mitochondria, pyruvate enters another pathway, variously referred to as the *tricarboxylic acid* (TCA) *cycle,* the *citric acid cycle,* or simply the *Krebs cycle,* after the man who discovered it. Metabolism of pyruvate in the mitochondria includes (1) decarboxylation by thiamin pyrophosphate (which explains the accumulation of pyruvate in blood during thiamin deficiency), (2) oxidation of the intermediate formed during decarboxylation, and finally (3) transfer of the 2-carbon acetyl group to coenzyme A, to form acetyl CoA. This condenses with oxaloacetate to form citrate, which in turn undergoes a series of transformations, the net effect of which is oxidation of acetate, yielding 2 moles of CO_2 and the restoration of oxaloacetate.

Acetyl CoA is also a common intermediate in the metabolism of fatty acids. In fact, the citric acid cycle is the final common energy pathway not only for carbohydrate and fat, but for the carbon fragments of protein when they are used for energy. There are many minor branches along the citric acid cycle, which are important in such interconversions as the formation of glucose from protein or the synthesis of fat from glucose.

Thus, at this point we shall interrupt our discussion of the citric acid cycle until we have described the metabolism of cellulose, hemicellulose, fat, and protein to the point where their metabolites enter this common pathway.

Suggested readings

Dickens, F., Randle, P. J., and Whelan, W. J. *Carbohydrate Metabolism and Its Disorders,* Vol. 1. Academic Press, London and New York (1968).

Dickens, F., Randle, P. J., and Whelan, W. J. *Carbohydrate Metabolism and Its Disorders,* Vol. 2. Academic Press, London and New York (1968).

Chapter 8
The carbohydrates and
their metabolism (continued)

Crude fiber and its component carbohydrates

Although the Weende analysis is not the only one that is in use or has been proposed to describe quantitatively the sum of the cellulose and hemicellulose of foods and feedstuffs, in this book the term *crude fiber* will always mean Weende fiber.

Many foods in the human dietary are rather low in fiber, if not completely devoid of it, and tables of composition giving their proximate analysis often omit figures for this fraction. Unfortunately, this practice has led to the erroneous impression that these carbohydrates are of no consequence in human nutrition, when in fact they play an important role because of their physical properties. In livestock rations, especially for herbivorous animals, the potential energy of cellulose and hemicellulose is of primary importance. In all species of animals, however, the mode of digestion and utilization of crude fiber differs from that of the components of nitrogen-free extract.

Makeup of Weende crude fiber

The general effects of the Weende analysis for crude fiber on a fat-free sample of food, or of other biological material are shown in Table 8-1. Since crude fiber is the ash-free residue of the acid-alkali treatment, it is evident that in any particular sample the crude fiber fraction contains most of the

Table 8.1
Effects of the Weende fiber analysis on the constituents of a fat-free sample

Constituent	Extraction on boiling with 1.25% H_2SO_4	Extraction on subsequent boiling with 1.25% $NaOH$
Protein	Partial	Complete
Starch and sugar	Complete	
Cellulose	Slight	Variable
Hemicellulose	Variable	Extensive but variable
Lignin	Slight	Extensive but highly variable

cellulose, variable proportions of the hemicelluloses, and a small proportion of the lignin, derived from lignocellulose.

Lignin itself is not a carbohydrate. It is a protective coating laid down on the cellulose-hemicellulose structure of plant tissues during their growth, apparently to protect them from bacterial attack. Wood is a highly lignified and hence a highly stable plant tissue; it is an extreme example of the stemmy material of plants used for foodstuffs. Because, nutritionally, lignin is always associated with cellulose and hemicellulose, it is appropriate to consider it one of the important components of crude fiber. It is in this sense that lignin is discussed in this book.

The same analytical procedure used for foods is applied to the fecal residues of those foods in order to compute coefficients of digestion for the proximate principles. In computing these coefficients, it is usually assumed that the portion of a food eaten that does not reappear in the feces has been digested. The difference between the measured intake of a nutritional component and the amount recovered from the feces over a corresponding period of time, expressed as a percentage of the intake, is by definition the *coefficient of apparent digestibility* for that component (discussed in detail in Chapter 23).

It is in measuring the digestibility of crude fiber that we see the effects of the variable extraction of hemicellulose, cellulose, and lignin that may occur in different samples analyzed according to this procedure. For example, of two different feeds having the same total amount of hemicellulose and cellulose, it is possible that in one the hemicellulose will be largely extracted in the Weende procedure, and consequently the crude fiber will be relatively high in cellulose. The other sample might contain a more resistant type of hemicellulose, so that the resulting crude fiber fraction would carry relatively less cellulose and more hemicellulose. If we assume that the hemicellulose from the feces will be extracted by the Weende procedure to the same extent as from the feeds themselves, then for these two samples we would get widely differing apparent digestibilities for the crude fiber. Some figures for a hypothetical example, shown in Table 8.2, will illustrate this effect.

Table 8.2
The effect of differing solubilities of hemicellulose in the Weende procedure on the apparent digestibility of crude fiber

Feed component	Actual amount in feed (g)	Insoluble in Weende treatment (%)	Weende fiber in feed (g)	Actual amount in feces (g)	Insoluble in Weende treatment (%)	Weende fiber in feces (g)	Apparent digestibility of crude fiber (%)
I							
Hemicellulose	10	10	1.0	1.5	10	0.15	
Cellulose	10	90	9.0	8.5	90	7.65	
Weende crude fiber			10.0			7.80	22
II							
Hemicellulose	10	50	5.0	4.0	50	2.00	
Cellulose	10	90	9.0	8.5	90	7.65	
Weende crude fiber			14.0			9.65	31

Table 8.3
Approximate makeup of the crude fiber
of alfalfa hay and of a cereal grain

Constituent	Alfalfa hay, mature (%)	Cereal grain, seed (%)
Cellulose	40	70
Hemicellulose	10	15
Lignin	50	15

The probable explanation for the variable extraction of lignin and hemicelluloses by the crude fiber procedure is that these substances are not of constant chemical makeup, but vary according to the kind of plant and perhaps also according to the part of the plant from which they come. Certainly we have sufficient evidence that the makeup of the crude fiber of different feeds is not the same, as can by seen from the data of Table 8.3.

Digestion of crude fiber

Crude fiber that is actually digested yields to an animal about the same amount of energy per gram as digested starch or sugar. Thus, the difference between nitrogen-free extract and crude fiber as sources of useful energy to an animal is one primarily of digestibility. It is generally believed that hemicellulose is more completely digested than cellulose. However, for most foodstuffs, cellulose is the major component of the crude fiber. Consequently, the digestibility of crude fiber depends largely on the digestibility of the cellulose in it.

The digestion of cellulose and hemicellulose by any species of animal with which we shall be concerned in this book is unique among the energy-yielding substances, in that it is not accomplished by enzymes of the animal body. Rather, the digestion of these carbohydrates depends upon the enzymes of symbiotic microorganisms that inhabit one or more parts of the digestive tract of all species of animals for which fibrous plant material constitutes a major portion of the diet. Under the attack of the microorganisms, cellulose and hemicellulose are degraded primarily to such volatile fatty acids as acetic, propionic, and butyric acids. In addition, considerable quantities of carbon dioxide and methane are produced by the fermentation that takes place in the digestive tract.

The role of lignin in the digestion of cellulose   The total amount of lignin and its sites of deposition in the stems of cured hay have been reported to affect the digestibility and nutritive value of forage. Botanists consider as lignin that group of substances which impart stiffness and durability to the plant cell wall. S. H. Clarke regarded the plant cell wall as a continuous interpenetrating system of cellulose and lignin; he likened the structure to reinforced concrete, in which the iron rods represent the cellulose framework, and the concrete represents the lignin and the other constituents of the structure.[*]

The chemist contends that lignin, isolated from plants, is not a single compound but a group of somewhat similar substances. These contain methoxyl and phenolic groups and aromatic "nuclei," and have carbon/hydrogen/oxygen ratios different from those of true carbohydrates. (A typical structural unit of lignin has the molecular formula $C_{10}H_{11}O_2$.)

Nutritionists find that lignin in forage plants not only is useless as a nutrient, but may have an adverse effect on the availability of nutrients within lignified cells. Data on the digestibility of lignin vary, perhaps because methods for its chemical isolation have yet to be perfected.

The cellulose of unlignified cell walls of forage is quickly attacked *in vivo* by cellulolytic microflora of the digestive tract of herbivorous animals. Because lignified cell walls are not attacked as readily, lignin inhibits the digestion of cellulose in forage. When we consider that cellulose can make up 90%–95% of dietary crude fiber, it is evident that difficulty in digesting crude fiber is in fact difficulty in digesting cellulose; this in turn is related to the degree to which the forage has become lignified.

The rate at which cellulose from a feedstuff is fermented (i.e., degraded or digested) by cellulolytic microflora can be measured *in vitro*, using rumen inoculum as a source of the microflora. Given sufficient time (36 hours), all of the cellulose of the forage is degraded in normal digestion. The rate, however, is not constant. Before fermentation of lignified cellulose begins there is a time lag, which depends on the degree of lignification. Measurements of this lag have been used to establish the comparative effective feeding values of forages for ruminant animals.[†]

Extent of fiber digestion   Species differ in the extent to which they can digest cellulose. In fact, the digestibility is not constant even among individuals of a species, because their microfloral population varies in size and composition. The latter depends importantly on the type of food eaten by the host animal, since not all intestinal tract microorganisms attack cellulose or hemicellulose.

---

[*]Clarke, S. H., *Nature* **142**(1958):899.

[†]Crampton, E. W., Donefer, E., and Lloyd, L. E., *J. Animal Sci.* **19**(1960):538.

The following list gives the digestibility of crude fiber by various species of animals:

Species	Where digested	% Digested
Ruminants	Rumen, colon	50–90
Horse	Caecum, colon	34–40
Pig	Caecum, colon	3–25
Rabbit	Caecum	16–18
Guinea pig	Caecum	34–40
Dog	Caecum	10–30
Human	Small and large intestine	25–35
Poultry	Caeca	20–30

It is evident that crude fiber digestion may be of sufficient magnitude in any of these species to necessitate its consideration in estimating the net energy of foods or diets. Only recently have we realized that cellulose digestion may be considerable in the human.

These digestibility figures are applicable only to the crude fiber typical of a diet normally eaten by the species named. For example, it should not be assumed that a human is necessarily able to digest any portions of the crude fiber in alfalfa hay. The cellulose in a human diet is more likely to come from cereals and leafy vegetables.

Products of crude fiber digestion   The end products of cellulose and hemicellulose digestion are volatile fatty acids and gases. Present evidence indicates that these short-chain fatty acids are absorbed primarily from that portion of the intestinal tract at which they are formed. It is well known that the volatile fatty acids formed in the rumen are absorbed rapidly and almost completely through the walls of the rumen into the bloodstream. Thus, in the ruminant the degraded carbohydrates do not necessarily travel through the digestive system proper, as is normally the case with nonruminants. The fate of the metabolized end products of carbohydrate digestion in the ruminant is summarized graphically in Table 8.4.

For most diets there is a residue of undigested and unabsorbed dietary components, "spent" microflora, and/or by-products of intermediary metabolism (e.g., calcium, iron) normally eliminated in the feces, which ultimately reaches the caecum and large intestine. Here, the organic components of the fecal mass undergo fermentation, to a degree that depends on the nature of the diet and the species of animal.

Fermentation of crude fiber and gas losses   The formation of carbon dioxide and methane gas in fermentation of the cellulose in the digestive tract complicates the determination of the useful energy the animal derives

Table 8.4
**Principal changes and ultimate fate of carbohydrate components
of the ration during their passage through the rumen and
small intestine of an adult ruminant**

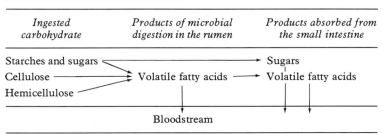

Ingested carbohydrate	*Products of microbial digestion in the rumen*	*Products absorbed from the small intestine*
Starches and sugars		Sugars
Cellulose	Volatile fatty acids	Volatile fatty acids
Hemicellulose		
	Bloodstream	

from crude fiber. These gases escape from the digestive system either through belching or by entrapment in the feces. Since neither is recorded with the fecal output of crude fiber they are usually counted as digestible portions of the crude fiber ingested.

In some species, the quantities of these gases may be very large: a well-fed dairy cow may produce 300 liters each of carbon dioxide and of methane. This represents an energy loss of about 4000 kcal per day, which is equivalent to about one-third of the maintenance energy cost of a 550-kg cow and is more energy than is normally consumed daily by most adult humans.

In practice it is commonly assumed that the energy loss from fermentation gases amounts to about 10% of the digestible energy of the mixed diet of herbivorous animals. It is considerably less in diets that do not contain cellulose or hemicellulose. In calculating metabolizable energy of human diets, gas loss is omitted as being quantitatively unimportant. However, gas loss cannot be disregarded in an accurate assessment of the useful energy of the diets of herbivorous animals.

Digestible, metabolizable, and net energy from cellulose

Species differ in the energy yield of the cellulose in their diets. If we define useful energy as the metabolizable energy, taking account of incomplete digestion of the energy-yielding components as well as the fermentative gas losses, then losses in one category by one species may be counterbalanced by losses in the other category by the other species. For example, it has been shown that, whereas cattle and rabbits digested quite differently the gross energy of experimental diets containing 4400 kcal per kilogram, the metabolizable energy they obtained from this diet was actually the same. Cattle suffered less loss from incomplete digestion than rabbits did, but rabbits suffered considerably less fermentation gas loss than the cattle did. The heat loss of the two species on this diet was the same, with the end result that both the metabolizable energy and the net energy yielded by the diet was the same for both species. A summary of the data from these experiments is shown in Table 8.5.

Table 8.5
Species differences in utilization of cellulose

Species	Gross energy of food (kcal/kg)	Fecal loss (%)	Digested energy (kcal/kg)	Gas loss (%)	Metabolizable energy (kcal/kg)	Heat loss (%)	Net energy (kcal/kg)
Cattle	4400	29	3124	15.5	2442	16.5	1716
Rabbit	4400	35	2960	9.5	2442	16.5	1716

Factors affecting the utilization of fiber energy

The very obvious differences between species of animals in their ability to digest cellulose or crude fiber have already been pointed out earlier. These differences are in part traceable to the anatomical structure of the digestive tracts: those species with simple digestive systems have insufficient capacity for storing large quantities of the bulky cellulose-containing diets or for housing a large active microflora that can attack the cellulose to produce end products utilizable by the host animal. But in addition to these species differences there are marked differences between individuals within a species. Age is an important factor—in general, young animals are less able to digest cellulose than adults are. There is no precise explanation of these differences due to age, but their existence is common knowledge in livestock feeding practice.

Another factor is the nutritional habits of the animal. It is easy to demonstrate increasing digestibility of crude fiber with an increasing length of time that fiber has been a part of the diet. This is evidence that a microflora capable of attacking cellulose and hemicellulose develops as a consequence of the continued ingestion of diets containing these materials.

There is also evidence that the nutrient makeup of the diet itself may have an effect on the extent to which cellulose is digested. The microflora of the digestive tract consists of a number of species, all of which appear to require certain inorganic elements and certain vitamins for their own sustenance. To a great degree, almost any source of nitrogen will suffice for their protein needs. With respect to energy needs, however, there appear to be differences among these microfloral species: some utilize starch and sugars from the host's diet, whereas others utilize cellulose. Apparently, those species of microorganisms that feed on starch or sugar begin their activity almost at once following the ingestion of food, and they draw the quantities of minerals and vitamins and nitrogen needed to support their growth.

The cellulose feeders, on the other hand, do not become fully active until two or three hours after the arrival of the swallowed food. As a consequence, they have available to them only the amounts of minerals and vitamins that the starch feeders have left. Thus, with diets deficient in minerals, vitamins, or nitrogen the growth and multiplication of the cellulose-splitting bacteria may be curtailed, so that cellulose digestion is much reduced.

This has been offered as an explanation for what has been called the *associative effects between foods*. It is believed that certain foods or products may furnish supplementary amounts of some nutrients sufficient to permit increased bacterial activity, and consequently to alter the amount of energy yielded by the mixture from that which would be yielded by some other combination of equivalent energy content, or which might be predicted on the basis of the chemical content of the individual foods.

It might be supposed that cellulose would be more completely digested if it were finely ground before ingestion. This is probably true in the case of monogastric animals, but in the case of ruminants fine grinding usually results in a more rapid passage of the material through the rumen. This reduces the length of time the material stays in the area where microfloral activity is most active. Consequently, it could cause the completeness of the attack on the cellulose to be reduced, and thus decrease the completeness of digestion. In addition, finely ground material will not be regurgitated to the same extent, resulting in a change in rumen pH and a consequent change in the character of the microfloral population in the rumen. The effect of finely grinding the roughage in ruminant diets is often underestimated. The average digestibility by steers of the dry matter of pasture herbage clippings has been reported as about 80%; if these dried clippings are ground for feeding, digestibility may drop to 66%. Most of this reduction can be ascribed to a reduction in the digestibility of the crude fiber portion.

The nature of the cellulose itself may have an effect on the extent of its digestibility. Under normal environmental conditions, cellulose-splitting bacteria attack this carbohydrate readily and promptly. However, cellulose as it appears in typical foodstuffs may be not pure cellulose, but a combination of cellulose and lignin, the latter in various concentrations and distributions in the plant tissues. Lignin, perhaps because of its phenolic nucleus, is not readily attacked by microorganisms; consequently, lignification of cellulose tends to interfere with its digestibility by these agents.

Lignification of plant tissue usually starts in the main stalk at the base portions and, with increasing maturity, gradually affects tissues farther removed from the base. However, the very young stems of plants will not have become lignified even after the plant is nearly mature, and these are usually quite readily digested by any animal species that has a suitable microflora. Thus, although forages tend to decrease in digestibility of carbohydrate with advancing maturity, the degree of depression of digestibility may be related more to the extent of the lignification than to its concentration at any one point. This makes the measurement of total lignin in a feed an uncertain index of the digestibility of the crude fiber.

Hemicellulose

Hemicellulose is found chiefly in the leafy parts of plants, and it may constitute up to 20% of the crude fiber in diets of herbivorous animals. The manner of its digestion and ultimate utilization appears to be analogous to that of cellulose. The end products of the bacterial attack are the short-chain volatile fatty acids. There is probably less fermentative gas loss from hemicellulose than from cellulose. However, since hemicellulose makes up a smaller fraction of crude fiber than cellulose does, the usefulness of crude fiber as a source of energy depends more on the behavior of cellulose than on the behavior of hemicellulose.

Physical role of fiber

In those species of animals with simple digestive systems, particularly those with nonfunctional caeca, the physical role of cellulose and hemicellulose may often be of greater importance than any contribution they make to the useful energy demand of the animal.

Bulk and energy intake   Since the bulkiness of the diet is determined largely by the quantity of nondigestible material it contains (which, for all practical purposes, depends on the quantity of crude fiber), it follows that bulky foods are of lower food value per unit of their weight than nonbulky foods. This must be considered when foods are chosen for specific purposes.

The energy and nutrients needed under conditions of heavy work or high production could be supplied by some foods only if the animal were fed quantities that would exceed the capacity of its digestive system. Thus, maintenance rations for livestock may contain bulky feeds in amounts that satisfy hunger but yield limited amounts of nutrients. When more nutrients are required, bulky feeds must be replaced by more concentrated ones, thus increasing the ingested nutrients without increasing the total volume of feed consumed. Conversely, when intake of excess calories is to be avoided, fiber-containing foods are introduced into the diet to dilute the energy per volume of food consumed; such diets, while still satisfying hunger because of their bulk, effect a reduction in the caloric intake of the individual.

An example of the use of bulky foods to restrict fattening is a practice sometimes followed to produce lean hogs. Here the cereal grains and their concentrated by-products that are normally a part of the growing ration of the young pig are partly replaced by feeds of high fiber content, such as bran, alfalfa meal, and oat hulls. This dilution of the energy component with fibrous carbohydrates reduces the fattening value of the ration, even though the animals continue to be "full-fed."

When cellulose or hemicellulose is added to the diet to increase the fiber content the effect is to dilute the potentially useful energy of the ration. Naturally occurring cellulose in foods is part of the cell wall of the plant structure. Unless this cell wall is ruptured, the cell contents will be protected from digestive fluids, which results in a depression of the digestibility of the contained starch, sugars, nitrogen, and lipid material. Whenever cooking or grinding increases the digestibility of the food it is probably because the "envelope" enclosing the cell contents has been ruptured, thus exposing them to digestive action.

Laxative properties of fiber   The bulkiness of the fecal mass encourages the peristaltic action by which food residues are propelled through the intestinal tract. Some of this bulkiness is probably due to entrapped gas, but usually absorbed water is more important. The ability of fecal material to hold water depends more on the nature of the crude fiber components of the diet than on the total quantity of the indigestible material in it.

R. O. Williams and coworkers have found a high degree of correlation between the weight of the stool and the composition of the "indigestible residue" in the intestine.* "Indigestible residue" was defined as the total of the cellulose, hemicellulose, and lignin. For a standard, the experimenters used a residue-free diet, to which they added, in different tests, certain quantities of indigestible residue in various foods. The quantities of these added residues were such that in each case there was a daily intake of 10 grams of cellulose, hemicellulose, and lignin. The feces were analyzed for indigestible residue and for volatile fatty acids. The weight of the indigestible residue in the stool from the experimental diet and the weight of the stool formed on the residue-free diet were subtracted from the total weight of feces to give a figure for the increment of stool weight (i.e., the extra weight due to the cellulose, lignin, and hemicellulose) on the experimental diet.

A selection of the data from some of these tests shown in Table 8.6 illustrates the relation between the water-holding property of the fiber of some foods and their laxative property. These data make it evident that the laxative values of the indigestible residues from the various foods are not the result of the original bulk of the diet. There is, however, a correlation between the extra weight of the stool, the amount of the carbohydrate that has been digested, and the laxative value. This indicates that fatty acids produced from the microbial digestion of the fiber might be the irritants responsible for the laxative value. Certainly those residues that have the highest fatty acid indices are the most laxative.

It is notable that lignin itself appears to be costive: whenever the indigest-

*Williams, R. O., Wicks, L., Bierman, H. R., and Olmsted, W. H., *J. Nutr.* **19**(1940):593.

Table 8.6
Effects of the carbohydrate–lignin–hemicellulose complex on the behavior of foods in the digestive tract

Source of fiber	Cellulose (%)	Lignin (%)	Hemicellulose (%)	Total ingested with diet in 6 days (g)	Extra stool weight over fiber-free control (g)	Cellulose digested (%)	Fatty acid index of stool	Relative laxative action (on scale of 8)
Alfalfa	32	15	19	80	240	6	28	1
Agar-agar	0	0	81	80	666	49	90	5
Cellu flour	79	0	17	71	93	7	3	2
Carrots	23	3	29	107	541	74	97	7
Cottonseed hulls	19	21	32	106	97	15	28	3
Cabbage	30	3	28	96	625	63	135	8
Wheat bran	17	8	35	146	475	41	101	4
Corn germ	16	2	31	155	578	89	110	6

ible residue added had a high lignin value the laxative value of the ration was low. It is particularly notable that carrots and corn germ meal—two products the indigestible residues of which have nearly the same proportions of cellulose, hemicellulose, and lignin—produced nearly equal laxation values in the diets to which they were added.

It is not known whether the increment in stool weight is due to the nature of the indigestible residue or to greater water secretion due to stimulation of the intestine by the extra fatty acids.

Intermediary metabolism of digested cellulose and hemicellulose

Cellulose and hemicellulose, as we have already stated, are not digested to sugar but to volatile fatty acids. These are absorbed at the site of their formation; that is, they are absorbed through the walls of the rumen, the caecum, or the colon, depending on the species of animal and sometimes also on the nature of the products.

Of the volatile fatty acids in the rumen, caecum, or colon of the species listed in Table 8.7, acetic acid is the most abundant, and propionic acid second. Under normal conditions, the quantity of butyric acid formed is

Table 8.7
Fatty acids derived from the digestion of fiber (cellulose)

Species	Site of formation and absorption	Percentage of total acid as		
		Acetic	*Propionic*	*Butyric*
Sheep	Rumen	64	19	17
Ox	Rumen	69	18	13
Ox	Caecum	72	18	10
Pig	Caecum	62	28	10
Rat	Caecum	56	31	13
Dog	Colon	51	36	13

relatively small. Butyric acid is ketogenic; consequently it is normally not used to form carbohydrate in intermediary metabolism. Propionic acid is a precursor of glycogen, which is the only soluble product of cellulose digestion that is known with certainty to be a carbohydrate precursor. Acetic acid, on the other hand, does not form carbohydrate. In any case, the end products of the digestion of cellulose and of hemicellulose—or, for practical purposes, of crude fiber—enter intermediary metabolism as fatty acids, not as sugars. Consequently, they do not proceed through the glycolytic pathway from

Box 8.1   The role of fiber in the human diet

Dietary fiber has long been considered an inert part of the human diet, primarily because it contributes only negligible amounts of nutrients to the diet. However, recent clinical and epidemiological observations suggest that dietary fiber may play an important physiological role in the maintenance of health and general well-being.

Dietary fiber is not synonymous with crude fiber. It is a generic term that includes all plant constituents that are not digestible by secretions of the human digestive system. It includes the nondigestible carbohydrates—such as cellulose, hemicellulose, pectin, and gums—and the noncarbohydrate constituent lignin. Crude fiber, on the other hand, is the ash-free material that remains after rigorous digestion with hot sulfuric acid and with hot sodium hydroxide. It has been suggested that crude fiber amounts to only 20%–50% of the total dietary fiber in most diets.

All foods of vegetable origin contribute to the fiber content of the diet. Whole grain cereals and cereal by-products, such as bran, are rich sources of dietary fiber. Dry beans and roasted nuts also contain appreciable quantities of fiber. The amount of fiber in plant foods varies with the maturity of the fruit or vegetable and the degree of processing it has received. Owing to the lack of a satisfactory analytical method, it is not possible to determine accurately the amount of fiber in our diets. However, there is little question that there has been a precipitous drop in the fiber content of Western diets during the present century. The per capita consumption of whole wheat bread and other cereal products has declined by about 40% since 1900. There also has been a slight decline in the consumption of fruits and vegetables. It has been estimated that the fiber contributed to the diet by fruits and vegetables has declined about 20% since 1900, and that contributed by breads and cereals about 50%.

The effectiveness of fiber for relieving constipation has been recognized for some time. In fact, some breakfast cereals have been promoted on the basis of their high fiber content. The ingestion of increased amounts of fiber is associated with larger, wetter stools, decreased transit time for food, and decreased pressure within the colon. The success of high-fiber diets in the treatment of diverticulitis—a disorder characterized by inflammation of the small protrusions, or diverticula ("sacs"), that form on the large intestine—is thought to be due primarily to the laxative effect of the fiber. It is ironic that, until recently, the traditional treatment for diverticular disease, which is virtually endemic in Western societies, has been the use of low-fiber diets.

A considerable number of unrelated noninfectious diseases—such as diverticulosis, appendicitis, coronary-artery disease, and cancer of the colon—have been associated with the low fiber content of Western diets.[*] However, many of these associations have been questioned.[†] The importance of fiber in the human diet will finally be determined only by clinical and experimental observations.

---

[*]Burkitt, D. P., Walker, A. R. P., and Painter, N. S., *Lancet*, No. 2 (1972):1408.
[†]Mendeloff, A. I., *Nutr. Rev.* **33**(1975):321.

sugars to pyruvate. Instead, acetic acid proceeds directly to acetyl CoA, while propionic acid enters the citric acid cycle as succinyl CoA. These considerations are of some importance in the normal feeding of certain herbivorous animals, especially when the diet may consist entirely of roughage. Under these conditions there may be a large production of acetyl CoA from the acetate derived from cellulose, but a relatively smaller production of propionate and hence succinate and oxaloacetic acid. This could reduce the rate of formation of citrate, with a consequent increase in the rate of formation of acetoacetic acid and acetone. Indeed, this may be one of the ways in which secondary acetonemia occurs. It is significant that one of the treatments for acetonemia is the injection of glucose; it may be that this treatment is effective because it increases the amount of pyruvate and hence the ratio of oxaloacetate to acetyl CoA.

Suggested readings

Crampton, E. W., and Harris, L. E. *Applied Animal Nutrition* (2nd ed.). W. H. Freeman and Company, San Francisco (1969): Chapter 2.

Dehority, B. A. "Hemicellulose Degradation by Rumen Bacteria," *Federation Proceedings* **32**(1973):1819.

Eastwood, M. A. "Vegetable Fibre: Its Physical Properties," *Proceedings of the Nutrition Society* **32**(1973):137.

Hungate, R. E. *The Rumen and Its Microbes.* Academic Press, New York (1966).

Kistner, A. *Physiology of Digestion in the Ruminant.* Butterworths, Washington, D.C. (1965).

van Soest, P. J. "The Uniformity and Nutritive Availability of Cellulose," *Federation Proceedings* **32**(1973):1804.

van Soest, P. J., and McQueen, R. W. "The Chemistry and Estimation of Fibre," *Proceedings of the Nutrition Society* **32**(1973):123.

Chapter 9
Fats and their utilization

In Chapter 2 we pointed out the relation between the neutral fats of foodstuffs and the Weende proximate principle called ether extract. The ether extract of plant seeds and of foods of animal or marine origin is mostly neutral fat. However, plant materials other than seeds usually contain considerable quantities of complex lipids and pigments that are extractable with ether but do not yield energy to an animal. Nevertheless, because the useful energy of ether extract is contained in the triglyceride portion, we can discuss the metabolism of ether extract as though it were neutral fat.

Dietary fat—amount and type

Before we proceed to the metabolism of fat it may be worthwhile to consider the overall importance of fat in the diets of animals and to describe in general terms what is meant by dietary fat. Fats are concentrated sources of energy, which makes them especially valuable in certain diets, such as those of broiler chickens. Some fat in the diet is necessary for practically all species, and for some, such as humans, it appears to be of considerable importance. However, the amount of fat that is necessary or desirable in the diet, particularly the human diet, remains uncertain.

Dietary fat is a source of linoleic acid, an essential fatty acid. Dietary fats also serve as "carriers" of fat-soluble vitamins, and some fat is necessary for absorption of these vitamins. In fact, impairment of the absorption of fat-soluble vitamins is the most serious consequence of a dietary deficiency of fat or fatty acids. Fat is also important to the palatability of food, especially in the human diet, where fat for frying food, as a spread, and as a base for salad dressing increases the taste appeal of meals. The part that fats play in the palatability of foods will be considered in greater detail at the end of this chapter.

It is estimated that fats supply about 40% of the calories in the average North American diet. About 45% of this total is from pure fat, such as butter, margarine, shortenings, and cooking oils. Meats supply slightly more than 30% and dairy products other than butter about 15% of the total. Although there has not been much change in per capita fat consumption since 1940, there has been an appreciable change in the source of dietary fat. Fat from animal sources has decreased from nearly 75% of the total in 1940 to slightly less than 60%, whereas vegetable oils, margarines, and shortenings increased their share from about 17% in 1940 to over 30% of the total. These changes have been accompanied by a lowered consumption of saturated fatty acids and oleic acid and an appreciably increased consumption of polyunsaturated fatty acids, particularly linoleic acid. It is difficult, however, to determine accurately the fatty acid content of foods. Lipid from animal sources, especially from nonruminants, can vary considerably in fatty acid composition, depending on the diet of the animal. The fatty acid composition of margarine and shortenings also may vary considerably, depending both on the source of the fats and on the method and degree of hydrogenation to which the fats have been subjected.

The data from which fat consumption by humans is calculated are not obtained from dietary surveys, but from surveys of the types and quantities of retail foods on the market. Thus, the figures contain, in addition to fat actually eaten, the total of all fat wastage, including meat trimmings at the sales counter, cooking losses, discarded fats from deep-fat frying, and plate losses. Nevertheless, the data indicate the direction of the changes that have occurred in the pattern of fat consumption. The major shift since 1940 has been an increase in the proportion of vegetable-based fats and oils at the expense of animal fats.

The average daily intake of fat from all sources by adults in North America is about 130 grams, and fats account for over 20%, by weight, of the human diet there. Livestock rations, on the other hand, seldom contain anywhere near 20% fat. Grain feeds normally average less than 5% fat, and the forages that make up a large proportion of the ration of herbivores contain only half this amount of ether extract. Poultry rations are frequently fortified with edible fats, but seldom to a level greater than 5% fat.

The proportion of fat in the diet is of interest to the dietitian for the same reasons that it interests the livestock feeder. The higher the proportion of fat, the more "fattening" each unit weight of diet or ration. The livestock feeder may wish to avoid fat in pig rations in order to produce lean bacon, whereas he may prefer fat in rations for broiler chickens and turkeys so as to produce a more acceptable carcass. Similarly, the dietitian dealing with problems of overweight will recommend a reduction in energy intake, which may be accomplished by a reduction in fat intake. On the other hand, the recommendation for the active child or adult engaged in heavy work may be an increase in fat intake in order to meet energy needs without unduly increasing the total quantity (bulk) of food that must be eaten. The dietitian and the livestock feeder are also concerned with the nature of fat in the diet. Many nutritionists advocate a shift from saturated to polyunsaturated fatty acids in the diet of humans because of the implication of dietary fat in heart disorders, although knowledge of the nutritional antecedents of disorders such as atherosclerosis is at present far from conclusive. The livestock feeder, by contrast, may wish to avoid polyunsaturated fatty acids in pig rations, because these fatty acids lower the melting point of carcass fat, thereby producing a soft, flabby carcass.

It should be mentioned that food processors also are concerned with food fats. As mentioned above, fat contributes to the palatability of foods. However, it also may create problems for the food processor. Fats, particularly those containing a high proportion of polyunsaturated fatty acids, are very susceptible to oxidation. This is a major cause of food spoilage; unless special precautions are taken, such as the addition of antioxidants or storage at low temperature, the shelf life of foods containing fat is very short. Fats also have a tendency to absorb odors and flavors that can render a food unpalatable.

Essential fatty acids

Complete removal of fat from the diet of an animal results in poor growth and the onset of dermatitis. These symptoms can be reversed by feeding small amounts of the polyunsaturated fatty acids linoleic acid and arachidonic acid. Linoleic acid is an 18-carbon acid with double bonds at the 9 and 12 positions, and arachidonic acid is a 20-carbon acid with double bonds at positions 5, 8, 11, and 14.

Since fatty acids are straight-chain, aliphatic monocarboxylic acids, the position of a double bond is designated by its distance from the carboxyl end of the molecule. However, in discussing the biological chemistry of fatty acids it is convenient to identify the position of a double bond by its distance from the methyl end of the molecule. The methyl carbon is designated the n-carbon irrespective of the length of the chain. Thus, linoleic acid ($C_{18:2n6}$)

and arachidonic acid ($C_{20:4n6}$) belong to the same class of fatty acid because in both of them the first double bond from the methyl end is between the 6th and 7th carbons. This feature, a double bond at the n-6 position, distinguishes the essential fatty acids as a group, and is illustrated for linoleic acid in Figure 9.1.

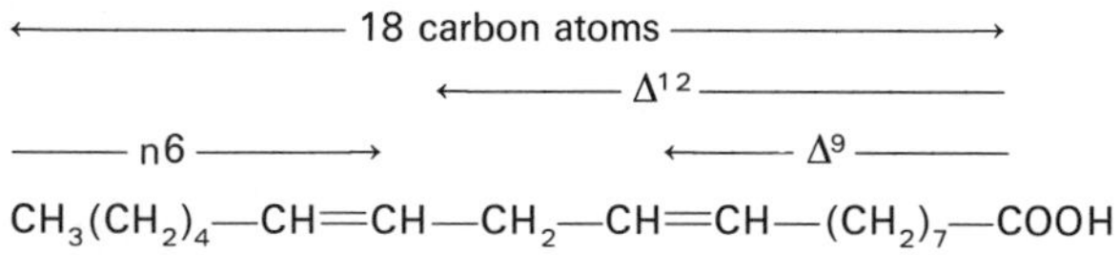

$$\overset{\longleftarrow \text{18 carbon atoms} \longrightarrow}{\underset{\text{CH}_3(\text{CH}_2)_4\text{—CH}=\text{CH—CH}_2\text{—CH}=\text{CH—(CH}_2)_7\text{—COOH}}{}}$$

(18 carbon atoms; Δ^{12}; n6 →; ← Δ^9)

CH$_3$(CH$_2$)$_4$—CH=CH—CH$_2$—CH=CH—(CH$_2$)$_7$—COOH

Figure 9.1
A schematic presentation of the formula for the essential fatty acid, linoleic acid, $C_{18:2n6}$ or cis,cis-$\Delta^{9,12}$-octadecadienoic acid.

Linolenic acid, which has double bonds at positions 3, 6, and 9 from the n-carbon, will restore growth in animals deficient in fatty acids, but has no antidermatitic action. Thus it appears that the presence of a double bond at the n-3 position interferes with one aspect of the metabolic functions of linolenic acid. However, in spite of these observations, there is considerable evidence that in brain lipids linolenic acid and its higher homologs perform a specific function not shared by members of the linoleic series, thus making linolenic acid a dietary essential.

Mammals and birds are able to synthesize oleic acid, an 18-carbon fatty acid with a double bond at the Δ^9 position. They are also able to convert linoleic acid to arachidonic acid by inserting double bonds between the carboxyl group and the Δ^9 double bond. However, essential fatty acids must be included in the diets of these species because of an inability to add a double bond beyond carbon 9 from the carboxyl end.

There is seldom a deficiency of essential fatty acids in practical diets and rations. Thus, for practical purposes, neutral fats are primarily nonspecific sources of energy in the diet.

Digestion and absorption of fat

In recent years, considerable advances have been made in understanding the digestion and absorption of fats. These advances include elucidation of events that occur in the lumen of the intestine and those that occur during the uptake and transport of lipid by the mucosal cells. A general scheme depicting the major steps in digestion and absorption of triglycerides by nonruminants—such as the pig, mouse, and human—is shown in Figure 9.2.

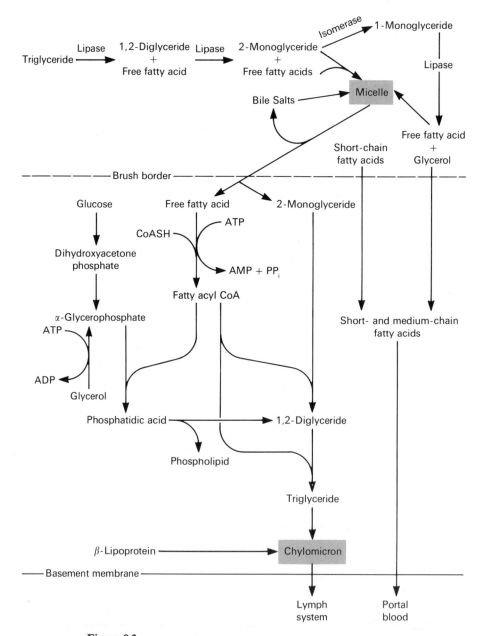

Figure 9.2
A schematic presentation of the major steps in the digestion and absorption of triglycerides in nonruminants.

Digestion of fats and absorption of fats are distinct, although intimately related processes. Digestion, which takes place in the lumen of the intestine, splits large lipid molecules into moieties that can be absorbed—that is, taken up from the lumen and transported to the lymphatic or the portal circulatory systems. Triglycerides are hydrolyzed to free fatty acids and 2-monoglycerides by the action of pancreatic lipase and bile salts. Pancreatic lipase acts only at an oil–water interface, which explains why emulsification is required for the digestion of some fats. Emulsification of triglyceride is aided by the detergent properties of bile salts, which also play a fundamental role in the formation of *micelles*. These are tiny particles formed by the combination of bile salts with the free fatty acids and monoglycerides produced during digestion. The net result of fat digestion is conversion of triglycerides in an emulsion phase to free fatty acids and monoglycerides in a micellar phase, which can be absorbed by the mucosal cells of the intestine. It is estimated that each emulsion particle gives rise to nearly 1 million micelles. Although the formation of micelles is essential for normal fat absorption, bile salts (which are reabsorbed and recycled via the liver) are not absorbed at the same site as fatty acids and monoglycerides. Bile salts are absorbed in the ileum, whereas fat absorption occurs primarily in the duodenum and upper jejunum.

During transport from the lumen to the lymphatic system, free fatty acids with chain lengths greater than 10 carbons are resynthesized to triglycerides by either the monoglyceride pathway or the L-α-glycerophosphate pathway. In both pathways the free fatty acids are first converted to their coenzyme A derivatives. In the monoglyceride pathway, the 2-monoglyceride acts as an acceptor of activated fatty acids, whereas L-α-glycerophosphate is the fatty acid acceptor in the pathway bearing its name. Esterification of L-α-glycerophosphate yields phosphatidic acid, which can be converted either to triglyceride or to phospholipid. The relative quantitative importance of these two pathways varies but, in general, the monoglyceride pathway predominates in nonruminants.

The mechanism of fat digestion and absorption in ruminants, however, varies with age. The mechanism in newborn calves or lambs, where the rumen is nonfunctional, is characteristic of that in nonruminants. In adult ruminants, on the other hand, virtually all of the dietary fat is hydrolyzed to free fatty acids and glycerol by the microflora of the rumen. Considerable hydrogenation of unsaturated fatty acids also takes place in the rumen. Thus, the fat entering the small intestine contains a high proportion of saturated free fatty acids and little monoglyceride. As in nonruminants, micelle formation is important for fat absorption in ruminants, but lysolecithin takes over the function of monoglyceride. Resynthesis of triglyceride in the intestinal epithelium takes place via the L-α-glycerophosphate pathway. (See Figure 9.3.)

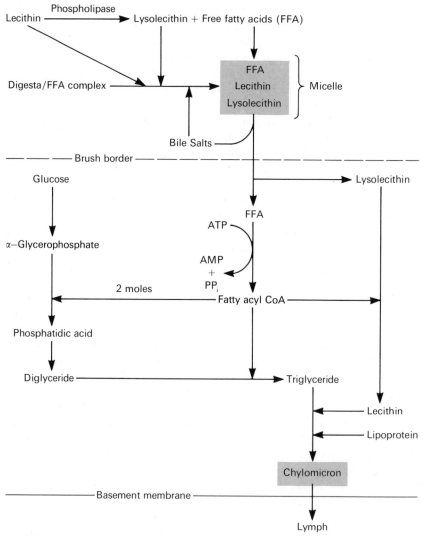

Figure 9.3
Schematic presentation of the major steps in the absorption of dietary fat in the small intestine of ruminants.

In both ruminants and nonruminants, triglycerides synthesized in the intestinal epithelium during fat absorption are secreted into the lymph in the form of *chylomicrons*. These are low-density lipoproteins that are approximately 86% triglyceride together with small amounts of protein, cholesterol, phospholipid, and the fat-soluble vitamins. Incorporation into chylomicrons prepares dietary fat for transport to various tissues in the body.

The synthesis of triglycerides, their incorporation into chylomicrons, and their subsequent secretion into the lymph occurs only for the long-chain fatty acids. Fatty acids with chain lengths of less than 10 carbons are not reesterified into triglyceride in the intestinal mucosa. These short- and medium-chain fatty acids are released unesterified into the portal blood-stream rather than into the lymph.

Fat digestibility and metabolic fecal fat   Apparent digestibility of fat, taken to be the difference between the amount of fat ingested and the amount excreted in feces, is usually high, although it varies with the fatty acid com- position of the dietary fat and the age of the animal. Digestibility is a compos- ite expression of the processes of digestion and absorption; any defect in either of these processes will be reflected in depressed digestibility.

Long-chain saturated fatty acids are poorly absorbed, especially by young animals. Thus the digestibility of palmitic acid and stearic acid is appreciably

---

Box 9.1   Protected fats in the rations of ruminants

Widespread interest, among not only animal nutritionists but also dietitians and cardiologists, met reports in 1970 that the polyunsaturated fatty acid content of meat and milk could be appreciably increased by feeding *protected fats* to ru- minants.* Protected fats are simply polyunsaturated oils—such as linseed, sunflower, or corn oil—that have been encapsulated in an envelope of for- maldehyde-treated casein. Encapsulation of the fats protects them from hy- drogenation by rumen microorganisms. The protected-fat complex is hy- drolyzed under the acid conditions of the abomasum, thereby releasing the fat, which is digested and absorbed almost unchanged from the small intestine. Feeding of protected fats to ruminants results in the incorporation of large amounts of polyunsaturated fatty acids into the triglycerides of plasma, milk, and depot fats. The proportion of polyunsaturated fatty acids in milk fat has been found to increase from the 2%–3% found in normal milk to 20%–30% in the milk of cows fed protected fat. The effect of protected fat on the fatty acid composition of milk fat was apparent within 1 to 2 days of its feeding. A longer time is necessary to induce changes in the fatty acids of depot fat.

Coating fats with formaldehyde-treated casein not only protects the polyun- saturated fatty acids from microbial hydrogenation in the rumen but also makes possible the feeding of greater than normal quantities of fat to ruminants. The net result of such a regimen is an increase in milk yield and in the fat content of the milk.

*Scott, T.W., Cook, L.J., and Mills, S.C., *J. Am. Oil Chem. Soc.* **48**(1971):358.

lower than that of oleic acid or linoleic acid. In fact, the presence of one or more double bonds in the fatty acid is equivalent to shortening the carbon chain by 6 carbons; thus the digestibility of oleic acid is approximately the same as that of lauric acid. However, configuration of the dietary triglyceride can have an effect on digestibility of individual fatty acids. For example, it has long been known that fat of human milk is better absorbed by human infants than butterfat from cow's milk. Recent work has shown that this difference is primarily due to the fact that palmitic acid, the principal fatty acid in both fats, is esterified at the 2-position in human milk, whereas it is randomly distributed in the triglyceride molecule of butterfat. Digestion of fat from human milk yields 2-monopalmitin, whereas hydrolysis of butterfat produces free palmitic acid. It also has been shown that fat in an infant formula is more readily absorbed when the fat fraction contains lard, where palmitic acid is principally in the 2-position, than when it has the same fatty acid composition with palmitic acid randomly esterified.

Ingestion of large quantities of fat slows the rate of passage of digesta through the digestive tract: presence of fat in the duodenum suppresses the muscular activity of the stomach and thus slows gastric emptying. Thus, fatty meals are said to be more "staying" than low-fat meals. This feedback mechanism encourages optimum digestion and absorption of fat.

Apparent digestibility underestimates the true digestibility of fat because some of the fecal fat is not of direct dietary origin. This nondietary component is referred to as *metabolic fat* and is composed of unabsorbed bile secretions, fats from sloughed and desquamated mucosal cells, and lipids synthesized by intestinal microorganisms. Figure 9.4 shows an example of the effect of metabolic fat on the estimation of the digestibility and the consequent metabolizable energy yield of fat.

Fat eaten: 100 units

Undigested fat in feces: 5 units   Digested and absorbed fat: 95 units

Metabolic fecal fat: 3 units

Total fecal fat: 8 units

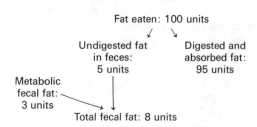

$$\text{True digestibility} = \frac{100 - 5}{100} = 95\%$$

$$\text{Metab. kcal} = 0.95 \times 9.45 = 9 \;\frac{\text{kcal}}{\text{g}}$$

$$\text{Apparent digestibility} = \frac{100 - 8}{100} = 92\%$$

$$\text{Metab. kcal} = 0.92 \times 9.45 = 8.7 \;\frac{\text{kcal}}{\text{g}}$$

Figure 9.4
Effect of metabolic fecal fat on the apparent digestibility of dietary fat and the yield of metabolizable energy from fat.

Effect of calcium on digestion of ether extract   The estimation of the digestibility of fats from high-calcium diets can require special methods. If, in the digestive tract, there are free fatty acids and also calcium ions, calcium soaps may be formed. These are not absorbed, but are voided as soap in the feces. However, if the fecal fat is estimated by ether extraction, the soaps will be undetected, because they are not ether-soluble. In that case the digestibility of the fat, and hence its yield of metabolizable energy, will be overestimated. The data in Table 9.1 illustrate the effect of excess calcium on digestion of ether extract.

To ensure accurate determination of fat in feces, extraction should be carried out under acidic conditions, whereby calcium soaps are converted to free fatty acids. From a nutritional point of view, however, the formation of calcium soaps in the digestive tract is of more concern because of its effect on calcium absorption than because of its effect on fat absorption.

Protein–energy ratio   There is a popular belief that animals have a rather low tolerance for fatty meals. However, this appears not to be true in general, but to depend somewhat on the balance between energy and protein in the diet. The necessity of maintaining some minimum ratio of protein to nonprotein calories is easily demonstrated experimentally. We have found in our laboratory that, whenever the protein calories fed to rats fall below about 16% of the total ingested calories, there is prompt appetite failure.

The effect of adding fat on the proportion of protein calories in the diet is shown by the data of Table 9.2. These figures show that for each 4% of extra fat in the diet the protein must go up 1% by weight to maintain a constant protein to nonprotein caloric ratio.

The necessity of maintaining optimum ratios of nutrients to energy is a fact now commonly observed in diet and ration formulation. There are many examples in practical feeding that illustrate the fact. For example, the use of a chocolate bar to boost the energy of an army field ration was found to result in appetite failure by the troops. Egg as a snack between meals for convalescents is satisfactory because of the extra protein, which balances the high fat content. Poultry rations to which fat has been added in order to increase the energy also require an increase in protein to maintain feed intake and feed efficiency.

Transport and metabolism of fat

Most of the lipid that is absorbed by the small intestine is incorporated into chylomicrons, which are released into the lymph and carried by way of the thoracic duct to the bloodstream. As a result, blood plasma has an opaque appearance following a fatty meal. Although chylomicrons are normally cleared fairly rapidly from blood, elevated blood lipid levels persist for some time after a meal, owing to a fairly constant influx of chylomicrons from the intestine as well as to the release from the liver of another moiety, known as

SOURCE: After Ward, G. M., and Reid, J. T., *J. Nutr.* 35(1948):249.

Table 9.1
Effect of excess calcium on the estimation of the apparent digestibility and metabolizable energy of fat in the rations of dairy cows

Group	Ca intake (g)	Feces fat measured under acidic conditions			Feces fat measured as ether extract		
		In feces (%)	Apparent digestibility (%)	Metabolizable energy (kcal/g)	In feces (%)	Apparent digestibility (%)	Metabolizable energy (kcal/g)
1	48	33	67	6.0	24	76	7.2
2	99	30	70	6.3	12	88	8.3

Table 9.2
Effect of replacing carbohydrate with fat on the percentage of protein calories of a diet

Fat in diet (%)	Protein in diet (%)	Carbohydrate in diet (%)	Calories from fat (%)	Calories from protein (%)
1	14.5	69.5	2.6	17
9	14.5	61.5	20.3	15
25	14.5	45.5	48.5	12
1	14.5	69.5	2.6	17
9	16.5	59.5	20.3	17
25	20.0	40.0	48.5	17

very-low-density lipoprotein (VLDL). Both liver and adipose tissue play an important role in the uptake and processing of plasma chylomicrons. In both tissues, uptake of triglyceride from chylomicrons requires that the triglycerides be hydrolyzed to free fatty acids and glycerol. In the liver, fatty acids and glycerol can be utilized directly for energy or converted to triglycerides and phospholipid and released back into the bloodstream as VLDL particles. In adipose tissue, most of the fatty acids released by lipoprotein lipase enter the *adipocyte*, or fat cell, to be stored as triglycerides. All of the glycerol is carried away for use by liver and other tissues, because adipose tissue does not contain the enzyme glycerokinase, which is necessary to convert glycerol to L-α-glycerophosphate.

During periods of fast or excessive energy demand, fat is mobilized from storage. Fat mobilization is initiated by a hormone-sensitive lipase that hydrolyzes triglyceride to free fatty acids and glycerol. These products diffuse into the blood, where the fatty acids form a water-soluble complex with albumin for transport throughout the body. All tissues are capable of utilizing free fatty acids for energy. Utilization of fatty acids for energy entails degration of the fatty acids to substances that can be oxidized to CO_2 and H_2O via the tricarboxylic acid cycle. This process, which is known as the *β-oxidation pathway*, is generally believed to convert fatty acids containing an even number of carbon atoms totally to two-carbon acetyl CoA units. Thus, β-oxidation of a molecule of stearic acid yields 9 molecules of acetyl CoA. The degradation of unsaturated fatty acids also yields acetyl CoA units. Degradation of fatty acids containing an odd number of carbon atoms gives rise to propionyl CoA as well as acetyl CoA. Propionyl CoA, after it is converted to succinyl CoA, also is metabolized via the TCA cycle.

Storage of energy as fat is highly efficient because of the magnitude of the free energy change ($-\Delta G°'$) that occurs when fatty acids are catabolized—9 kcal per gram when fatty acids are completely oxidized to CO_2 and H_2O.

Influence of diet on the regulation of fat synthesis

In the last two decades, there has been a remarkable increase in knowledge about fat synthesis, or *lipogenesis*. Interest in lipogenesis has been stimulated by the implication of aberrations of fat metabolism in disorders such as cardiovascular disease and obesity. Thus, the effect of diet and eating patterns on fat synthesis has been the object of many studies.

The recognition that adipose tissue is a metabolically active tissue and not just a repository for excess energy led to studies of the relative importance of adipose tissue and liver in *de novo* fatty acid synthesis. It is now known that there are marked species differences in the relative importance of these two tissues in lipogenesis. Fatty acid synthesis in the pig, cow, and sheep is restricted almost exclusively to the adipose tissue, whereas *de novo* synthesis in man and birds occurs in the liver. In rats and mice, both liver and adipose tissue are important sites of fatty acid synthesis. These observations may be important to an understanding of the control of fat synthesis and the effect of diet and eating patterns on this process.

Control of the entry of glucose into the adipocytes plays a major regulatory role in the conversion of glucose to fat by adipose tissue. On the other hand, the *hepatocytes*, or liver cells, are freely permeable to glucose; hence the control of substrate entry has no part in the regulation of fat synthesis in the liver.

Much research has been conducted on the effect of dietary components, especially carbohydrates, on lipogenesis. Studies with rats have shown that sugars promote lipogenesis more than starch does. Furthermore, in the liver, sucrose and fructose stimulate lipogenesis more than glucose does, whereas the reverse is true in adipose tissue. In general, however, dietary manipulation affects both tissues in a similar fashion: whereas sugars enhance lipogenesis, polyunsaturated fats (but not saturated fats) have been found to suppress induced hyperlipogenesis.

Not only the composition of the diet, but also the pattern of food intake, has an effect on the rate of lipogenesis.* Restricting rats who were on a nibbling regimen to one or two meals per day has been found to result in an appreciable increase in fatty acid biosynthesis. The degree of increase depended on the composition of the diet. The enzyme systems associated with fatty acid synthesis were found to adapt fairly rapidly (9 days) when nibbling rats were switched to a meal-eating regimen, while the speed at which they returned to normal rates of fatty acid synthesis when the rats were returned to a nibbling regimen was much slower (40 days).

Composition of body fat

Fatty acid composition and triglyceride configuration vary among species. In general, body fats are characteristic of the species. Chicken fat, for example, is readily distinguished from very hard white mutton fat. However, there are exceptions to this general rule; in carnivora and omnivora especially, it is possible to modify body fat by dietary means. For example, feeding processed soybeans to pigs produces a soft fat, which can be hardened by lowering the fat content of the ration. The melting point of the body fat of the dog normally is about 20° C; it can be increased to 40° C by feeding mutton tallow, or reduced to 0° C by feeding linseed oil. The iodine number of body fat in rats can be varied from 35 to 122 by feeding coconut and soybean oils having iodine numbers of 8 and 132, respectively.

---

*Leveille, G.A., *Nutr. Rev.* **30**(1972):151.

Body fat not static

One might think that, once formed, body fat is static except when it is mobilized for use as energy. This is not the case, as has been clearly shown by feeding ^{14}C-labeled fats. It appears that there is a continual and concurrent mobilization and resynthesis of body fat. This explains the changes in the nature of the adipose tissue when the ration is altered. In the rat it seems that body fat is "turned over" about once a month. With hogs, two months is long enough to accomplish the cycle because, when unsaturated fats have been fed to growing pigs, the carcass fat can be hardened by feeding the pigs rations of low fat content for two months.

Stability of dietary and body fats

The stability of dietary and body fats to oxidative degradation is related to their content of unsaturated fatty acids. The polyunsaturated fatty acids are especially susceptible to oxidation through an autocatalytic mechanism by which free radicals are formed; these readily react with molecular oxygen to form peroxides. Thus, the stability of fats depends on the amount of peroxidizable lipid they contain.

Oxidation of unsaturated fatty acids is inhibited by the presence of antioxidants, which are frequently added to foods (such as potato chips) and to animal feeds. Rancidity in foods and rations is of particular concern to the nutritionist because oxidation destroys vitamins A, E, and C. Alpha-tocopherol (vitamin E) is an important inhibitor of oxidation of polyunsaturated fatty acids in tissue lipids. In fact, the level of α-tocopherol required to prevent symptoms of vitamin E deficiency varies with the quantities of polyunsaturated fatty acids in the diet and in the tissues. Fortunately, the body is not easily depleted of vitamin E.

Palatability of fats

Fats are of interest to those preparing rations, whether for the table or for farm animals, for reasons that have nothing to do directly with their nutritive properties, unless we wish to include under nutritive properties the ill-defined quality of acceptability. We may define acceptability as the degree to which an offered food is willingly eaten by a regularly well-fed animal or human.

It is not easy to demonstrate this property, especially in the case of humans. Food selection is so much a matter of habit, and perhaps of attitude, that it may be impossible to establish that the use of a fatty spread on breads or on dry biscuits adds to their acceptability because of the fat itself.

What is the effect of variations in the fat level on the acceptability of livestock rations whose components are air-dry meals that are mixed together for feeding? Feed manufacturers have found that increasing the percentage of oil to as much as 2% tends to make the mixture more acceptable, but this probably is because the oil tends to reduce dustiness. We have seen that increasing the fat may cause a *decrease* in voluntary intake unless the protein level is also adjusted upward so that it is in the same proportion to the energy-yielding nutrients as it is in the lower-fat mixture.

Box 9.2   Dietary fat and coronary heart disease

Coronary heart disease (CHD) is the main cause of death among persons over forty years of age in Canada and the United States. Although heredity can contribute a predisposition to CHD, there is little question that individual habits, such as diet and cigarette smoking, are also potent contributors to its development. Nevertheless there is considerable debate about the precise role diet, and in particular the fat components, plays in the development of CHD.

Atherosclerosis, the primary condition causing CHD, is a multifactorial disease, and for this reason it is difficult to ascertain the precise effect of a single variable on its development. The main case for a causal relationship between dietary fat and atherosclerosis is based on world-wide epidemiological findings of a correlation between the type and amount of fat in the diet and the incidence of atherosclerosis and CHD. This general relationship between dietary fat and atherosclerosis has been confirmed by experiments with laboratory animals. Level of serum cholesterol, which is a major risk factor in CHD, can be altered by diet manipulation—in particular, by changing the amount of saturated fatty acids and of cholesterol in the diet. Yet a direct causal relationship between saturated fatty acid intake and CHD has not been found in long-term research studies, such as the Framingham Study. This lack of agreement in so-called "scientific data" is unsettling to the public. People want answers, many of which have not been found in spite of a quarter-century of intense research into this disease. As a consequence, the whole question of diet and CHD is fraught with emotionalism.

The relative effects of cholesterol, saturated fatty acids, and polyunsaturated fatty acids (PUFAs) on serum cholesterol level are of practical and theoretical importance. The bulk of the evidence suggests that saturated fat has the dominant influence on serum cholesterol level. In fact, saturated fatty acids appear to be about twice as effective in elevating serum cholesterol level as PUFAs are in decreasing it. Thus, the effectiveness of a particular vegetable oil in decreasing serum cholesterol level depends not only on the amount of PUFA it contains, but also on the ratio of PUFAs to saturated fatty acids in its makeup. In addition, there appear to be distinct differences in the ability of saturated fatty acids

But the everyday use of fatty spreads in the home adds such small amounts of extra fat and the diet is usually so abundant in protein that no effect on the nutritive value of the diet will be apparent. The fact remains that in an efficient diet there is a maximum ratio of metabolizable energy to protein, to the vitamin B complex, and to some minerals. Increase in energy by the addition of fats must be balanced by similar increases in the levels of those other nutrients to maintain the nutritive efficiency of the diet.

to bring about an elevation in serum cholesterol level. Lauric, myristic, and palmitic acids are hypercholesterolemic, whereas stearic acid does not cause an increase in serum cholesterol level. Thus fats that contain high levels of stearic acid, such as beef tallow or cocoa butter, although highly saturated, are not hypercholesterolemic. There is general agreement that dietary cholesterol intake influences serum cholesterol level, but the magnitude of this influence remains undetermined.

The relationship of dietary fat to atherosclerosis and CHD is further obscured by the fact that a large proportion of the vegetable oil consumed in the developed countries is hydrogenated, principally in products such as margarines and shortenings. Since PUFAs are much more readily saturated than monounsaturated fatty acids, the primary effect of hydrogenation is an appreciable reduction in the level of PUFA. Confusion also arises between the preventive and the therapeutic approaches to dietary management of atherosclerosis. Although the rationale is similar in both approaches, the importance of strict control of the type and amount of fat in the diet differs a great deal.

Dietary factors other than type and amount of fat have also been implicated in CHD. Protein source (animal vs plant), level of purified carbohydrate (in particular, sugar), amount of fiber, and hardness of the drinking water are but a few of the dietary variables that have been studied. Probably the best-validated observation is that soft-water communities have a higher incidence of CHD than hard-water communities. However, none of these other dietary factors has nearly the amount of research and epidemiological support that exists for dietary fat.

There is little question that an individual with a serum cholesterol level above 225 mg/100 ml has a greater chance of suffering a heart attack than an individual with a serum cholesterol level below this figure. Diet modification, particularly of the fat component, usually restores serum cholesterol levels to normal. Although similar modifications of other suspected factors may not of themselves prevent a heart attack, they probably are sound preventive measures, in view of the fact that diet manipulation seems to be most effective when other risk factors (such as diabetes and cigarette smoking) are known to be present.

Suggested readings

Call, D.L., and Sanchez, A.M. "Trends in Fat Disappearance in the United States 1909–1965," *Journal of Nutrition* **93**(1967):1.

Gurr, M.I., and James, A.T. *Lipid Biochemistry: An Introduction* (2nd ed.). Chapman and Hall, London (1975).

Harrison, F.A., and Leat, W.M.F. "Digestion and Absorption of Lipids in Non-ruminants and Ruminant Animals: A Comparison," *Proceedings of the Nutrition Society* **34**(1975):203.

Johnston, J.M. "Mechanism of Fat Absorption." In *Handbook of Physiology, Section 6: Alimentary Canal, Volume III: Intestinal Absorption*. Edited by C.F. Code and W. Heidel. American Physiological Society, Washington, D.C. (1968):1353–1375.

Scheig, R. "What Is Dietary Fat?" *American Journal of Clinical Nutrition* **22**(1969):651.

Vergroesen, A.J. *The Role of Fats in Human Nutrition*. Academic Press, New York (1975).

Chapter 10
Protein and its metabolism

We have now seen something of the scheme by which carbohydrates and fats are involved in the nourishment of the animal. Digested carbohydrate and fat are usually considered merely as metabolizable energy, and they are frequently referred to in terms of calories. The metabolizable calories yielded by carbohydrate and fat are simply the total contained calories less the amount in the undigested food. In other words, the complete metabolism of these nutrients leaves no energy-containing residues. In spite of the fact that carbohydrate and fat contain many chemically different entities, eventually they all are degraded to CO_2 and H_2O. Since their main function is to supply energy to drive the processes of life, any surpluses are stored in the body primarily as neutral lipid in the adipose tissue.

Protein, on the other hand, although it may serve as a source of energy, is important primarily as a source of amino acids from which an organism can build its own structural and functional proteins. Some of the highly specific roles played by the body proteins were discussed in Chapter 4.

An excess of dietary protein or a deficiency of calories from carbohydrate and/or fat will cause part of the protein to be used for energy. When protein serves as a source of energy the carbon portion enters the same energy pathways that are followed by carbohydrate and fat, but a nitrogenous residue remains, which must be excreted from the body. In mammals the main nitrogenous residue is urea, whereas in birds it is uric acid.

Thus protein nutrition is somewhat more complex than that of either carbohydrate or fat. Not only are there a greater number of metabolic pathways involved, many being specific to an individual amino acid, but attention must be given to providing optimum levels of certain amino acids in the diet. There is no amino acid storage comparable to depot fat for lipids or liver glycogen for carbohydrates; intake of amino acids in excess of current needs is followed by their rapid catabolism and the excretion of their nitrogen. Thus, all essential amino acids must be supplied together in the diet if optimum utilization is to be made of them for synthesis.

The nature of protein—its nutritional description

Proteins are made up of one or more chains of amino acids. These chains are termed *polypeptides* because the amino acids are linked together by amide bonds, known as *peptide linkages*, between the α-amino group of one amino acid and the primary carboxyl group of another amino acid. The particular way in which the 23 or so amino acids are combined in each protein determines its biochemical characteristics, but the amounts of the various amino acids present in a protein determine its nutritional value. Thus, for the nutritionist concerned with diets for nonruminants, the most important information about protein is its content of amino acids.

Quantitative determination of the amino acids is difficult, time-consuming, and expensive even with the aid of fully automated amino acid analyzers. The nutritionist therefore continues to make extensive use of Kjeldahl nitrogen determinations to assess the protein content of foods and feeds. In Chapter 2 we learned that, on the average, nitrogen makes up about 16% of the molecular weight of proteins.

Use is made of this fact in the Weende analysis scheme, in which protein is estimated as 6.25 times the nitrogen content. This estimate is based on an assumption that is only approximately true: depending on their amino acid composition, proteins vary in nitrogen content from 15% to 18%. Proteins of nonleguminous plant origin, as a group, show the greatest deviation from the commonly used value of 16%, averaging about 17.5% nitrogen. Milk proteins, on the other hand, average only 15.5%, while meat, egg, and fish proteins and those of leguminous plant seeds average 16% nitrogen.

The 6.25 factor   Tables dealing with the composition of foods are normally compiled with the assumption that the nitrogen content of the proteins is 16%, although on occasion it may be desirable to apply the specific factor for a food to convert its determined nitrogen value to its protein level. For example, the factor 6.38 is often used for milk, whereas the factor 5.70 is used for wheat and its by-products. The increased accuracy may be significant for low-fiber products, because the factor chosen affects not only the value for protein but also that for carbohydrate and nitrogen-free extract when these are determined by difference.

For example, the Weende proximate composition of cow's whole milk (dried) and of whole-wheat flour (as purchased) changes if the specific nitrogen values of the proteins of these foods are used instead of the typical 16% figure (see Table 10.1).

Table 10.1
Effect of the factor used for calculating crude protein on proximate composition

Proximate principle	Dried cow's milk		Whole-wheat flour	
	$N = 16\%$ (factor 6.25)	$N = 15.5\%$ (factor 6.38)	$N = 16\%$ (factor 6.25)	$N = 17.5\%\star$ (factor 5.70)
Water	4.0%	4.0%	12.0%	12.0%
Crude protein	25.4	26.0	13.2	12.4
Ether extract	27.0	27.0	2.3	2.3
Ash	6.0	6.0	1.7	1.7
Carbohydrate (by difference)	37.6	37.0	70.8	71.6

$\star$See Jones, D. B., USDA Circular No. 183 (1931).

However, the gain in accuracy by the use of a specific factor may be more apparent than real, particularly if the information is to be used to calculate the protein digestibility of a food or feed. There is no easy way to distinguish fecal nitrogen of dietary origin from endogenous fecal nitrogen. Hence, it is necessary to fall back on some average value to convert fecal nitrogen to protein equivalents, and the factor 6.25 is the logical choice. In fact, many nutritionists simply express protein digestibility in terms of nitrogen digestibility. This practice probably should be encouraged, particularly in the case of ruminant animals whose protein requirements are being met with the help of considerable quantities of nonprotein nitrogen, such as urea.

Table 10.1 shows that an error of about one percentage unit in the calculated value for crude protein, and therefore also in the carbohydrate figure, may be introduced for some foods if the conventional equation ($N \times 6.25 =$ crude protein) is used. However, there is a further possible error, due to variations among different samples of a given food.$\star$ Tabulated composition figures are arithmetic averages, and the "normal" variation among samples on which these averages are based may be expressed by a coefficient of variation of about ±8% for crude protein. Thus, if a food is analyzed as 12% crude protein (i.e., $N \times 6.25$), we may expect other samples of this food to

$\star$Crampton, E. W., and Harris, L. E., *Applied Animal Nutrition* (2nd ed.), W. H. Freeman and Company, San Francisco (1969):226.

range from about 10% to about 14% protein. (12% $\times$ $\pm$8% = $\pm$1.9 percentage units, or values from 10.1% to 13.8%.)

The coefficient of variation in digestibility of the complete diet by different human subjects is about $\pm$1.0%. However, the digestibility of most foods of the human dietary is, of necessity, determined indirectly, because each food constitutes 20% or less of the diet. The probable variation in the measured digestibility of each foodstuff is seldom less than 5 percentage units.

Refinement of the proximate analysis by computing crude protein according to a specifically correct nitrogen concentration is of much less importance in the proximate description of most foods and feeds than the chemist might like us to believe, and it probably will decrease further in importance as the amino acid values themselves come into wider use. Meanwhile, estimation of a protein equivalent by the use of the conventional factor 6.25 is justified by practicability if not by chemical accuracy.

True versus crude protein   Leafy parts of plants (particularly of those grown on heavily fertilized soils) and roots and tubers (such as cassava or potatoes) often contain considerable amounts of nonprotein nitrogen. Yeasts, which have been suggested as a source of protein, also contain appreciable amounts of nonprotein nitrogen—particularly, nucleic acids. In these materials crude protein, estimated by multiplying the nitrogen content by the conversion factor, may deviate considerably from what is called *true protein*. On the other hand, the nitrogen of plant seeds and of animal and marine tissues is chiefly in the form of protein; in these cases crude protein closely approximates true protein.

Protein quality

It is evident that the Weende method of arriving at the protein content of a feed or of some biological product gives no indication of the component parts of the product. As was mentioned previously, chemically the protein molecule is a combination of amino acids, the numbers and molecular arrangement of which are unique for each specific protein. With few exceptions, protein molecules of the diet are hydrolyzed or digested to their component acids before being absorbed. Thus, it is not protein but amino acids that are the nutrients of this Weende fraction. It follows that if an individual's nutrient requirement is for some particular number and proportion of the 23 different amino acids, proteins as they occur in foods may have different nutritive values. This leads to the concept of *protein quality*.

In general usage, the term *quality* as applied to food proteins refers to the assortment and proportions of amino acids: the more complete the assortment and the more nearly the proportions approach the physiological needs of a species for amino acids, the higher the quality of the protein.* Thus, description of foods and feeds in terms of their amino acid composition will probably eventually supersede information based on nitrogen content. However, the amino acid composition of a foodstuff is not the final measure of protein quality, because some of the amino acids may be biologically unavailable to animals. We shall discuss amino acid availability in greater detail later in this chapter. It is sufficient at this point to mention that, according to many studies, excessive heat during the processing of a foodstuff can render some amino acids, especially lysine, unavailable for metabolism.

Classification of amino acids

Before discussing some of the specific aspects of protein and amino acid metabolism, we should point out some of the chemical and nutritional classifications applied to amino acids. With the exception of proline and hydroxyproline, all amino acids found in organisms have a primary amino group and a carboxyl group attached to the same carbon (the α carbon); thus, they are called *α-amino acids*. All amino acids except glycine are optically active, because the α carbon of each is asymmetric. With few exceptions, natural amino acids are of the L configuration. Synthetic amino acids, however, are racemic mixtures of the L and D forms. The D form of an amino acid can be utilized by an organism only if it can be converted to the L configuration.

Since the general structure $NH_2\text{-}\overset{\displaystyle R}{\underset{|}{C}H\text{-}COOH}$ is the same for all α-amino acids, what distinguishes one amino acid from another is the composition and structure of R, the side chain. Thus, amino acids are frequently classified as basic, acidic, or neutral, as well as according to whether their side chain is branched or whether it contains sulfur. Table 10.2 classifies the amino acids commonly found in protein hydrolysates according to the composition and structure of their side chains.

Dispensable and indispensable amino acids   For nutritional purposes, amino acids may be divided into two groups—dispensable and indispensable.† *Indispensable* amino acids are those that cannot be synthesized in the body at a rate sufficient to meet the physiological needs of the body, and must

---

*The term *quality*, as used here, is almost but not fully equivalent to the term *biological value*, as we shall see later in this chapter.

†The terms *dispensable* and *indispensable* are preferred to *nonessential* and *essential*, even though the latter terms are frequently found in the literature [Harper, A.E., *J. Nutr.* **104**(1974): 965].

Table 10.2
Classification of amino acids according to the composition and structure of the side chain

General class	Subclass	Amino acid
Basic		Arginine
		Histidine
		Hydroxylysine
		Lysine
Acidic (and their amides)		Asparagine
		Aspartic acid
		Glutamic acid
		Glutamine
Neutral	Aliphatic	
	Straight chain	Alanine
		Glycine
	Branched chain	Isoleucine
		Leucine
		Valine
	Hydroxy	Serine
		Threonine
	Sulfur-containing	Cysteine
		Cystine
		Methionine
	Aromatic	Phenylalanine
		Tryptophan
		Tyrosine
	Imino	Hydroxyproline
		Proline

therefore be furnished preformed in the diet. *Dispensable* amino acids, on the other hand, are those that can be synthesized in the body from a suitable carbon source and amino groups from other amino acids or simple compounds such as diammonium citrate; they obviously need not be in the diet. This means that they are dispensable as dietary components, but not that they are dispensable to the animal.

In a sense, all amino acids found in animal tissues are physiologically indispensable. As one research philosopher put it, "Some are so essential the body ensures an adequate supply by synthesis." As we use the term, indispensable amino acids are those that the body cannot synthesize fast enough, or cannot synthesize at all. Thus, high-quality proteins are those that supply an abundance of indispensable amino acids.

The classic definition of an indispensable amino acid as one that must be furnished preformed in the diet is not completely correct. The α-hydroxy analogue of methionine, for example, will meet an animal's requirement for methionine. In fact, the hydroxy analogue of methionine is commonly used as a dietary supplement in livestock rations. Studies with rats[*] and humans[†] have shown that the α-hydroxy- or α-keto-substituted derivatives of the indispensable amino acids, except those of lysine and threonine, can substitute for the indispensable amino acids. Thus, it appears that the requirement is for the preformed carbon skeleton of the indispensable amino acids, except in the case of lysine and threonine. Apparently, most birds and mammals have lost the ability to synthesize the carbon skeletons of about half the 23 amino acids that make up proteins.

The metabolic pathway by which the hydroxy and keto analogues are converted to the corresponding indispensable amino acids is illustrated for methionine in Figure 10.1. The dietary requirement for preformed lysine and

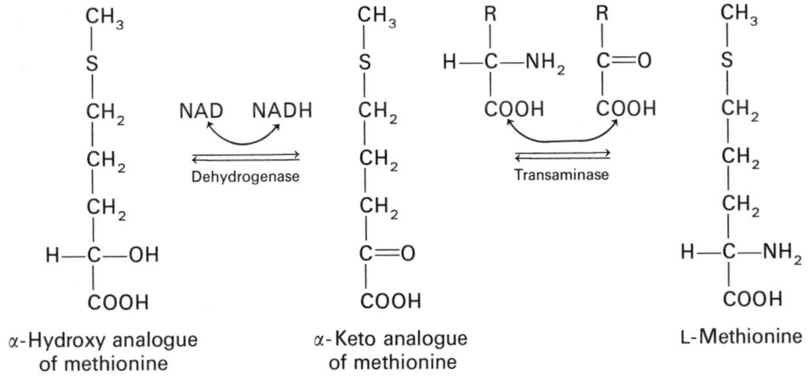

Figure 10.1
Conversion of the α-hydroxy analogue of methionine to L-methionine.

threonine appears to stem from the fact that higher animals lack the specific transaminases that convert the α-keto analogues of these two amino acids to the L-amino acids.

---

[*]Pond, W.G., Breuer, L.H., Jr., Loosli, J.K., and Warner, R.G., *J. Nutr.* **83**(1964):85; Clow, K.W., and Walser, M., *J. Nutr.* **105**(1975):372.

[†]Walser, M., Coulter, A.W., Dighe, S.V., and Crantz, F.R., *J. Clin. Invest.* **52**(1973):678; Sapir, D.G., Owen, O.E., Prozefsky, T., and Walser, M., *J. Clin. Invest.* **54**(1974):974.

For a nutritionist, the important question is whether an amino acid (or a suitable analogue) must be supplied in the diet. There is considerable evidence about which amino acids are indispensable in diets, although the number and amount may vary, depending on the age and species of animal, as Table 10.3 shows.

Table 10.3
Requirement for each indispensable amino acid when all other amino acids of nutritive importance are provided (*figures are precentages of total diet, except for man*)

Amino acid	Young rat	Starting chicken	Laying hen	Growing pig	Adult man
Arginine	0.20%	1.20%	0.80%	0.22%	—
Glycine	—	1.00	?	—	—
Histidine	0.30	0.40	?	0.22	—
Isoleucine	0.50	0.75	0.50	0.53	0.70 g/day
Leucine	0.80	1.40	1.20	0.64	0.98
Lysine	0.90	1.10	0.50	0.75	0.84
Methionine	0.60*	0.75*	0.53*	0.52*	0.91†
Phenylalanine	0.90‡	1.30‡	?	0.52§	0.98‖
Threonine	0.50	0.70	0.40	0.45	0.49
Tryptophan	0.15	0.20	0.15	0.13	0.24
Valine	0.70	0.85	?	0.48	0.70
Total protein	20%	20%	15%	16%–18%	0.55 g/kg body weight

*About ½ of the requirement can be met by cystine.
†About ¾ of the requirement can be met by cystine.
‡About ⅓ to ½ of the requirement can be met by tyrosine.
§About ⅓ of the requirement can be met by tyrosine.
‖About ¾ of the requirement can be met by tyrosine.

Amino acid composition and protein quality

Proteins that contain an abundance of indispensable amino acids are commonly considered high-quality proteins. Furthermore, it is generally accepted that the more closely the indispensable amino acid composition of a protein approximates an animal's requirements for indispensable amino acids, the more efficiently the protein will be utilized by that animal. Inherent in this principle, however, is the assumption that the protein contains a reasonable ratio of indispensable to dispensable amino acids. Thus, in addition to the minimum daily required intake of indispensable amino acids, we must concern ourselves with *amino acid balance*—the intake of each indispensable amino acid relative to the intakes of other amino acids.

In practice we are seldom concerned with a single isolated protein source; the nutritive value of a particular protein must be considered in relation to all other proteins in the diet. The proteins of cereal grains are likely to be deficient in lysine and threonine (and tryptophan, in the case of maize), whereas the proteins of seeds of legumes, such as soybeans, are relatively well supplied with lysine and threonine but lack the sulfur-containing amino acids. Thus, soybean meal is commonly added to cereal-based rations for livestock and poultry with the object of improving the pattern of amino acids. Meat, milk, fish, and eggs are rich sources of both lysine and methionine. Hence we are prone to apply the term *high quality* to proteins of high lysine and/or methionine content in spite of the fact that they also contribute other amino acids to the diet.

It is generally believed that surplus amino acids contributed by a protein have no adverse effect on the animal ingesting such a protein. This appears to be true for most diets composed of natural feedstuffs. Nevertheless, there is some question of whether excess amino acids can be metabolized without affecting those in limited supply. The facts that amino acid requirements increase as the protein content of a diet is increased and that a large excess of an amino acid is toxic emphasize the importance of a balance among dietary amino acids.

Although the concept of amino acid balance is relatively simple, our knowledge is still too fragmentary to assign a nutritive value to proteins simply on the basis of amino acid composition.

Amino acid availability

A satisfactory level and balance of amino acids in a diet does not guarantee that ingestion of the diet will satisfy the amino acid requirements of an animal. Under certain conditions, some of the amino acids may be unavailable because the proteins in the diet are incompletely digested. In mucoproteins, for example, some sections of the peptide chain adjacent to sugar residues are totally resistant to digestive attack. The celluloses and hemicelluloses in the cell walls of plants also may render the proteins in the cell inaccessible to the digestive enzymes. In other cases, digestion may be impaired by the presence of inhibitors of the digestive enzymes. Perhaps the best-known example of the latter is the trypsin inhibitor found in soybeans; it is heat-labile, which explains why the digestion of soybeans is markedly improved by heat processing.

Although heat processing may have beneficial effects, such as the heat denaturation of trypsin inhibitor in soybeans, if not properly controlled it can have deleterious effects. One of the more common causes of heat damage to proteins is the Maillard reaction, whereby reducing sugars react with the ε-amino group of lysine, thus rendering the lysine biologically unavailable. Heat damage depends on the degree of heat and the moisture content of the food. The greatest hazard of heat damage arises in the heat processing involved in making milk powder, fish flour, and oil-seed meals.

Substances other than reducing sugars also may interact with the lysine in proteins, thus rendering the amino acid biologically unavailable. A classic example is the combination of gossypol with the ε-amino group of lysine during the production of cottonseed meal from cottonseeds: rupture of the gossypol-containing pigment glands by moist heat and pressure releases free gossypol, which binds with cottonseed proteins. Although this markedly reduces the toxicity of gossypol, its combination with lysine diminishes the nutritive value of cottonseed protein. Two approaches have been used to overcome this problem: selective breeding for glandless cottonseed and the removal of the pigment glands during processing.

Studies of the inactivation of the trypsin inhibitor in soybeans and of the effects of heat treatment on amino acid availability have shown that the nutritive value of a protein can be altered without any appreciable change in gross amino acid composition. Thus, it should be evident that there are limitations on the use of amino acid determinations in assessing protein quality.

Evaluation of protein quality in nonruminants

The primary function of dietary protein is to supply the amino acids required by an animal for maintenance and for productive purposes such as growth, gestation, and lactation. It follows that evaluation of protein quality will be most accurate if it is determined with the species for which the protein is intended and with the conditions under which it will be used. However, biological assays with humans and large animals are expensive and difficult to carry out. For this reason biological assays usually are carried out under standardized conditions and with laboratory species, although the chicken and the pig also are popular choices. Regardless of species, all animal tests for evaluating food proteins measure, directly or indirectly, the degree to which these proteins meet amino acid needs for protein synthesis and body maintenance.

Biological value (BV)   One of the first concepts used to describe protein quality was *biological value*. Technically the term is defined as the proportion of absorbed nitrogen that is retained by the body. Since the primary paths for the elimination of dietary nitrogen are the feces and urine, ingested nitrogen not recovered from these outlets presumably has been retained and used by the body to meet its amino acid needs. Biological value is, in fact, the percentage of the true digestible protein that is utilized by the body.

In determining biological value, the logical assumption is made that the retained nitrogen reflects a perfect assortment of amino acids. Amino acids not utilized by the body for protein synthesis and body maintenance are immediately deaminated and the nitrogen excreted in the urine.

Biological value can be expressed by the Thomas–Mitchell equation:*

$$\% \, BV = 100 \times \frac{N \text{ intake} - [(\text{feces N} - \text{metabolic N}) + (\text{urine N} - \text{endogenous N})]}{N \text{ intake} - (\text{feces N} - \text{metabolic N})}$$

It will be seen that total fecal nitrogen is corrected for metabolic fecal nitrogen (that portion not of direct dietary origin). Likewise, endogenous urinary nitrogen is deducted from total urinary nitrogen to distinguish urinary nitrogen that would appear even in the absence of dietary protein intake (as a result of nitrogen loss from "wear and tear") from that which represents unutilized dietary amino acids.

In order to determine the metabolic fecal nitrogen and the endogenous urinary nitrogen of a test animal, it must be fed a nitrogen-free diet and its fecal and urinary nitrogen output must be measured during that regimen. Except for rats, few animals will consume protein-free diets long enough for such a digestion trial to be completed. Thus, although a determination of biological value yields valuable results when properly carried out, it is laborious and time-consuming and is seldom used to assess protein quality. However, biological value is commonly used to describe protein quality, so that it is important to understand the concept expressed by this term.

Nitrogen balance   *Nitrogen balance* is the difference between nitrogen retention and nitrogen output:

$$B = I - (U + F)$$

where B is the balance, I the nitrogen intake, and $(U + F)$ the nitrogen excreted in urine and feces. The nitrogen balance method has been widely used to evaluate protein foods in human diets. It has also been extensively used to test standard amino acid mixtures for humans. Like biological value, nitrogen balance is laborious and time-consuming to determine and varies with nitrogen intake.

An extension of the nitrogen balance that is one of the best methods of determining the nutritive value of proteins for humans is the *nitrogen balance index*, which at submaintenance levels of protein intake is essentially the same as biological value, except that endogenous nitrogen losses are not explicitly considered. The nitrogen balance index simply compares the slopes of the regression lines for nitrogen balance versus nitrogen absorbed

---

*Mitchell, H. H., *J. Biol. Chem.* **58**(1924):873.

Box 10.1   H. H. Mitchell and the biological value of proteins

Harold Hanson Mitchell (1886–1966) is most famous as the co-originator of the Thomas–Mitchell method for determining the biological value of proteins. Although the concept of biological value originated with the German scientist Karl Thomas, it was Mitchell who developed and applied the method. He also confirmed, through animal experiments, the usefulness of the amino acid index for assessing the nutritive value of proteins. In addition to his outstanding contributions to our knowledge of the nutrition and metabolism of proteins, H. H. Mitchell made significant contributions to our knowledge of the calcium requirements of human adults and to our knowledge of the effect of climatic stress, particularly environmental temperature, on the nutritional requirements of humans.

H. H. Mitchell was born in Evanston, Illinois. He received his Bachelor's, Master's, and Ph.D. degrees from the University of Illinois and spent his entire career as a chemist and nutritionist at his alma mater. One of his closest collaborators was Tom S. Hamilton, who obtained his Ph.D. under Mitchell. They published together extensively on methods of evaluating the nutritive quality of proteins and on the assessment of the protein requirements of animals.

The tremendous achievements of H. H. Mitchell are truly amazing, considering the fact that he was handicapped by extremely poor vision. He was unable to read without the aid of special lighting and a large magnifying glass on a stand on his desk. His inability to read signs at a distance, to cross busy intersections, or to recognize familiar faces prevented him from attending many professional meetings other than those held on the University of Illinois campus. In spite of this severe handicap he was a prolific reader, well known for his meticulous and astute approach to scientific literature. He always claimed books were his teachers, and the extensive library he maintained, largely at his personal expense, attested to this claim.

H. H. Mitchell proudly referred to himself as a nutritionist. He believed very firmly that there were no nutritional experiments in which food intake was not an important parameter. His career culminated with the writing, during the early years of his retirement, of two volumes entitled *Comparative Nutrition of Man and Domestic Animals*. [For further information, see *J. Nutr.* **96**(1968):1.]

at intakes below and slightly above nitrogen equilibrium. The validity of the index is based on the fact that the relationship between nitrogen balance and nitrogen absorbed is linear in the regions of negative nitrogen balance and of slight positive balance. The main deterrent to the use of the nitrogen balance index is the fact that it is even more laborious and time-consuming than either the biological value or the nitrogen balance methods, because nitrogen retention must be determined at three or four levels of nitrogen intake.

Net protein utilization (NPU)   NPU combines in a single index both the digestibility and the biological value of a protein (NPU = BV × digestibility). Nitrogen retention estimated by carcass analysis can be used to estimate NPU as follows:

$$NPU = \frac{p - o}{I}$$

where p is the carcass nitrogen of animals fed a diet containing protein, o is the carcass nitrogen of comparable animals fed a protein-free diet, and I is the nitrogen intake of animals fed the diet containing protein.

The method is much less laborious and time-consuming than determining biological value or nitrogen balance, but it is limited to those species that lend themselves to analysis of the total carcass. NPU of humans can be determined by using fecal and urinary excretion values to estimate the gain in body nitrogen.

Growth   The rate of growth of an animal is a fairly sensitive index of protein quality. Under controlled conditions, weight gain is proportional to the supply of essential amino acids. In fact, the correlation between body weight gain and gain in body nitrogen by rats is very good. The growth trial is an extremely simple test and has been used extensively in the livestock industry. The method also has been used with children. Furthermore, there is evidence that, in general, results of rat growth studies may be applied to the evaluation of human diets.

Protein efficiency ratio (PER)   PER, which is defined as the grams of weight gained per gram protein consumed, is probably the most widely used of all methods for evaluating protein quality. Although the method can be undertaken with any species, it is basically a rat growth assay. Several recommendations have been made for standardizing the method, such as fixing the age of rat, number of rats per test group, length of the study, and composition of the diet.*

The PER assay is subject to a number of criticisms. Probably the most fundamental is that it assumes all protein is used for growth, so that no allowance is made for maintenance. In spite of this criticism, the method continues to be widely used, because it is extremely simple.

Net protein ratio (NPR)   The NPR assay represents an attempt to avoid the fundamental criticism of PER by making allowance for maintenance. NPR is simply the weight gain of a group of rats fed the test diet plus the weight loss of a similar group fed a protein-free diet, the total divided by the weight of protein consumed by the first group.

---

*Campbell, J. A., Evaluation of Protein Quality, NAS-NRC Publ. 1100 (1963):31.

Chemical methods   Determination of protein quality with animals is time-consuming and expensive. Thus, it is not surprising that considerable effort has been expended in search of chemical methods for the evaluation of proteins. R. H. Block and H. H. Mitchell were the first to introduce a reasonably successful chemical method, which they termed *chemical score.** The method is based on the concept that the nutritive value of a protein depends primarily on the amount of the essential amino acid in greatest deficit in that protein, compared to a reference protein. The quantity of each essential amino acid in the test proteins is compared with the quantity in whole egg protein. The chemical score of the protein is taken to be the percentage of the essential amino acid in greatest deficit relative to that of whole egg protein. Such an analysis of wheat protein, whose lysine is in greatest deficit, is shown in Table 10.4.

Table 10.4
Calculation of the chemical score of Block and Mitchell for wheat

Amino acid	% in egg protein	% in wheat protein	% deficiency in wheat
Arginine	6.4	4.2	34
Cystine	2.4	1.8	25
Cystine + methionine	6.5	4.3	34
Histidine	2.1	2.1	0
Isoleucine	8.0	3.6	55
Leucine	9.2	6.8	26
Lysine	7.2	2.7	63
Methionine	4.1	2.5	39
Phenylalanine	6.3	5.7	10
Threonine	4.9	3.3	33
Tryptophan	1.5	1.2	20
Tyrosine	4.5	4.4	2
Valine	7.3	4.5	38

NOTE: Chemical score for wheat, based on amino acid in greatest deficit (lysine), is $100 - 63 = 37$.

Chemical scores such as that of Block and Mitchell assume the pattern of amino acids available to an animal to be the same as that obtained by chemical analysis. This assumption is not always correct, as we pointed out when we discussed amino acid availability. Decreased lysine availability appears to be one of the most common causes of the reduced nutritive value of processed and stored proteins. For this reason the *Carpenter test*† for available lysine

---

*Block, R. H., and Mitchell, H. H., *Nutr. Abstr. and Revs.* **16**(1947):249.
†Carpenter, K. J., *Biochem. J.* **77**(1960):604.

has received considerable attention in the food and feed industry as a rapid screen for losses in protein quality from processing and storage. The method involves the reaction of fluoro-2,4-dinitrobenzene (FDNB) with the free ϵ-amino groups of lysine in intact protein; it is assumed that reduced biological availability of lysine is due to the reaction of the ϵ-amino group with other active groups to form linkages that are stable to enzyme hydrolysis. The method is reasonably satisfactory for animal proteins but has questionable applicability to plant protein materials, which contain large amounts of carbohydrate.

Many other *in vitro* methods for the nutritional evaluation of proteins have been proposed, and great strides have been made since the early attempts, which were based solely on the Kjeldahl determination of nitrogen. Unfortunately, *in vitro* methods often yield values that bear little relationship to protein quality as established by animal tests. Nevertheless, considerable effort undoubtedly will continue to be expended on the refinement of chemical methods presently in use and on the development of new *in vitro* methods, because of the enormous need for simple, direct methods for the evaluation of protein quality.

Protein quality and the ruminant

The preceding discussion of protein quality and its relationship to the level and availability of the essential amino acids applies to the nonruminant animal. Ruminants, by contrast, can utilize both protein and nonprotein nitrogenous substances because microorganisms in the rumen use both sources of nitrogen to synthesize proteins for their own growth and reproduction. We have already seen that the extensive utilization of cellulose and hemicellulose by herbivora depends on the breakdown of these materials by the microflora of the rumen and/or caecum. Similarly, the utilization of nonprotein nitrogen sources—such as urea, biuret, ammonium salts, and ammoniated molasses—by ruminants depends on the rumen microorganisms that use the nitrogen from these materials for synthesis of microbial protein. The amino acids of the microbial protein become available to the host animal by the normal processes of digestion and absorption in the abomasum and small intestine.

It is now recognized that there is considerable variability in the proportion of dietary protein that escapes degradation in the rumen. In general, the proportion of dietary protein that passes through the rumen unchanged depends on the source of the protein. E. L. Miller has suggested the following percentages for an assortment of proteins.*

---

*Miller, E. L., *Proc. Nutr. Soc.* **32**(1973):79.

Source of protein	% Protein escaping degradation
Barley	10
Cottonseed (soluble)	20
Groundnut meal	20
Sunflower seed meal	25
Soybean meal	45
Dried grass	50
White fish meal	70
Peruvian fish meal	70

The overall effect of the rumen on the amino acid composition of the digesta reaching the intestine of the ruminant can be either an advantage or a disadvantage, depending on the source of dietary nitrogen and, if it is protein in origin, the quantity and quality of this protein. The availability of dietary nitrogen to the ruminant is only to a limited extent determined by the form in which it is ingested. The ruminant, unlike the nonruminant, does not depend on dietary protein to satisfy its protein requirements. Although many potential sources of nonprotein nitrogen have been tested for their protein replacement value, most of the work has been devoted to urea. Experiments have shown that urea can meet a significant proportion of the protein requirement of ruminants for growth, milk production, and other body functions; the usual practice is to supply 40%–50% of the total nitrogen as urea. On the other hand, if the diet contains protein of high quality, the advantages of ruminal fermentation may be lost by the wastage of nitrogen as ammonia and by the conversion of the dietary protein into microbial protein, which is of relatively low biological value and poor digestibility.

Several methods have been proposed to reduce the fermentation of dietary protein in the rumen. Heat treatment of various protein sources has been found to reduce the solubility of their proteins and thus decrease their susceptibility to ruminal fermentation; however, extended heating also renders these proteins less digestible, thus making the heated versions inferior to the untreated products. Treatment of proteins with aldehydes, such as formaldehyde, also reduces their solubility, presumably through the formation of complexes between the aldehyde and the free amino groups of the protein as in the Maillard reaction. The formaldehyde-protein complex is fairly stable at the pH of the rumen but readily decomposes at the acid pH of the abomasum. Excess formaldehyde, however, tends to inhibit the cellulolytic activity of the rumen microorganisms. In general, the response of ruminants to formaldehyde-treated proteins is highly variable. Another method that theoretically should be effective in protecting proteins against ruminal fermentation is encapsulation with a material that is insoluble in the rumen but readily soluble in the abomasum or small intestine. One of the protective agents that has been used to encapsulate methionine is hydrogenated fat, which is readily broken down by the action of lipase and bile in the duodenum.*

*See Box 9.1 for a discussion of the similar method of protecting *un*saturated fats from ruminal fermentation.

The merits of protecting proteins or individual amino acids to increase the efficiency of their utilization by ruminants are fairly obvious. However, it may be asked whether it would be more desirable to use the ruminants' built-in protein-synthesizing system to the fullest advantage, particularly if the ever-increasing demand for protein for human consumption is to be met.

Protein digestion and absorption

Proteins are large polymers of amino acids joined together in peptide linkages. Utilization of dietary proteins in metabolism requires that the protein molecules be degraded to their constituent amino acids. Digestion of protein is simply the hydrolysis of the peptide linkages; it may be diagramed as follows:

This reaction, which (if carried out to completion) yields free amino acids, is catalyzed by a group of enzymes referred to collectively as the *proteolytic* enzymes. The action of these enzymes is rather selective. Investigations have shown that, although peptide bonds between amino acid pairs seem identical, they vary considerably in their susceptibility to cleavage by the different proteolytic enzymes. In fact, the different enzymes preferentially split peptide bonds adjacent to particular amino acids. This selectivity appears to depend upon the nature of the side chains of the amino acids.

Protein digestion takes place in the stomach and upper small intestine. It is very rapid, and the products (the amino acids) are rapidly absorbed from the digestive tract. The proteolytic enzymes are themselves proteins, and it is perhaps ironic that their action is directed against substances of like composition. The bulk of the proteolytic enzymes also is digested and absorbed but, unlike digestion and absorption of dietary proteins, the process probably occurs along the full length of the intestine, with the tendency toward autolysis increasing with distance from the stomach. Dietary protein not only stimulates the secretion of proteolytic enzymes but it protects the enzymes against proteolysis, apparently because dietary protein denatured in the stomach is the preferred substrate for proteolytic enzymes.

The proteolytic enzymes are initially secreted as inactive precursors called *zymogens*; activation entails cleaving off a peptide chain that presumably shields the active center of the enzyme. For example, pepsinogen, the inactive precursor of pepsin, has a molecular weight of 42,000, whereas the active enzyme, pepsin, has a molecular weight of 35,000. Broadly speaking, the proteolytic enzymes may be classified as *endopeptidases*, which attack peptide bonds in the interior of a peptide chain, and *exopeptidases*, which attack terminal peptide linkages. The exopeptidases may be further classified as *amino*peptidases or *carboxy*peptidases, depending on whether they specifically attack N- or C-terminal bonds. Some basic information about the source and action of proteolytic enzymes is summarized in Table 10.5.

Trypsin, which participates directly in the breakdown of dietary protein, as indicated in Table 10.5, activates not only its own precursor, trypsinogen, but other zymogens as well. Evidently, this is why foods containing trypsin inhibitors have such a pronounced depressive effect on protein utilization unless precautions, such as heating, are taken to denature these inhibitory substances. On the other hand, trypsin hydrolyzes peptide bonds adjacent to lysine or arginine, and lysine, in particular, is rendered biologically unavailable by heating during the processing of protein foods and feeds.

Although the digestion of proteins is fairly well understood, knowledge of the absorption of the products of digestion still is largely theoretical. Apparently the intestine is an efficient and selective filter, since only free amino acids reach the portal bloodstream. It is generally accepted that proteins are absorbed primarily as free amino acids; dipeptides also can be absorbed from the lumen but they are hydrolyzed in the wall of the intestine, and the amino acids thus liberated are transferred to the portal blood. The nutritional importance of this phenomenon is unclear. That the products of digestion rapidly disappear from the intestinal lumen is evidenced by the fact that digesta contain very low levels of free amino acids. In general, absorption is considered to be an active transport process (i.e., the amino acids can be concentrated against a concentration gradient). This view is supported by three observations: (1) there is an elevation in the postprandial concentration of plasma amino acids, (2) L isomers of amino acids are absorbed more rapidly than D isomers, and (3) high concentrations of certain amino acids will inhibit the absorption of other amino acids.

Although the intestine of adult mammals is a selective filter, in newborn mammals it is permeable to proteins, especially the γ-globulins. This is particularly important to the calf, piglet, and lamb, as well as the newborn human infant, because the colostrum is the sole source of immunoglobulins, the maternal placenta being impermeable to these proteins. Most newborns rapidly lose the ability to absorb intact proteins, but there is some evidence that this ability, or at least the ability to absorb large peptides, is retained to some small degree by certain individuals. It is for this reason that some persons are allergic to marine foods and that doctors caution against the feeding of eggs to some infants.

Proteins and other dietary nitrogenous materials that resist or escape digestion eventually leave the body in the fecal waste. Also eliminated in the feces are endogenous proteins (e.g., digestive enzymes, mucoproteins secreted into

Table 10.5
The source and action of the proteolytic enzymes

Enzyme	Source	Precursor	Activator	Action
Endopeptidases (proteases)				
Pepsin	Stomach (chief cells)	Pepsinogen	H⁺, pepsin	Hydrolyzes peptide bonds adjacent to aromatic amino acids and other bulky nonpolar residues
Trypsin	Pancreas	Trypsinogen	Enterokinase, trypsin	Hydrolyzes peptide bonds in which a dibasic acid (lysine or arginine) contributes the carboxyl group
Chymotrypsin	Pancreas	Chymotrypsinogen	Trypsin	Hydrolyzes peptide bonds in which an aromatic acid (or perhaps methionine) contributes the carboxyl group
Exopeptidases				
Carboxypeptidase A	Pancreas	Procarboxypeptidase A	Trypsin	Hydrolyzes C-terminal aromatic residues
Carboxypeptidase B	Pancreas	Procarboxypeptidase B	Trypsin	Hydrolyzes C-terminal basic residues
Aminopeptidases	Intestine			Split off terminal amino acids with free NH₂ groups
Dipeptidases	Intestine			Split dipeptides to amino acids

the alimentary canal, and desquamated mucosal cells) that escape digestion and absorption.

A third component of the fecal nitrogen is contributed by the microflora. It has been estimated that of the human fecal nitrogen, 40% is bacterial, 40% is dietary, and 20% is from spent enzymes. These proportions vary with species and also with diet, as does the total quantity of nitrogen excreted. In farm animals on normal rations, the fecal nitrogen typically amounts to 20%–25% of the total dietary nitrogen intake; in humans it amounts to 4%–8%. Because a considerable portion of fecal nitrogen is not of direct dietary origin, the actual digestibility of food protein cannot be accurately estimated from the total fecal nitrogen. The error is usually not serious in most applied nutrition, but for the sake of clarity the difference between the quantity of dietary nitrogen consumed and the quantity subsequently found in the feces is referred to as the *apparent digestible protein* (or nitrogen). By feeding a protein-free diet, the amount of the nondietary residual protein (the metabolic fecal protein) can be determined and the total output adjusted accordingly, to calculate the true digestibility of the protein. This is almost never done, and practically all figures tabulated for protein digestibility are for apparent digestibility.

Figure 10.2 depicts the path of dietary protein (nitrogen) through the stages of digestion and absorption.

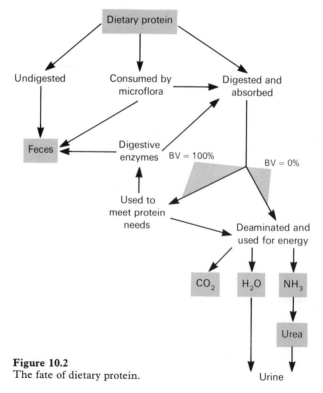

Figure 10.2
The fate of dietary protein.

Metabolic fate of dietary protein (amino acids)

Dietary protein enters the portal bloodstream as free amino acids. These amino acids mix with those of endogenous origin to produce the amino acid patterns that are found in physiological fluids after ingestion of a protein-containing meal. Free amino acids within the body may follow three different metabolic pathways: (1) they can be used for protein synthesis; (2) they can serve as precursors in the synthesis of nitrogen-containing compounds such as nucleic acids, creatine, choline, and thyroxine; or (3) they can be degraded, the nitrogen being excreted as urea and the carbon skeleton entering energy metabolism. These three pathways compete with each other; equilibrium among them is constantly regulated in such a way that changes in the rate of disposal of amino acids along one route are often compensated for by reciprocal changes along one or both of the other pathways. It has become evident during the past few years that a more complete understanding of the relationships among these pathways and the effects of both internal and external factors on them will be necessary if the ever-increasing demand by the world's population for protein is to be met.

These interrelationships may be illustrated by the influence of carbohydrate and fat on protein metabolism. Since protein, carbohydrate, and fat all may serve as dietary sources of energy, it is not surprising to find that restriction of carbohydrate or fat in a diet otherwise adequate for an adult results in a decrease in nitrogen retention. A similar effect has been observed in growing animals, although the combined influence of protein intake and energy intake on nitrogen retention is somewhat more complex. Nevertheless, optimum calorie/protein ratios have been defined for the growing chicken. Since the growing animal, as well as the adult, eats primarily to meet its requirement for energy, food intake is governed primarily by the energy content of the diet. Thus, suboptimal calorie/protein ratios result in the degradation of amino acids to meet the energy needs of the body, whereas calorie/protein ratios much higher than the optimum result in an inadequate intake of protein.

The importance of recognizing the effect of just one factor, such as energy, on amino acid metabolism can be illustrated by a brief discussion of protein malnutrition in humans. One of the widespread human deficiency diseases in the developing world today is protein malnutrition. The disease is particularly prevalent among young children because their rapid rate of growth results in a high protein requirement per unit of body weight. Although varying degrees of combined protein and calorie malnutrition are found, protein deficiency frequently is observed even among children whose diets are adequate or even excessive in calories. In such cases, the children's diets are composed predominantly of cereals or starchy roots and fruits. Not only are these diets low in protein, but the protein is of low biological value, so that the children satisfy their appetite and their requirement for energy without meeting their protein requirements.

Any attempt to assess the quantitative requirements of protein for maintenance and for productive purposes—such as growth, lactation, and egg production—requires a knowledge of the factors governing the metabolic pathways that amino acids follow in the body. Although proteins may serve as a source of energy, the primary reason for including protein in the diet is to provide amino acids for the synthesis of essential tissues and fluid components, and to meet other specific needs for nitrogen. Consequently, we shall consider first the fate of amino acids that are used in ways other than as energy sources.

Protein synthesis

Protein synthesis in the cell has been studied exhaustively in the past few years. An outline of the details as they were understood at the time of writing this text is given in this section. Students who wish a more detailed discussion of the biosynthesis of protein are advised to consult a recently published biochemistry text.

The nucleic acids participate intimately in the process of protein synthesis. In general, protein synthesis takes place in cells that are rich in *ribonucleic acid* (RNA). *Deoxyribonucleic acid* (DNA) in the nucleus of the cell contains the entire code for the formation of all proteins synthesized in an organism. The information present in DNA is transcribed to a particular kind of ribonucleic acid known as *messenger RNA* (mRNA). The mRNA, which is formed in the nucleus, moves out into the cytoplasm, where it directs protein synthesis. Within the cytoplasm are the various constituents of the so-called *amino acid incorporating system*. Included among the components necessary for peptide synthesis are the following:

> microsomal fraction (mRNA and ribosomes),
> transfer RNA,
> amino acid activating enzymes,
> various factors for initiation and elongation of peptide chains,
> guanosine triphosphate (GTP) and amino acids, and
> an ATP-generating system.

Information contained in the mRNA is translated by a specific ribonucleic acid known as *transfer RNA* (tRNA). The tRNA units are relatively small, and there is at least one specific tRNA for each of the amino acids. A particular tRNA with its attached amino acid will combine with mRNA only when the code on the mRNA specifies the tRNA bearing that amino acid.

Synthesis of protein begins with the attachment of a special tRNA, designated fMet-tRNA, to a ribosomal subunit (40S).* This complexing occurs on a molecule of mRNA at a specific site referred to as the *initiation codon* (or *initiation site*). A second ribosomal subunit (60S) then attaches to the complex to complete the formation of a ribosome. The ribosomal subunits are comprised of a single strand (40S) or triple strand (60S) of ribosomal RNA and a large number of proteins. Some of the proteins are required for structural purposes, whereas others function as binding sites and as enzymes. The ribosomes are compact structures, and there are generally several of them attached to a single mRNA. In fact, protein synthesis occurs only when several ribosomes attach to a single mRNA to form what is known as a *polyribosome*, or simply a *polysome*.

The completed ribosomes move along the mRNA, and the various amino acid–tRNA units successively attach to the mRNA as each ribosome passes the site corresponding to the amino acid carried by its tRNA. As each amino acid–tRNA unit binds to the mRNA, the growing peptide chain is transferred from the previously bound tRNA to the amino group of the newly attached tRNA. The previously bound tRNA now returns to solution in the cytoplasm, where it can again combine with the appropriate free amino acid. Thus, the polysome can be visualized as a series of ribosomes building longer and longer peptide chains as they move along a strand of mRNA. When the final amino acid residue has been added, the peptide chain is somehow released and the ribosome liberated from the mRNA.

The protein-synthesizing process is essentially an "all-or-nothing" mechanism. For protein synthesis to take place, all of the amino acids must be available simultaneously. Since the body is able to synthesize the dispensable amino acids, protein synthesis is appreciably impaired only when the diet lacks one or more of the indispensable amino acids. Studies by H. N. Munro and his associates have shown that the feeding of a tryptophan-deficient amino acid mixture results in the disaggregation of liver polysomes and a concomitant impairment in protein synthesis by the liver.† They have also shown that the addition of a complete amino acid mixture to an *in vitro* cell-free protein-synthesizing system stimulates polysome aggregation, whereas omission of any one amino acid removes this stimulus. Similar effects of amino acid pattern have been postulated for other tissues, although no other tissues have been as actively investigated as liver has. The rapidity with which polysome aggregation and disaggregation can occur in response to changes in amino acid supply may explain why the feeding of imbalanced

---

*Particles of this size are not referred to in terms of molecular weight but in terms of their sedimentation coefficients in a centrifugal field; these are expressed in *Svedberg units* (S).

†Munro, H. N., *Proc. Nutr. Soc.* **28**(1969):214.

amino acid mixtures has such an immediate and devastating effect on an animal.

Not only are observations such as those by Munro important in our understanding of protein metabolism, but they may prove valuable in the biochemical determination of protein requirements and in understanding the internal and external factors affecting protein needs.

Nonprotein nitrogenous constituents of animals

Amino acids are important not only as building units of proteins and peptides but as the primary constituents of many nonprotein nitrogen-containing compounds or as sources of nitrogen for them. In many cases the amino acids undergo only slight changes to yield important physiological compounds. In other cases they are practically unrecognizable in their new forms. A few nonprotein nitrogenous compounds that originate from amino acids are listed with their physiological functions in Table 10.6.

Table 10.6
Nonprotein nitrogenous constituents formed from amino acids in animals

Biological compound	Amino acid precursor	Physiological function
Purines and pyrimidines	Glycine and aspartic acid	Constituents of nucleotides and nucleic acids
Creatine	Glycine and arginine	Energy storage as creatine phosphate in muscle
Glycoholic and taurocholic acids	Glycine and cysteine	Bile acids, aid in fat digestion and absorption
Thyroxine, epinephrine, and norepinephrine	Tyrosine	Hormones
Ethanolamine and choline	Serine	Constituents of phospholipids
Histamine	Histidine	A vasodepressor
Serotonin	Tryptophan	Transmission of nerve impulses
Porphyrins	Glycine	Constituent of hemoglobin and cytochromes
Niacin	Tryptophan	Vitamin
Melanin	Tyrosine	Pigment of hair, skin, and eyes

Amino acids are sources of energy

Unlike the carbohydrate and lipid of a ration, the catabolism of the protein component leaves a nitrogenous residue to be disposed of, in addition to any CO_2 and H_2O arising from the oxidation of its carbonaceous portion. Following the paths of the dietary nitrogen to excretion is complicated by the fact that protein breaks down into twenty or more amino acids, each a metabolically separate entity. The molecular rearrangements that intervene between the ingestion of an "intact" amino acid and the ultimate disposal of the amino group on the one hand and the carbon-chain residue on the other are numerous and complicated. Rather than dealing with the detail of these events we shall depict the overall scheme of operation of the metabolic machinery.

General pathways of amino acid degradation   Amino acids have been found to undergo four general reactions in: their transformation into other nitrogen-containing compounds, such as some of those listed in Table 10.6; the formation of the dispensable amino acids; and the transfer of nitrogen to urea when the amino acids are used as sources of energy. These general reactions are (1) transamination, (2) oxidative deamination by amino acid oxidases or dehydrogenases, (3) nonoxidative deamination by amino acid dehydratases, and (4) decarboxylation.

Transaminations, which were mentioned when we discussed the essential amino acids, involve the transfer of the amino group from one carbon skeleton to another:

$$H-\underset{\underset{COOH}{|}}{\overset{\overset{R^1}{|}}{C}}-NH_2 + \underset{\underset{COOH}{|}}{\overset{\overset{R^2}{|}}{C}}=O \overset{Transaminase}{\rightleftharpoons} \underset{\underset{COOH}{|}}{\overset{\overset{R^1}{|}}{C}}=O + H-\underset{\underset{COOH}{|}}{\overset{\overset{R^2}{|}}{C}}-NH_2$$

Pyridoxal phosphate is the coenzyme that catalyzes these reactions. It will be recalled that transaminations are involved in the conversion of the α-keto analogues of the indispensable amino acids, except lysine and threonine, to the corresponding L-amino acids. Transaminases are found in most animal tissues, and their presence in high concentrations in the plasma is an indication of tissue damage such as that accompanying myocardial infarction.

Oxidative deamination by amino acid oxidases results in the liberation of ammonia and the conversion of the amino acid to the corresponding α-keto acid:

$$H-\underset{\underset{COOH}{|}}{\overset{\overset{R}{|}}{C}}-NH_2 + \tfrac{1}{2}O_2 \overset{\overset{\text{Amino acid}}{\text{oxidase}}}{\longrightarrow} \underset{\underset{COOH}{|}}{\overset{\overset{R}{|}}{C}}=O + NH_3$$

In mammals, amino acid oxidases are found primarily in the liver and kidneys. Oxidative deamination by NAD- or NADP-linked dehydrogenases also results in the formation of ammonia and an α-keto acid. Animal tissues possess only one powerful amino acid dehydrogenase, glutamic acid dehydrogenase, which is specific for glutamate. This is a fairly important enzyme, however, because it is by this reaction that the nitrogen residues from many of the amino acids are transferred to urea (details of this pathway are presented in Figure 10.3).

Nonoxidative deamination by a group of dehydratases results in the removal of amino groups from serine, homoserine, threonine, cysteine, and possibly homocysteine; for example,

$$\text{Serine} \xrightarrow{\text{Serine dehydratase}} \text{Pyruvate} + H_2O + NH_3$$

Decarboxylation reactions are responsible for the formation of important biological compounds, such as serotonin, taurine, and histamine; for example,

$$\text{Histadine} \longrightarrow \text{Histamine} + CO_2$$

Disposal of nitrogen—the urea cycle   Nearly all of the nitrogen released during the catabolism of amino acids in mammals is excreted as urea. The formation of urea is a very important process in terrestrial animals because they are extremely intolerant to the presence of ammonium ion in their cells.

Urea is produced by the hydrolysis of arginine. The other product of the hydrolysis is the amino acid ornithine. Thus, urea synthesis simply requires a mechanism for the formation of arginine. This is achieved by a cyclic process known as the *urea cycle*, the details of which are presented in Figure 10.3.

The urea cycle, which is active in the liver and kidneys, begins with the condensation of ornithine and carbamyl phosphate to form citrulline. Citrulline then picks up a second nitrogen from aspartic acid eventually to yield arginine. Hydrolysis of arginine by the enzyme arginase produces urea and restores the ornithine originally used to initiate the cycle. The overall reaction accomplished by the urea cycle can be summarized in the following equation:*

$$NH_4^+ + CO_2 + 2H_2O + 3ATP + \text{Aspartic acid} \longrightarrow$$
$$\text{Urea} + 2\,ADP + AMP + 2P_i + PP_i + 5H^+ + \text{Fumarate}$$

---

*P_i represents inorganic phosphate; PP_i represents pyrophosphate.

This equation reveals in part why the gross energy value of protein is 5.65 kcal per gram, whereas the physiological energy value is usually taken to be 4.00 kcal per gram. Utilization of protein for energy purposes results in a direct energy expenditure of 32–34 kcal (i.e., 4 mole equivalents of high-energy phosphate) for each mole of urea formed. During the catabolism of protein, energy is also lost in the rather complex series of reactions involved in the degradation of the individual carbon skeletons of the amino acids.

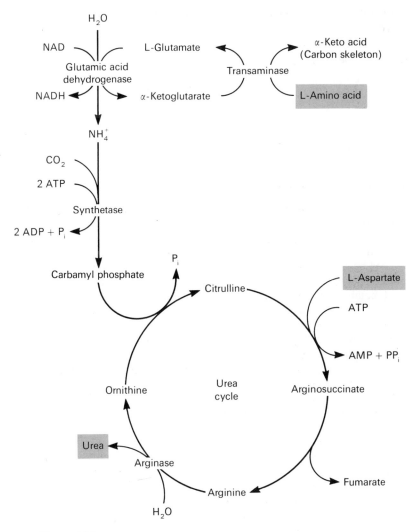

Figure 10.3
The pathway of urea synthesis in the excretion of amino acid nitrogen.

Fate of the carbon skeleton The overall degradation of amino acids in animals is the result of two basic processes: the removal and disposal of the amino nitrogen and the breakdown of the carbon skeleton. We have just seen that the body rids itself of the nitrogenous part of amino acids by a series of general reactions (transaminations, deamination by glutamate dehydrogenase, and urea formation). On the other hand, disposal of the carbon skeletons of the amino acids is the result of several series of reactions, the great majority of which are specific for each amino acid. We shall not discuss the details of these degradative pathways. It is sufficient for our purposes simply to show the major intermediates in the catabolism of the carbon skeletons (Table 10.7). These intermediates enter the citric acid cycle, which is the common final pathway of energy metabolism, whether of carbohydrate, fat, or protein.

Box 10.2   Inborn errors of amino acid metabolism

Over 250 inborn errors of metabolism have been described in man. Many of these congenital defects have been identified during the past decade by modern biochemical and clinical diagnostic techniques. Fortunately, most of these defects are extremely rare, and several of the more common disorders can be treated by dietary management.

Phenylketonuria (PKU) is one of the better-known inborn errors of amino acid metabolism. Failure to diagnose and treat PKU results in mental retardation, as is the case with many of the inborn errors of metabolism. In fact, it was estimated in 1954 that 1% of all institutionalized mental defectives in America suffered from PKU. Fortunately, the disorder can easily be detected, and most hospitals now routinely test all newborn infants for PKU, thus practically eliminating the tragedy and heartache that so often attended this disorder a quarter-century ago.

Phenylketonuria is transferred by an autosomal recessive gene. In North America, the disease occurs in 1 out of every 14,200 births. Owing to a lack of the enzyme phenylalanine hydroxylase, the liver fails to hydroxylate phenylalanine to tyrosine. As a consequence, the plasma level of phenylalanine is elevated and phenylalanine—together with phenylpyruvate, phenyllactate, and other products of the minor pathways of phenylalanine metabolism—is excreted in the urine.

Elevation of serum phenylalanine levels can be controlled effectively by feeding phenylketonurics special formulae from which phenylalanine has been removed and to which tyrosine (as essential amino acid for these patients) has been added. In many cases the diet of the phenylketonuric must be carefully

Table 10.7
Major intermediates in metabolism of amino acids, with their amino acid precursors

Acetate	Pyruvate	α-Ketoglutarate	Oxaloacetate	Succinate
Leucine	Alanine	Arginine	Aspartic acid	Valine
Lysine	Cysteine	Glutamic acid		Threonine‡
Phenylalanine*	Cystine	Hydroxyproline		Methionine‡
Tyrosine*	Glycine	Histidine		Isoleucine§
Tryptophan†	Serine	Proline		

*Part of the molecule is also converted to fumarate.
†Part of the molecule is also converted to pyruvate via alanine.
‡Converted to succinyl CoA via propionyl CoA.
§Part of the molecule is also converted to acetate.

controlled for years. Although strict dietary control is possible, it is difficult to maintain with children because of the extreme monotony of the diet and the well-meant but poorly placed kindnesses of neighbors and relatives. Extreme care on the part of the parents and education of all those with whom the PKU child has contact are the only ways of solving this problem.

Other inborn errors of amino acid metabolism that can be treated by careful diet management include tyrosinemia, maple sugar urine disease, homocystinuria, and cystathioninuria. Tyrosinemia is a particularly interesting condition because it is basically of two forms—hereditary and neonatal. Hereditary tyrosinemia is an autosomal recessive metabolic disease that results in a marked decrease in the activity of the enzyme p-hydroxyphenylpyruvic oxidase. Treatment of the disease entails restriction of dietary tyrosine and phenylalanine to levels compatible with the normal growth and development of the patient. Neonatal tyrosinemia is characterized by a transient deficiency of p-hydroxyphenylpyruvic oxidase. The disorder is particularly prevalent among premature infants. Unlike hereditary tyrosinemia, neonatal tyrosinemia disappears within a few weeks of birth. The correction of the biochemical defect can be hastened by the administration of vitamin C. The Canadian Dietary Standard recommends an intake of 100 mg of vitamin C daily during the first week of life, because it is not known whether neonatal tyrosinemia is harmless.

Early detection and careful dietary management have largely eliminated the mental retardation that almost invariably accompanied phenylketonuria and tyrosinemia only a few years ago. Although these advances in treatment have not eliminated the diseases themselves, they have certainly reduced the anguish and frustration that once attended these disorders.

Suggested readings

Chalupa, W. "Utilization of Nonprotein Nitrogen in the Production of Animal Protein," *Proceedings of the Nutrition Society* **32**(1973):99.

Gitler, C. "Protein Digestion and Absorption in Nonruminants." In *Mammalian Protein Metabolism*, Vol. 1. Edited by H. N. Munro and J. B. Allison. Academic Press, New York and London (1964):35.

McLaughlan, J. M., and Campbell, J. A. "Methodology of Protein Evaluation." In *Mammalian Protein Metabolism*, Vol. 3. Edited by H. N. Munro. Academic Press, New York and London (1969):391.

Munro, H. N. "A General Survey of Mechanisms Regulating Protein Metabolism in Mammals." In *Mammalian Protein Metabolism*, Vol. 4. Edited by H. N. Munro. Academic Press, New York and London (1970):3.

Ørskov, E. R. "Nitrogen Digestion and Utilization by Young and Lactating Ruminants." In *World Review of Nutrition and Dietetics*, Vol. 26. Edited by G. H. Bourne. S. Karger, Basel.

Swaminathan, M. "Availability of Plant Proteins." In *Newer Methods of Nutritional Biochemistry*, Vol. 3. Edited by A. A. Albanese. Academic Press, New York and London (1967):197.

Wright, K. N. "Methods Used in Evaluating Protein Quality in High Protein Feed Stuffs," *Nutrition Reports International* **3**(1971):221.

Chapter 11
The final common pathway
of energy metabolism and
the energy transfer system

In Chapters 7–10 we followed carbohydrates, fats, and proteins through the stages of digestion and metabolism characteristic of each. We saw that the carbon atoms of each eventually give rise to intermediates in the citric acid cycle. Because this cycle plays such a central role in energy metabolism, it has been aptly called the final common pathway of energy metabolism. More than two-thirds of the carbon atoms of ingested food enter the citric acid cycle as acetyl groups to be catabolized in processes such as oxidation of acetyl CoA. The reactions and substrates of this cycle are also important in synthetic (anabolic) processes such as the conversion of protein to carbohydrate or the synthesis of metabolites such as purines, pyrimidines, and dispensable amino acids. Figure 11.1 is a skeleton of the cycle, showing where substrates enter the cycle, which molecules are formed at each step of the cycle, and the points at which molecules of CO_2 are split off and pairs of electrons are transferred to NAD and FAD.

The citric acid cycle

The citric acid cycle is localized in the mitochondria of the cell. The reason for the localization of some metabolic pathways in the mitochondria and others in the cytoplasm is not completely understood but it appears to be founded in the need for orderly integration of energy production with other processes in the body. The importance of compartmentalization of metabolism is illustrated by fatty acid metabolism, in which acetyl CoA is both the starting material for synthesis and the major product of β-oxidation. Synthesis of fatty acids takes place in the cytoplasm, whereas degradation takes place in the mitochondria. Thus, the pathways do not compete directly, and the dominance of one over the other depends on the balance between the supply of energy-yielding compounds and the need for energy.

Metabolites may enter the citric acid cycle at any point, although the cycle is usually represented as beginning with the condensation of acetyl CoA and oxaloacetate to yield citrate. Citrate stands at a major branching point in the metabolism of acetyl CoA because it can either undergo rearrangement to form isocitrate or it can diffuse out of the mitochondria into the cytoplasm, where it is cleaved to acetyl CoA and oxaloacetate. In the cytoplasm, acetyl CoA is utilized for fatty acid synthesis, whereas the oxaloacetate is converted via malate to pyruvate. The pyruvate thus formed can diffuse back into the mitochondria, where it undergoes either recarboxylation (the pathway represented by a dashed line in Figure 11.1) to form oxaloacetate or decarboxylation to yield acetyl CoA. The net result of this side branch from citrate is the transfer of acetyl CoA formed in the mitochondria to the cytoplasm, where it can be synthesized into fatty acids.

The isocitrate formed in the mitochondria undergoes oxidative decarboxylation to produce α-ketoglutarate. The CO_2 is released into solution and two electrons are transferred to NAD. Conversion of α-ketoglutarate to succinyl CoA entails a second oxidative decarboxylation and is brought about by a complex of enzymes analogous to that catalyzing the decarboxylation of pyruvate to acetyl CoA; thiamin pyrophosphate is a coenzyme in both processes. This reaction produces the second and final mole of CO_2 released in the citric acid cycle.

The remaining steps in the citric acid cycle include hydrolysis of succinyl CoA and two more oxidations. The potential energy of the thiol ester of succinyl CoA is recovered directly as the high-energy phosphate GTP (guanosine triphosphate). Oxidation of the succinate formed upon the hydrolysis of succinyl CoA involves FAD as a cofactor. As mentioned in Chapter 7 in connection with the oxidation of glycerol-3-phosphate, direct transfer of a pair of electrons to oxygen via FAD (or coenzyme Q) yields only 2 molecules of ATP because it bypasses the first site of oxidative phosphorylation. Oxidation of malate by NAD restores the oxaloacetate that initiated the citric acid cycle.

Oxaloacetate is important not only as an intermediate in the citric acid cycle but as an intermediate in *gluconeogenesis*. Synthesis of glucose in the body is carried out primarily by the liver and kidneys, and is basically a reversal of glycolysis (Chapter 7). Pyruvate or any components that can be catabolized to pyruvate, such as lactate or certain amino acids, can be used

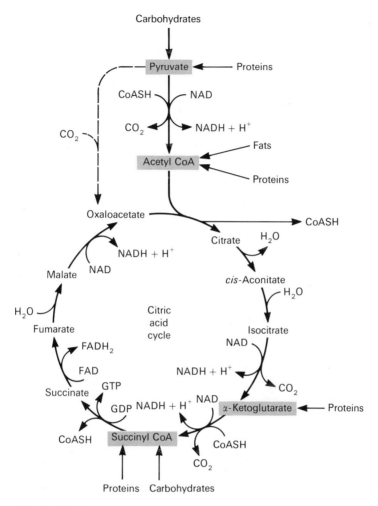

Figure 11.1
The common pathway of carbohydrate, fat, and protein energy metabolism. The compounds in boxes are major metabolites formed directly from ingested nutrients.

for glucose synthesis. However, glycolysis is not directly reversible from pyruvate because the conversion of pyruvate to phosphoenolpyruvate is a thermodynamically unfavored reaction: in other words, it is essentially unidirectional, because the equilibrium lies strongly on the side of the formation of pyruvate from phosphoenolpyruvate. The importance of oxaloacetate in gluconeogenesis is explained by the pathway that circumvents this thermodynamically unfavored reaction. We mentioned above, when discussing the metabolic side path that begins with citrate, that pyruvate can be carboxylated to form oxaloacetate. Oxaloacetate can either condense with acetyl CoA to give citrate or be converted to phosphoenolpyruvate and, in turn, glucose by reversal of glycolysis. Thus, glucose can be synthesized from any components that give rise to oxaloacetate. Among these are pyruvate and its precursors and any of the citric acid cycle intermediates and their precursors. The primary precursors of glucose in the nonruminant are the glucogenic amino acids—that is, the amino acids whose carbon skeletons are metabolized via pyruvate, oxaloacetate, succinate, and α-ketoglutarate.

Gluconeogenesis is particularly important in certain physiological conditions, such as diabetes and starvation. It also is important in the dairy cow: high-producing dairy cows may synthesize as much as 1.8 kg of lactose daily. All of this sugar is derived from gluconeogenesis because the primary sources of energy for the ruminant are the short-chain fatty acids. Of particular significance in the formation of lactose is propionate, which, as we mentioned in Chapter 9, is converted to succinyl CoA. Thus, propionate can serve as a precursor of oxaloacetate and, if necessary, of glucose.

The importance of the citric acid cycle in the integration and control of metabolism cannot be overemphasized. Not only is it a common pathway of energy metabolism for carbohydrates, fats, and proteins, but many of its reactions and substrates play a crucial role in biosynthetic processes. Some of the biosynthetic functions of the citric acid cycle in birds and mammals are charted in Figure 11.2. It is important to remember, however, that any time an intermediate is "bled off" from the cycle for synthetic purposes it must be replenished by a molar equivalent amount of material at the same or at a different site in the cycle if equilibrium is to be maintained.

Oxidative phosphorylation—the generation of ATP.   Oxidation of substrates in the citric acid cycle results in the production of carbon dioxide and the transfer of electrons to oxygen. We learned in Chapter 7 that the transfer of electrons to oxygen is accompanied by the phosphorylation of ADP to ATP and that the process is called oxidative phosphorylation. Electrons are transferred from substrate to oxygen by a series of intermediate carriers that are themselves reduced by the addition of electrons and then reoxidized when the electrons are transferred to the next intermediate. Figure 11.3 shows the intermediaries of the flow of electrons and the possible points of phosphorylation. NAD is the primary acceptor of electrons from the various substrates, although certain substrates transfer electrons directly to flavoproteins. It is important to know which is the case, because 3 moles of ATP are generated for each mole of NADH oxidized, but only 2 moles for each mole of FADH oxidized.

The initial carriers of electrons in the oxidative phosphorylation pathway are of particular interest to the nutritionist because they are derivatives of the

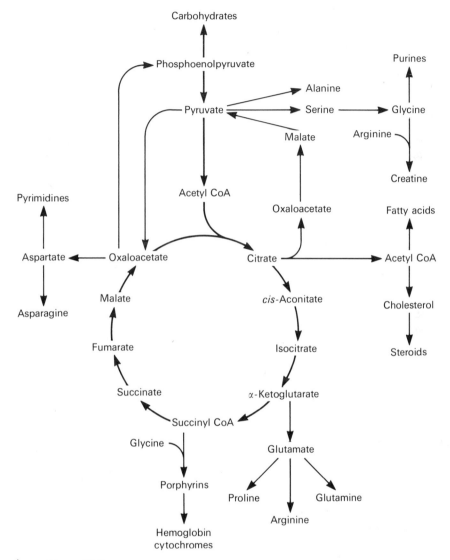

Figure 11.2
Some biosynthetic functions of the citric acid cycle in mammals and birds.

vitamins niacin and riboflavin, in the form of NAD and FAD. In fact, the requirement for these vitamins is frequently given in terms of energy requirements, in recognition of the close association of these vitamins with energy metabolism.

We have repeatedly referred to the oxidative process as a transfer of electrons through a succession of intermediaries, with the final acceptor being oxygen. On the other hand we have represented reduced NAD as NADH. In fact, reduction of NAD entails the addition of a hydride ion—that is, a proton

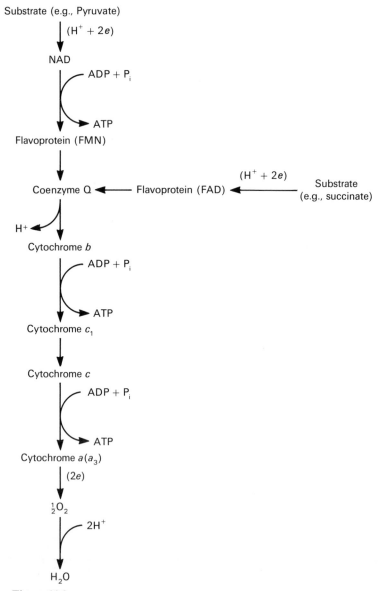

Figure 11.3
The sequence of intermediaries of the flow of electrons and the possible points of phosphorylation in the oxidative phosphorylation pathway in mitochondria.

and two electrons. In the electron transport chain as depicted in Figure 11.3, the pair of electrons is passed from one carrier to another, whereas the proton is released to aqueous solution in the mitochondria.

Although our discussion has been somewhat oversimplified, it can be seen that the important features of oxidative phosphorylation are these: (1) some of the free energy that is released in the successive oxidation-reduction reactions is recaptured as high-energy phosphate, and (2) oxygen, the final acceptor of electrons, picks up a pair of protons to form water. Thus, complete oxidation of one mole of acetate results in the formation of two moles of CO_2 and two moles of H_2O:

$$CH_3COOH + 2O_2 \rightarrow 2CO_2 + 2H_2O$$

Elimination of CO_2 and H^+   The CO_2 that is formed is eliminated from the body, in the ordinary course of respiration, in the exhaled air. The hydrogen ions released during electron transport are in equilibrium with other H^+ ions in the mitochondria, and, potentially, with all H^+ ions throughout the body. In general, equilibrium is maintained because a pair of H^+ ions combines with a half-molecule of O_2 to form a molecule of H_2O for each pair of electrons transferred. This H_2O leaves the body in the urine and the sweat. If the nature of a food or the pattern of an animal's internal metabolism causes a net formation or removal of H^+ ions, the shift in H^+ ion concentration must be compensated for to avoid a lethal change in internal pH. Usually the body is confronted with too much H^+; the main mechanism for correcting this entails exchange of H^+ for Na^+ by the kidney tubules. The capacity for concentrating H^+ ions in the urine is not unlimited, but the kidney is capable of coping with mild acidosis for short periods of time.

Caloric value of oxygen in metabolism   In the discussion of ATP in Chapter 7 we mentioned that the transfer of electrons from substrate to oxygen is accompanied by phosphorylation of ADP to ATP and that the two processes are essentially inseparable. This relationship is illustrated in Figure 11.3, and it is evident from Figures 11.1 and 11.3 that rate of energy metabolism is proportional to the amount of oxygen used to form water. The rate of energy metabolism is also reflected in the total heat lost from the body. Thus, by simultaneously measuring oxygen consumption and the heat escaping from the body we can establish the energy equivalent of oxygen in metabolism. Actual determinations with healthy animals fed a mixed diet containing carbohydrates, fats, and proteins have shown that 4.825 kcal is produced per liter of oxygen consumed. The use of this figure for calculating energy needs of the body will be dealt with in Chapter 28.

Recapitulation   The carbohydrates, fats, and proteins of the diet supply the body with molecules consisting principally of carbon, hydrogen, oxygen, and nitrogen. Each of these molecules contains a complement of energy associated with the particular valence bonds of its structure. This energy is made available to the body by a series of orderly reactions whereby the original molecules are recast into 2-, 3-, and 4-carbon molecules that can be metabolized in the citric acid cycle. The fact that metabolism of carbohydrates, fats, and proteins culminates in a common pathway, the citric acid cycle, permits the ready interconversion of these constituents without any need for an elaborate system of separate reactions. It also guarantees the integrated control of energy metabolism and synthetic processes in the body, and the coordination of energy storage with the supply and needs for energy.

Complete metabolism of substrates to CO_2 and H_2O in the citric acid cycle results in the energy being captured by the formation of ATP—the equivalent of 12 molecules for each molecule of acetyl CoA converted to CO_2 and H_2O. The CO_2 leaves the body in respiration. The hydrogen atoms are split off in pairs, one as a hydride ion, the other as a proton. The hydride ion is transferred to NAD or FAD, its pair of electrons is transferred to oxygen, and the oxygen combines with a pair of protons to form H_2O. Water is eliminated as urine or as perspiration.

Utilization of protein for energy purposes requires the elimination of nitrogen as urea. Protein metabolism involves a more extensive series of reactions than the metabolism of either carbohydrate or fat, but eventually the carbon skeletons of amino acids also enter the citric acid cycle.

The main pathways of carbohydrate, fat, and protein metabolism are presented as a unit in Figure 11.4.

Energy storage and utilization

In Chapter 7 we stated that the chemical transformations of intermediary metabolism provide the cell with chemical substances from which it can build its structural and functional components and with the energy needed for its many functions. We have considered something of the pattern and sequence of these molecular changes but we have said nothing about the mechanisms by which energy is accumulated, stored, and finally used to perform work.

We have noted that the principal way energy is transferred from one chemical reaction to another in biological systems is by the high-energy intermediary ATP. Most of the ATP is formed in the mitochondria by biological oxidation of substrates in the citric acid cycle and the oxidative phosphorylation pathway. ATP is the principal driving force in the energy-requiring biochemical processes of life. The innumerable individual transformations involving ATP will not be considered in this book, but some knowledge of the overall scheme of energy transfer and use is needed to understand the general functioning of the body machine.

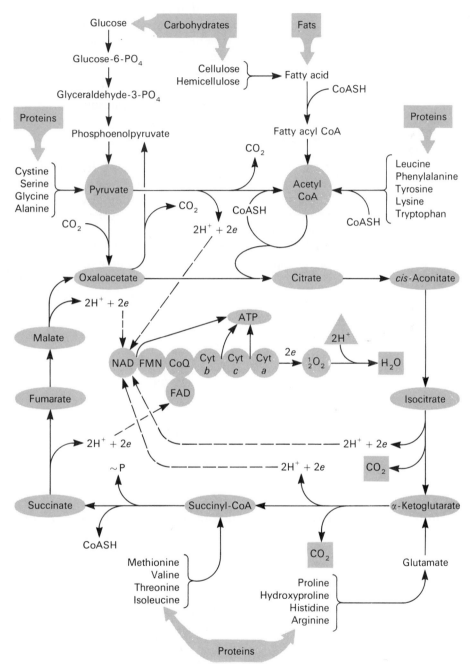

Figure 11.4
The "oxidation" of carbohydrate, fat, and protein.

Energy storage   Energy for muscle contraction is provided by the cleavage of ATP to ADP and P_i. Muscles such as the heart muscles, which are capable of steadily repeated contractions over a long period of time, have the capacity to continuously generate ATP as it is needed. However, sudden short bursts of violent contraction, such as those which characterize skeletal muscle, use up ATP faster than it can be produced by mitochondrial oxidations. Thus, the skeletal muscles depend upon stores of high-energy phosphate that can be readily transferred to ADP and also upon the conversion of glycogen to glucose with the generation of ATP in glycolysis.

CREATINE PHOSPHATE   High-energy phosphate is stored in muscle as creatine phosphate, the phosphoric amide of creatine. Creatine is readily phosphorylated by ATP in a reaction that is freely reversible. Any temporary excess of ATP is relieved by transfer of the high-energy phosphate from ATP to creatine. The creatine phosphate, in turn, is readily available to replenish ATP when it is being rapidly consumed. This relationship between "stored" and "active" high-energy phosphate is depicted in the following equation:

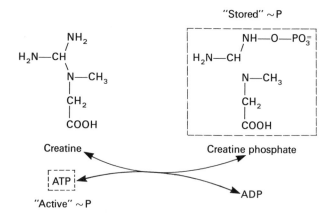

About two-thirds of the creatine in resting muscle is in the form of creatine phosphate.

Creatine phosphate continuously undergoes a slow, spontaneous cyclization to form *creatinine*, which is excreted in the urine. Creatinine formation takes place at a constant rate that is proportional to muscle mass. Thus the urinary creatinine excretion rate frequently is used as a baseline for measuring the rate of urinary excretion of other metabolites, such as those of the water-soluble vitamins.

GLYCOGEN   The ability of an organism to store transitory excesses of energy, particularly as *glycogen*, permits it to eat sporadically and still meet the constant demand for high-energy phosphate. The main stores of glycogen are in skeletal muscle and liver, with the amount present dependent on the activity of the animal and the nature of its diet. The amount of glycogen in the liver varies considerably with diet composition and feeding pattern, whereas the amount in muscle depends more on immediate past activity, because exercise rapidly depletes glycogen in skeletal muscle. The liver in a normal resting animal on a typical diet will contain about 5% glycogen and the muscle 1% glycogen, although the total quantity in muscle will be 5 to 6 times that in the liver because of the difference in the total masses of the two tissues.

Glycogen is a branched polymer of glucose. Its formation and breakdown are summarized in Figure 11.5. Glycogen is synthesized from glucose-1-phosphate by the transfer of glucose from UDP-glucose to terminal glycogen chains.* It is degraded by phosphorolysis of terminal glucosidic bonds to form glucose-1-phosphate. Since glycogen is formed from and broken down to glucose-1-phosphate, the two pathways are competitive and the enzymes catalyzing these processes are intricately controlled. Regulation is accomplished by the alteration of the catalytic activity of phosphorylase and glycogen synthetase. Adrenalin in skeletal muscle and glucagon in liver initiate a series of changes that bring about the phosphorylation of these enzymes, resulting in conversion of phosphorylase from the inactive *b* form to the active *a* form and conversion of glycogen synthetase from the active I form to the inactive D form. The net result of these changes is a stoppage of glycogen synthesis and an acceleration of glycogen breakdown. Removal of adrenalin and glucagon reverses the entire chain of events; the phosphate groups are removed from the enzymes by the action of phosphatases, thereby rendering glycogen synthetase active and phosphorylase inactive. This encourages glycogen formation and inhibits glycogen breakdown.

Storage of glucose as glycogen is energetically very efficient. Very little ATP is needed to activate the various enzyme systems involved in glycogen metabolism, compared to the amount of ATP generated by the metabolism of glycogen in glycolysis and the citric acid cycle. One high-energy phosphate is used in the storage of glucose as glycogen; that is, for conversion of UDP to UTP. Thus 97% of the energy that would have been produced by direct metabolism of glucose-6-phosphate is obtained when glucose has been stored as glycogen and later used in the same tissue.

FAT   Neutral fats and triglycerides are a major source of fuel for animals. They may come directly from dietary sources or they may be synthesized in the body from other dietary components. Nearly all tissues are capable of synthesizing fat, although the primary sites of synthesis appear to be the liver and adipose tissue, depending on the species concerned. In the rat, adipose tissue is the major site of *de novo* synthesis (lipogenesis) of fatty acids from

---

*UDP = uridine diphosphate.

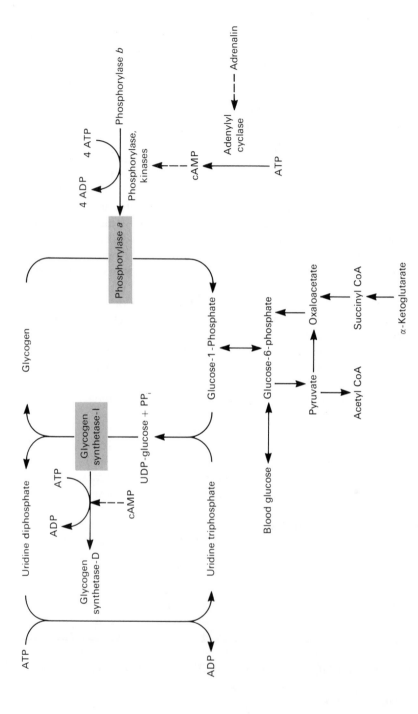

Figure 11.5
Summary of glycogen synthesis and breakdown.

carbohydrate, although the liver also is capable of synthesizing appreciable quantities of fat. The primary site of lipogenesis in the pig is adipose tissue, whereas in the chicken and man the bulk of the fatty acids is synthesized by the liver.

When carbohydrate is present in excess of immediate metabolic needs, fat is laid down, primarily in adipose tissue. In the postabsorptive phase the stored triglycerides are mobilized by the action of a hormone-inducible lipase that hydrolyzes the triglycerides to free fatty acids and glycerol. The free fatty acids, bound to albumin, are transported by the blood to the energy-requiring tissues, such as muscle. Fatty acids are oxidized in the mitochondria of the cell. Muscles that are continuously active, such as those of the heart or diaphragm, are well equipped for using fatty acids as fuel.

Breakdown of fat is under the same sort of control as that described for glycogen. Control is maintained by a lipase that is activated by cyclic AMP, the same compound that brings about activation of phosphorylase. Formation of cyclic AMP in adipose tissue is stimulated by adrenalin, glucagon, and ACTH, just as it is in the liver. However, the stimulus for cyclic AMP formation can be overridden by insulin, which is secreted in response to high concentrations of glucose in the blood, the net effect being the storage of fat under the same conditions that favor glycogen accumulation in skeletal muscle.

Storage of energy as fat is somewhat less efficient than storage as glycogen. Recovery of utilizable energy when glucose is stored as glycogen is about 97%, whereas only about 80% of the potential energy is realized when glucose is stored as fat. Nevertheless, there are distinct physical advantages of the storage of fat rather than glycogen. Not only is the potential energy of fat per unit weight much greater, approximately 2.25 times that of glycogen, but less water is associated with stored fat than with glycogen. Thus, storage of energy as fat can be achieved with about one-tenth the body-weight increase that would be necessary for storage of an equivalent potential of high-energy phosphate as glycogen.

Use of energy   In the normally active animal a large part of the daily energy requirement is for muscle activity or the production of some product such as milk. During maintenance living, there is smooth-muscle and heart-muscle activity, and during work or play there are added the needs of skeletal muscle. For lactating individuals, the energy in milk and also that used in its synthesis are a further demand. Table 11.1 compares energy requirements of adults for maintenance with those for "work." The data are calculated from current dietary and feeding standards.

Table 11.1
Approximate daily energy requirements for adult maintenance and for activity or production

Species	Adult maintenance requirement	Activity or production		
		Type (daily)	Energy requirement	Activity req't as % of total
Man, 68 kg	2400 kcal	Light work	768 kcal*	23
		Maximum work	2400 kcal†	50
Cow, 450 kg	14.2 Mcal	25 kg milk	30.0 Mcal	68
Horse, 630 kg	17.6 Mcal	3 hr work	6.5 Mcal	27
		6 hr work	13.0 Mcal	42

*1.6 kcal/min for 8 hours.
†5.0 kcal/min for 8 hours.

ENERGY TRANSMISSION   The energy transmission scheme as a whole is illustrated, albeit greatly over-simplified, in Figure 11.6. It must be remembered that muscular activity demands an increase in total energy metabolism, so that in addition to the increased use of ATP for muscle contractions required for activity beyond that of idle living, there is a speed-up of the whole machine. In Figure 11.6 the energy-using reactions are grouped into several categories—not because they act as independent units, but because this makes clearer the difference between maintenance and production needs.

Because not all the energy from exothermic reactions is recovered in metabolism, the efficiency of energy transfer is less than 100%. The total potential energy ($\Delta G^{o\prime}$) of one mole of glucose, for example, is 673 kcal. The energy content of the phosphate bonds formed per mole of glucose is 288 kcal; that is, there is a net formation of 36 moles of ATP. On this basis we calculate that the efficiency of energy transfer is 42%. The average efficiency of muscle has been found to be about 30%, both with excised muscle and by direct calorimetric determinations of external work for a number of species of animals.

ENERGY FOR MUSCLE ACTIVITY   In Chapter 4 the nature of skeletal muscle was discussed, with a brief description of the role of ATP in muscle contraction and relaxation. There often arises the question whether a given food is a preferred dietary source of energy for muscular work; it should now be evident that any food or food component that will contribute to the formation of ATP is acceptable fuel for work. Protein, because some 20% of its potential energy is excreted in the urine, is less efficient than either carbohydrate or fat. At the cellular level, however, the body shows no preference for its source of energy.

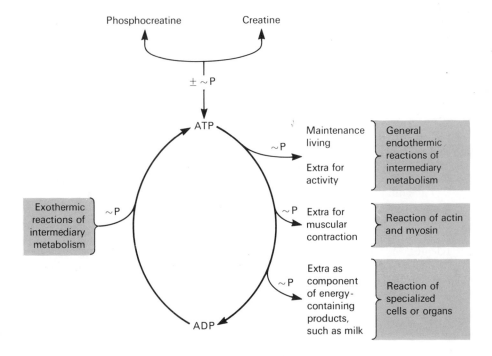

Figure 11.6
The energy transmission system.

Feeding standards have implied that the extra energy necessary for work need not require an increase in the protein intake. This view is to be questioned, if for no other reason than that, in order to metabolize carbohydrate or fat, the whole metabolic machine must increase its operations. Some activities of this increased operation require protein, for extra enzymes and hormones and for special molecules used in urea synthesis and other functions. For example, it is estimated that some 15% of the daily energy of resting metabolism in the rat is associated with protein turnover. Furthermore, there is an energy cost associated with the operation of the Na^+/K^+ pump mechanism. It has been estimated that Na^+ and K^+ transport accounts for some 17% of the energy expenditure of muscle.

Experiments with livestock and poultry, and with laboratory animals, make it clear that there is an optimum ratio of the digestible protein to the metabolizable energy of a ration. The precise value of this ratio varies among species but the concept is generally valid: increases in energy concentrations without appropriate increases in usable protein of a ration lead to a marked decline in ration efficiency, and often a decline in voluntary food intake.

The practical implications for applied dietetics or animal feeding are obvious. Demands for production or for muscular activity above maintenance levels require increased quantities of every component of the diet. The proportions in which the components should be supplied are determined by the useful energy intake. As energy needs increase, so also do the nutrient requirements, with the optimum ratio of nutrient to energy depending on the purpose for which the energy is used.

In Sections V and VI of this book we shall return to the subject of energy to consider quantitatively the requirements of the individual and how these requirements are determined by biological tests.

Suggested readings

Baldwin, R. L. "Estimation of Theoretical Calorific Relationships as a Teaching Technique: A Review," *Journal of Dairy Science* **51**(1968):104.

Blaxter, K. L., Kielanowski, J., and Thorbek, G. *Energy Metabolism of Farm Animals*. Proceedings of the 4th Symposium of the European Association of Animal Production, Publication 12. Oriel, Newcastle on Tyne (1969).

Kleiber, M. *The Fire of Life*. John Wiley & Sons, New York (1961).

Milligan, L. P. "Energetic Efficiency and Metabolic Transformations," *Federation Proceedings* **30**(1971):1454.

Section III
THE VITAMINS:
THEIR NATURE AND
ROLES IN METABOLISM

In Section II we described the animal organism as a metabolic machine whose chief function is to degrade organic food substances into molecules from which it can then manufacture some of its own "parts," and/or obtain the energy needed to perform work. We now turn our attention to the catalytic and regulatory mechanism essential to the operation of the machine.

This mechanism consists of the seemingly innumerable enzymes, which together with their cofactors and coenzymes form enzyme systems. The enzymes are specific combinations of amino acids—proteins of unique patterns. The cofactors, which usually serve to activate the enzymes, may be inorganic ions and/or coenzymes. Coenzymes are complex molecules, some being derived from one or another of the B vitamins.

The multiplicity of units in the catalytic and regulatory mechanism is evident from the figure below. The phases of energy metabolism pictured "adjacent" to pyruvate and acetyl CoA require four minerals and four vitamins. Because animals can synthesize no minerals and only a few vitamins, their diet must contain both minerals and vitamins.

We did not consider each amino acid separately in great detail because the amino acids normally combine to function as polypeptides or proteins. By contrast, the minerals and vitamins seem to maintain their identity throughout metabolism. Even though this invariance is more apparent than real, it necessitates a consideration of these nutrients as separate entities. This we shall do in Section III (the vitamins) and Section IV (the minerals.)

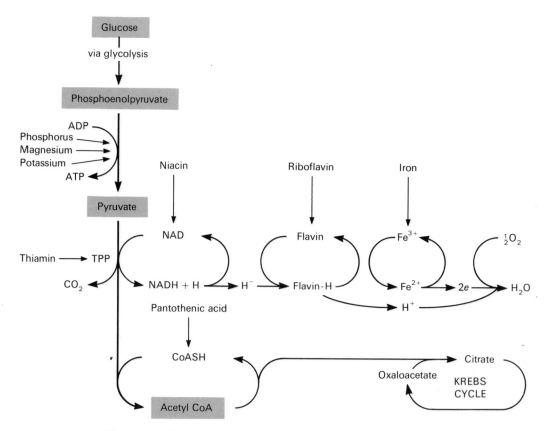

Illustration of vitamin and mineral involvement in energy metabolism.

Chapter 12
Vitamins—general

Until the turn of the twentieth century, nutritionists and lay people alike considered carbohydrates, fats, and proteins, plus certain minerals, to be the only dietary elements required for the normal functioning of the animal body. However, at that time it became evident that other organic compounds had to be present in the diet if health was to be maintained.

A number of observations had contributed to recognition of this fact. For example, it had been known for over 300 years that scurvy could be prevented or cured by eating fresh fruits or vegetables; it had also been known for some time that rickets could be cured by ingesting cod-liver oil. In 1897 the Dutch physician C. Eijkmann showed that beriberi, a disease which resulted from the prolonged consumption of polished rice, could be cured by adding back to the diet the rice polishings.

These observations suggested that natural foods contain substances which are indispensable for health but which are neither carbohydrate, fat, nor protein. In 1906 F. G. Hopkins* called these substances "accessory food factors," and in 1911 C. Funk† introduced the term *vitamine*. *Vitamin* became the accepted term to denote this group of organic compounds. Since about 1912, researchers have made remarkable advances in the study of vitamins; they have isolated, purified, synthesized, and elucidated the physiolog-

---

*Hopkins, F. G., *Analyst* **31**(1906):385; *J. Physiol.* **49**(1912):425.

†Funk, C., *J. Physiol.* **43**(1911):395.

Box 12.1 Casimir Funk and the *vitamine*

At the beginning of the twentieth century, Casimir Funk and F. G. Hopkins proposed that diseases such as beriberi and scurvy are caused by a deficiency of certain food components. This theory challenged the contemporary popular view that such conditions are either the result of food toxins or are in fact infectious diseases. Funk called these food components *vitamines*, implying they are amines required for life. The ideas of Funk and Hopkins generated interest in a new field of biochemistry, and resulted in the discovery (between 1915 and 1948) of all the vitamins known today.

Casimir Funk (1884–1967) was born in Warsaw, Poland. The son of a physician, he was not encouraged by his father to follow that profession. Sent to Switzerland to study biology, Funk eventually specialized in organic chemistry, passing his oral exams and defending his doctoral thesis at the age of twenty. As a result of his work at the Lister Institute in England during the post–World War I period, he received the degree of Doctor of Science from the University of London.

Funk's professional life spanned two world wars. This fact, along with the political unrest in his native Poland between those wars, perhaps accounts for his frequent moving from country to country. In chronological order, he held positions in France, Germany, England, the United States, Poland, France, and finally returned to the United States in 1939 to remain there for the duration of his life.

While at the Lister Institute, Funk was given the task of finding the substance in rice polishings that is associated with the prevention and cure of beriberi. In 1912, he succeeded in preparing thiamin-containing extracts, first from rice polishings and later from yeast, milk, and ox brain. At that time he claimed "the curative substance is a pyrimidine base, analogous to uracil and thymine."

Although he is known to historians of nutrition primarily for his early work with vitamins, Funk was also one of the pioneers of the American chemical industry. While employed by Metz and Co. during his first sojourn in the United States, he was one of the researchers responsible for the production of "Oscodal," a vitamin A and D concentrate which was the first vitamin preparation to be accepted by the American Medical Association as a product that could ethically be promoted as a source of vitamins. Funk also worked extensively on the chemistry of various hormones. From 1939 on, as a member of the U.S. Vitamin Corporation, he worked on the chemistry of carcinomas and on determining the cause of ulcers.

Casimir Funk, after a long and productive life, retired from the Vitamin Corporation in 1963 at the age of seventy-nine.

For further information, see *J. Nutr.* **102**(1972):1107.

ical action of many of these organic compounds. Today it is possible to state (for some vitamins) which chemical reaction in animal metabolism requires which vitamin(s).

Vitamins defined

Basing our description on H. R. Rosenberg's definition,* we can describe vitamins as organic compounds required for normal growth and the maintenance of animal life. Animals are unable to synthesize many of these compounds. Vitamins are effective in small amounts. Some are essential for the transformation of energy, but do not themselves supply energy to the body. Finally, some vitamins are essential for the regulation of the metabolism of structural units, but are not themselves used as building units for the structure of the body.

Nomenclature

By 1913 only two vitamins had been discovered; one was fat soluble and the other was water soluble. E.V. McCollum and M. Davis† proposed "fat-soluble A" and "water-soluble B" as names for these substances, which were otherwise known only by the consequences of their absence in the diet. Classification by solubility in water or fat is still in use.

In 1920, before scientists had determined the chemical composition of any of the vitamins, J.C. Drummond‡ proposed calling vitamins simply by letters of the alphabet. This system worked satisfactorily for a few years, and gradually nine vitamins appeared on the scene: A, B, C, D, E, F, G, H, I. However, scientists soon found that F was not a true vitamin because it supplied energy; they also learned that B was not a single vitamin but a mixture of several, which necessitated adding number subscripts to the letters, as in B_1, B_2, and so on. When vitamins B_2 and G turned out to be identical, G was dropped from the vitamin alphabet. Vitamin H was also dropped when biotin was identified as one of the B-complex vitamins.

Members of the vitamin B complex discovered after the identification of biotin were named according to their known chemical composition, and as researchers clarified chemical structures and biological function, it became possible to identify named vitamins with substances earlier given subscript

---

*Rosenberg, H. R., *The Chemistry and Physiology of the Vitamins*, Interscience, New York (1945).

†McCollum, E. V., and Davis, M., *J. Biol. Chem.* **15**(1913):167.

‡Drummond, J. C., *Biochem. J.* **14**(1920):660.

numbers. Many of the letter designations have now been dropped. This is true for all the vitamins of the B-complex except B_6 and B_{12}. Vitamin B_6 is found in nature in three forms—pyridoxine, pyridoxal, and pyridoxamine—all of which are biologically active in mammals. The original term "B_6" remains the official name for this multiform vitamin. Cobalamin has been suggested as the name for B_{12}, but the letter designation continues to be used.

In contrast to the B family, letters of the alphabet have been retained for fat-soluble vitamins A, D, E, K, and for water-soluble C.

Because there is still no universal agreement on the nomenclature of the vitamins, we will use the names adopted in 1977 by the American Institute of Nutrition.*

Solubility in water or fat is sometimes used as a basis for classifying vitamins into two broad groups; the several members of each group have some similar characteristics and functions. Vitamin C is the only member of the water-soluble group that is not a member of the B family. Moreover, it has characteristics and functions so different from the B vitamins that it requires separate consideration. Consequently, we shall exclude vitamin C from the following comparisons of fat-soluble and water-soluble vitamins and shall deal with it separately in Chapter 15.

Fat-soluble vitamins versus water-soluble B vitamins

These two groups of vitamins exhibit several differences that serve to distinguish them both chemically and biologically.

Chemical composition   Fat-soluble vitamins contain only carbon, hydrogen, and oxygen, whereas the water-soluble B vitamins contain these three elements plus either nitrogen, sulfur, or cobalt.

Occurrence   Vitamins originate primarily in plant tissues and are, with the exception of vitamins C and D, present in animal tissues only if an animal consumes foods containing them or harbors microorganisms that synthesize them. Fat-soluble vitamins can occur in plant tissue in the form of a provitamin (a precursor of vitamin), which can be converted into a vitamin in the animal body. No provitamins are known for any water-soluble vitamin. Tryptophan, which can be converted into niacin, is not considered a provitamin (see page 158). In addition, fat- and water-soluble vitamins differ in that the water-soluble B vitamins identified so far are universally distributed in *all* living tissues, whereas the fat-soluble vitamins are completely absent from some.

---

*Nomenclature Policy, *J. Nutr.* **107**(1977):7.

Box 12.2 E. V. McCollum and vitamins

Born on a Kansas farm, Elmer Verner McCollum (1879–1967) entered the University of Kansas in 1900 with the intention of becoming a physician, but his interests soon shifted to organic chemistry. After obtaining B.A. and M.S. degrees in 1903 and 1904, he studied at Yale University, where he completed his Ph.D. degree in 1906. McCollum financed his education at Yale by teaching elementary chemistry at a Y.M.C.A. evening school, tutoring students, and serving as a laboratory assistant.

After receiving his Ph.D., McCollum worked for a year as a postdoctoral fellow in the laboratory of Dr. L. B. Mendel before joining Professor E. B. Hart in 1907 at the Wisconsin Agricultural Experiment Station. There he also associated with Dr. Stephen Babcock, the inventor of the Babcock quantitative test for milk fat.

In the ten years he worked in Wisconsin, McCollum made a number of fundamental discoveries in the field of nutrition. Perhaps the most famous of these were the discoveries of "fat-soluble A" (1913) and "water-soluble B" (1915). He did not call these essential substances vitamins because he objected to the term *vitamine* coined by Funk. McCollum argued that the prefix "vita" was too all-encompassing to be applied to the substances in question, and that the evidence for the presence of an amino group was too meagre to warrant the use of the ending "amine." He of course lost his case.

From Wisconsin, McCollum went to The Johns Hopkins University in Baltimore as head of the Department of Chemical Hygiene. The proximity of the School of Medicine facilitated close collaboration with physicians and eventually led to the discovery of vitamin D and a solution to the mystery of rickets. From 1917 to his retirement in 1946, McCollum's work at Johns Hopkins resulted in the publication of some 150 papers on a wide variety of topics related to nutrition, including discussions of several minerals, as well as thiamin, riboflavin, and vitamin E.

Although described as having gentle humor, ready wit, dignity, kindliness, and interest and concern for others, McCollum was always willing to take unpopular stands on issues he considered critical to the improvement of nutritional practices. For example, he opposed the enrichment of white flour with thiamin, riboflavin, niacin, and iron, suggesting instead its enrichment with nonfat milk solids, defatted corn, and wheat germ. He also objected to the manufacture and sale of vitamin pills.

In 1918, E. V. McCollum published his famous textbook *The Newer Knowledge of Nutrition*, in which his use of the phrase "protective foods" did much to popularize the principles of sound eating. The fifth and last edition of this book appeared in 1939. After retirement, McCollum spent ten years researching and writing his famous *History of Nutrition*, a comprehensive review of nutrition findings up to 1940.

For more information, see *J. Nutr.* **100**(1970):3.

Physiological action   The water-soluble B vitamins almost collectively are concerned with the transfer of energy. Because they are present in every living tissue, they are all available as they become required. In contrast, fat-soluble vitamins are required for the regulation of the metabolism of structural units, and each vitamin appears to have one or more specific and independent roles.

Absorption   The division of vitamins as to solubility in fat or water is a particularly useful classification in a consideration of their absorption. Fat-soluble vitamins are absorbed from the intestinal tract in the presence of fat. Any factor that increases the absorption of fat, such as small particle size or the presence of bile, will also increase the absorption of fat-soluble vitamins. The absorption of the water-soluble vitamins is, in general, a simpler process because there is a constant absorption of water from the intestine into the bloodstream.

Storage   Fat-soluble vitamins and water-soluble B vitamins also differ in the extent to which they are stored in the body. Any of the fat-soluble vitamins can be stored wherever fat is deposited, the storage increasing with intake. The water-soluble B vitamins, on the other hand, are not stored in the same way or to the same extent. However, because all living cells contain all the B vitamins, deficiency symptoms do not appear immediately following their removal from the diet. The body conserves nutrients that are in short supply by using them only in vital reactions.

Excretion   Fat-soluble vitamins are excreted exclusively in the feces. The water-soluble B vitamins may also be present in the feces (though sometimes only because of bacterial synthesis), but their chief pathway of excretion following metabolic use is via the urine. This difference in pathway of excretion reflects the difference in solubility.

Determination of vitamins in foods

Many types of assays are available for estimating the vitamin content of foods. The oldest method, and one which is still used to check all other methods, is the bioassay.

The biological assay   In the most common method of bioassay, groups of animals are first depleted of a vitamin by being fed a diet lacking that substance. Then a series of specific doses of the vitamin are administered to the animals, with each group receiving only one of the doses in the series. The animals' response to intake, in growth and/or other appropriate criteria, is measured and recorded in a standard response curve. While the different groups of animals are receiving known amounts of the vitamin, other comparable groups are fed correspondingly increasing amounts of the vitamin carrier being assayed, and the responses of the second set of animals are recorded. The vitamin potency of the carrier is then estimated by comparing the responses of the second set of animals with the standard response curve. Such assays are based on the assumption that, under comparable conditions, animals will respond similarly to equal amounts of the vitamin.

Many criteria are used in this type of assay, but the most common is growth. It may be the growth of a population, an individual, an organ, a tissue, or a cell. The bioassay may also be based on the prevention or cure of some deficiency symptom known to develop in the absence of the vitamin.

The usefulness of biological assays is limited because of their high cost in terms of equipment, labor, and time. Their fundamental advantage is that they give positive proof of biological activity, and thus compounds that are chemically similar to the true vitamin but biologically inactive can be detected with certainty.

The microbiological assay   Assays of this type use microorganisms as the test subjects, and require much less time to complete than bioassays using animals. However, they have the disadvantage that the vitamin (or substance suspected of being a vitamin) must first be extracted from its carrier (foodstuff) before being added to the growth medium used for the microorganism.

The chemical assay   Chemical assays are based on some established chemical property (or properties) of the vitamins. They have the definite advantage of being much faster than bioassays, but they must be compared at intervals with bioassays in order to rule out the possibility of assaying as the vitamin any substances that do not function as a vitamin in the body.

Factors influencing the utilization of vitamins

There are several causes of vitamin deficiency. Most common is the lack of the nutrient in the diet being consumed. Metabolic variability is another crucial factor: adequate intake by one individual may in fact be insufficient intake for another. However, a number of the factors that may influence vitamin requirements are unrelated to the amount of vitamin consumed or to the metabolism of the individual.

Availability   Not all of the vitamins found in foods are in an absorbable form. For example, niacin in many cereals is bound to a protein and thus cannot be absorbed through the intestinal wall. Treatment with alkali releases the vitamin from this inaccessible complex. Fat-soluble vitamins cannot be absorbed under any condition that precludes the digestion and absorption of fats. Vitamin B_{12} requires a factor produced in the stomach (intrinsic factor) for its absorption.

Antivitamins   Antivitamins, also called "vitamin antagonists" or "pseudovitamins," are compounds that do not function as vitamins even though they are chemically related to the biologically active vitamins. Antivitamins cause vitamin deficiencies if the body is unable to distinguish between them and true vitamins, and incorporates them into essential body compounds.

Antivitamins have been used to produce vitamin deficiencies for experimental purposes. They have also been used medically to retard the undesirable growth of tissues; for example, an antagonist of folacin has been used to slow the growth of leucocytes in leukemia.

Provitamins   Substances that are not themselves vitamins but that can be converted into vitamins are referred to as provitamins. Perhaps the best known example is β-carotene, which is converted in the intestinal wall to vitamin A. Another example is cutaneous 7-dehydrocholesterol, which is converted to vitamin D by ultraviolet light. In plants, irradiation of ergosterol with ultraviolet light yields vitamin D_2. By means of a more complex, multistep reaction, the amino acid tryptophan can be converted to niacin; however, because of the poor efficiency of this reaction (60 mg of tryptophan required to produce 1 mg of niacin), the amino acid is not a true provitamin.

Microorganisms in the gut   The normal bacterial flora in the intestinal tract (as well as in the forestomach of ruminant species) is capable of synthesizing appreciable amounts of certain vitamins, including most members of the vitamin B complex as well as vitamin K. In fact it is virtually impossible to produce a folacin deficiency in normal experimental animals unless their gastrointestinal tract is sterilized by the oral administration of sulfa drugs.

Although some species of microorganisms can synthesize vitamins, other species compete with the host for these nutrients. These deleterious microorganisms predominate in certain diseases and appear to inactivate the vitamin(s) in the region where absorption normally occurs; as a consequence, the vitamins are excreted in the feces.

Suggested readings

Baker, H., Frank, O., Thomson, A. D., and Feingold, S. "Vitamin Distribution in Red Blood Cells, Plasma, and Other Body Fluids," *American Journal of Clinical Nutrition* **22**(1969):1469.

Bourne, G. H., and Kidder, G. W. "Structural Changes in Vitamin Deficiency." In *Biochemistry and Physiology of Nutrition*, Vol. 2. Academic Press, New York (1953):43.

Harginge, M. G., and Crooks, H. "Lesser-Known Vitamins in Foods," *Journal of the American Dietetic Association* **38**(1961):240.

Rosenberg, H. R. *Vitamins*. Interscience, New York (1951).

Sebrell, W. H., and Harris, R. S. *The Vitamins—Chemistry, Physiology, Pathology, Methods* (2nd ed.), Vol. 3. Academic Press, New York (1971).

Chapter 13
The water-soluble vitamin B complex

We have described the vital role of carbohydrates and fats in supplying energy to the body and outlined the pathways by which these nutrients, as well as proteins, are broken down to compounds capable of supplying energy. The members of the B-vitamin family appear to function primarily as parts of the enzyme systems that catalyze the metabolism of carbohydrates, fats, and proteins.

R. J. Williams has enlarged on Rosenberg's definition of a vitamin (see Chapter 12) by applying the following qualifications to members of the vitamin B complex: a B vitamin must be the simplest organic substance capable of carrying out the function ascribed to the vitamin; it must function nutritionally for at least some of the higher animals; it must be catalytically active (i.e., must function as a coenzyme) and present in catalytic (i.e., small) amounts; and it must be present in all living tissues.*

Eight vitamins meet these requirements, though others may eventually be found that also meet the specifications. According to Williams' definition, the following vitamins are members of the B complex:

Niacin	Biotin
Pantothenic acid	B_6
Riboflavin	Folacin
Thiamin	B_{12}

The distribution of the first five of these vitamins in various organs and tissues of the human body is shown in Table 13.1; the distribution throughout the whole organism of various animals and plants is given in Table 13.2.

---

*Williams, R. J., Eakin, R. E., Beerstecher, E., Jr., and Shive, W., *The Biochemistry of the B Vitamins, Section A*, Reinhold Publishing Corp., New York (1950).

Table 13.1
Relative amounts of five B vitamins in various human tissues
(*in mg/gram of wet weight*)

Tissue	Niacin	Pantothenic acid	Riboflavin	Thiamin	Biotin
Adrenal gland	24	8	8	2	0.4
Brain	20	15	3	2	0.6
Colon	13	5	2	1	0.1
Heart	41	16	8	4	0.2
Ileum	19	5	4	1	0.1
Kidney	37	19	20	3	0.7
Liver	58	43	16	2	0.7
Lung	18	5	2	2	0.2
Mammary gland	10	4	2	1	0.1
Ovary	18	4	4	1	0.1
Seminal ducts	9	2	1	1	0.1
Skeletal muscle	47	12	2	1	0.1
Skin	9	3	1	1	0.1
Smooth muscle	31	6	2	1	0.1
Spleen	23	5	4	1	0.1
Stomach	19	6	5	1	0.2
Testes	16	5	2	1	0.1
Total	412	163	86	26	4.0
Average	24.2	9.6	5.1	1.5	0.24

Table 13.2
Relative amounts of five B vitamins in various animals and plants
(*in mg/gram of dry weight*)

Organism	Niacin	Pantothenic acid	Riboflavin	Thiamin	Biotin
Brewer's yeast	126	42	15	9	0.1
C. butyricum	250	92	55	9	1.7
Chick embryo	405	370	13	8	1.8
Cockroach	120	65	26	16	0.5
Earthworm	48	10	25	8	0.3
Fish	78	24	5	10	0.3
Lima bean	12	9	1	6	0.1
Mold	60	15	5	1	0.1
Mushroom	540	138	26	9	1.4
Rat	180	38	11	5	0.3
Wheat seed	45	13	2	6	0.1
Total	1864	816	184	87	6.7
Average	169.4	74.2	16.7	8	0.6

These tables illustrate the universal distribution of niacin, panthothenic acid, riboflavin, thiamin, and biotin in various organs and tissues of the human body and in different animal and plant species. It is significant that, in most cases, the relative amounts of the five vitamins are roughly of the order of 20:10:2:1:0.1. It will be shown that the absence of a dietary source of thiamin can have a deleterious effect on a monogastric animal whose whole carcass contains only a small amount of thiamin relative to niacin, pantothenic acid, and riboflavin.

The B vitamins participate in a number of types of chemical reactions, most of which effect the transfer of energy. However, vitamins are not used directly in an enzyme system but must first be changed into more complex molecules called coenzymes. An enzyme system (holoenzyme) consists of an apoenzyme and its cofactors. The apoenzyme is a protein, and the cofactors are inorganic ions and/or coenzymes. Not every enzyme system requires both types of cofactors. There are three types of coenzymes (or prosthetic groups):

1. Adenylic acid or one of its phosphorylated derivatives.

2. A metallic complex of a porphyrin.

3. A derivative of one of the B vitamins.

Because each member of the B vitamin group takes part in a particular type of reaction and has its own unique metabolism, we shall discuss each member separately.

Thiamin

Beriberi in humans and polyneuritis in birds are well-known deficiency diseases caused by an inadequate dietary source of thiamin. This vitamin was known as vitamin B_1 until its synthesis by R. R. Williams and J. K. Cline[*] in 1936.

Physiological function   Thiamin is important as a component of the coenzyme thiamin pyrophosphate (TPP or ThPP). This coenzyme is also known as cocarboxylase. In the form of its coenzyme, thiamin is involved in the enzymatic decarboxylation of certain α-keto acids and in a transketolation reaction in the hexose monophosphate shunt pathway of glucose metabolism.

In the tricarboxylic acid cycle there are two oxidative decarboxylations of α-keto acids which require thiamin in the form of its TPP coenzyme:

---

[*]Williams, R. R., and Cline, J. K., *J. Am. Chem. Soc.* **58**(1936):1504.

1.   Pyruvate $\left.\begin{array}{c} \text{Pyruvate} \\ + \\ \text{Coenzyme A} \\ + \\ \text{NAD} \end{array}\right\}$ $\xrightarrow[\text{(TPP + lipoic acid)}]{\text{Pyruvic dehydrogenase}}$ $\left\{\begin{array}{c} \text{Acetyl CoA} \\ + \\ \text{NADH} \\ + \\ CO_2 \end{array}\right.$

2. $\left.\begin{array}{c} \text{α-ketoglutarate} \\ + \\ \text{Coenzyme A} \\ + \\ \text{NAD} \end{array}\right\}$ $\xrightarrow[\text{(TPP + lipoic acid)}]{\text{α-ketoglutaric dehydrogenase}}$ $\left\{\begin{array}{c} \text{Succinyl CoA} \\ + \\ \text{NADH} \\ + \\ CO_2 \end{array}\right.$

The third enzymatic function of the thiamin coenzyme is as an activator of transketolase, the enzyme involved in the oxidation of glucose via the pentose shunt or hexosemonophosphate (HMP) pathway:

$\left.\begin{array}{c} \text{Xylulose-5-}PO_4 \\ + \\ \text{Ribose-5-}PO_4 \end{array}\right\}$ $\xrightarrow[\text{(TPP)}]{\text{Transketolase}}$ $\left\{\begin{array}{c} \text{Sedoheptulose-7-}PO_4 \\ + \\ \text{Glyceraldehyde-3-}PO_4 \end{array}\right.$

It is of interest that the level of transketolase found in red blood cells can be used to establish the nutritional status of the body in respect to thiamin.

Metabolism   Thiamin is absorbed mainly from the upper intestinal tract. The phosphorylation of the vitamin to form the coenzyme occurs rapidly in liver and kidney cells, although all nucleated cells are apparently capable of bringing about this conversion.

Thiamin is the most poorly stored of all vitamins. For this reason, symptoms of thiamin deficiency precede those of any other vitamin deficiency. The one exception to this general rule occurs in pigs, which can store fairly large quantities of thiamin in their tissues; for this reason, pork is a reasonably rich source of the vitamin. Excess dietary thiamin is excreted soon after ingestion in the urine—as thiamin, thiamin disulfide, and about 16 other degradation products.

The vitamin is secreted into milk and eggs.

Sources   All plant and animal cells contain thiamin, but the primary sources of the vitamin are the outer coat and germ of cereals, nuts, pork products, organ meats, the legumes (i.e., peas and lima beans), enriched breads, and dried brewer's yeast and wheat germ.

Thiamin is readily destroyed by oxidation at elevated temperatures, especially in the presence of alkali. Thus the practice of adding baking soda to cooking water to preserve the color of fresh vegetables is not recommended because it promotes the destruction of both thiamin and ascorbic acid. In addition, because it is highly soluble in water, thiamin is readily leached out of foods during boiling, blanching, etc.

Thiamin is very susceptible to destruction by irradiation. For example, the thiamin content of pork is virtually depleted by the irradiation procedures sometimes used in food preservation.

Deficiency symptoms   The symptoms of a thiamin deficiency result primarily from the accumulation of pyruvate; lack of thiamin destroys the body's ability to convert pyruvate to acetate.* The symptoms are primarily those of dysfunction of the metabolically active tissues (i.e., muscle and nervous tissue). The fact that thiamin is required for several stages in the

---

*See the figure on page 150.

Box 13.1   R. R. Williams and thiamin

Robert R. Williams (1886–1965) was born in India to missionary parents and came to the United States with his family at the age of ten. Following schooling in Kansas and California, he earned B.S. (1907) and M.S. (1908) degrees in chemistry from the University of Chicago. Although he pursued further graduate studies, he never completed the Ph.D. degree; nevertheless, he eventually received eight honorary degrees—seven D.Sc.'s and one LL.D.

When he left the university, Williams went to work in the Philippines, where he was assigned the task of identifying the factor in rice polishings that had been shown to prevent beriberi in humans and polyneuritis in chickens. It took him over twenty years to identify and synthesize the vitamin we now know as thiamin, but his eventual success (in 1935) brought him international fame.

In 1915, Williams returned to the U.S. to work for the Food and Drug Administration in Washington, D.C. After World War I, he joined the Western Electric Company (which later became the Bell Telephone Laboratories) as a research chemist. During this period he continued his search for the antineuritic factor by experimenting at home with pigeons housed in his own garage. In this private work, Williams was aided by Robert E. Waterman, a fellow employee at Bell Laboratories who later became his son-in-law.

Williams and Waterman soon became associated with Columbia University and divided their time between their regular employment with Bell Laboratories and their evening research at Columbia. The detailed record of the steps they took to isolate, identify, and synthesize the pure form of the antiberiberi vitamin is worth reading; their research procedure is a model of sound techniques devised and implemented without the aid of elaborate, expensive equipment.

In his struggle to obtain a patent for the synthesis of thiamin, Williams ran into problems similar to those encountered by Harry Steenbock in his drive to

breakdown of carbohydrates explains why a deficiency of this vitamin develops rapidly when animals consume diets rich in carbohydrates.

Early symptoms* of thiamin deficiency in most species are anorexia, bradycardia, decreased rate of growth, and gastrointestinal troubles. Muscle weakness, incoordination, and hyperirritability can also occur. In foxes a deficiency of thiamin gives rise to Chastek paralysis. This condition, which can be brought on by eating raw fish, is due to an enzyme, thiaminase, which inactivates the thiamin molecule by splitting it into two parts. There is increasing evidence that thiaminases are widely distributed, being found in fish, ferns, bacteria, and related organisms.

*Williams, R. J., Eakin, R. E., Beerstecher, E., Jr., and Shive, W., *The Biochemistry of B Vitamins,* Reinhold Publishing Corp., New York (1950): Chapter VI, Section C.

---

irradiate foods in order to produce the antirachitic factor; they both incurred the antagonism of their peers. To simplify long and complicated negotiations, Research Corporation, a science-based philanthropic foundation in New York, finally agreed to accept his patents. The agreement was that only 25 percent of the resulting royalties would be shared by Williams, Waterman, and four other colleagues. The foundation would keep the remaining 75 percent, with about two-thirds of this being directed to the establishment of a Williams–Waterman Fund for the Combat of Dietary Diseases.

In 1945, Williams retired from the Bell Laboratories and became director of grants (until 1950) and chairman (until 1956) of the Williams–Waterman Committee. In 1950, he assumed a directorship of Research Corporation. Upon his retirement in 1956 at age seventy, he remained a director of Research Corporation and a member of the Williams–Waterman Committee. In 1968, when the resources provided by the thiamin royalties had been expended, the Research Corporation assumed the responsibility of funding the Williams–Waterman Program. Up to that time some six million dollars had been allocated for the combat of dietary diseases as a result of R. R. Williams' scientific ability and business foresight.

Williams returned to the Philippines in 1948 and helped set up the famous "Bataan Experiment" in which it was demonstrated that rice fortified with thiamin, niacin, and iron fostered the nutritional well-being of that portion of the population which consumed it. He thus carried beyond the U.S. his earlier recommendations that bread and cereal grains be enriched with vitamins and minerals. This accomplishment of Williams has received less attention than his role in the identification and synthesis of thiamin, or his efforts to provide funds and leadership for a grant program to combat nutritional diseases on an international scale.

For further information, see *J. Nutr.* **105**(1975):3.

Thiamin requirements   A dietary source of thiamin is required by all but the ruminant species. Ruminants, through microbial action in the rumen, are capable of synthesizing their total requirement for this vitamin. Although synthesis does take place in the caecum of such nonruminant herbivora as the horse, the extent of such synthesis is apparently not sufficient to meet requirements.

Because thiamin is closely associated with the transfer of energy, animal requirements for the vitamin vary in proportion to the intake of energy. For example, although an adult man generally requires 0.5 mg of thiamin per 1,000 kcal, the actual requirement is contingent on the composition of the diet. For example, high-fat diets decrease the body's thiamin requirements because fatty acids can enter the tricarboxylic acid cycle without going through pyruvic acid.

The thiamin requirements of animals that practice coprophagy (rat, pig, etc.) can be lowered by regulating the kind of carbohydrates in the diet (i.e., potato starch vs. sucrose or glucose), by assuring the presence of some carbohydrate derivatives such as sorbitol in the diet, and by orally administering antibiotics. These influences appear to foster bacterial synthesis of thiamin in the intestine and increase the amount of the vitamin excreted in the feces, which the animals can then ingest in that form. The sparing action of sorbitol and antibiotics disappears when coprophagy is prevented.

In North America, thiamin deficiency is confined mainly to alcoholics. Several clinical symptoms of alcoholism, previously attributed to alcoholic poisoning, have now been shown to be caused by nutritional inadequacies. To minimize the thiamin deficiency associated with alcoholism, it has been suggested that alcoholic beverages be fortified with thiamin, that alcoholics be frequently "immunized" with thiamin, or that bars make available thiamin-impregnated snacks.

Riboflavin

With the synthesis of riboflavin in 1935, nutritional scientists recognized that this vitamin was in fact the entity originally called either vitamin G or B_2. The greenish yellow, fluorescent pigments lactoflavin, ovoflavin, hepatoflavin, and verdoflavin (found in milk, eggs, liver, and grass, respectively) were also shown to be chemically identical to riboflavin.

Physiological function   Riboflavin forms a part of two flavoprotein coenzymes: flavine mononucleotide (FMN) and flavine adenine dinucleotide (FAD). The coenzymes are bound to the protein component of the enzyme, and the enzyme–coenzyme complex is often referred to as the flavoprotein. Functioning in close association with NAD and NADP, both riboflavin coenzymes serve to transport hydrogen. The riboflavin in flavoprotein coenzymes is required in the breakdown of energy-yielding nutrients, in the same places that NAD or NADP are required. Specifically, these "yellow" coenzymes are required for the completion of the following reactions (see Figure 13.1):

1. Pyruvate → Acetyl coenzyme A

2. Fatty acids → Acetyl coenzyme A

3. α-ketoglutarate → Succinyl coenzyme A

4. Glycerol-3-phosphate → Dihydroxyacetone phosphate (in mitochondria)

In addition to its role in energy transfer, riboflavin is a component of L-amino acid oxidase (via FMN) and of such enzymes as xanthine oxidase, glycine oxidase, and succinic dehydrogenase (via FAD). Flavine enzymes are also involved in reactions in which double bonds are introduced into such molecules as butyryl CoA.

Hence, as a component of two coenzymes, riboflavin is essential to the metabolism of carbohydrates, fats, and proteins.

Metabolism   Riboflavin is absorbed through the walls of the intestine by passive diffusion, which requires no expenditure of energy. It is phosphorylated in the intestinal wall and carried by the blood to the tissues where it may occur as the phosphate or as a flavoprotein.

Animal organs have a limited capacity for storing riboflavin; although higher concentrations are found in the liver and kidneys than in any other tissue. Excretion is primarily via the urine, but unabsorbed vitamin is found in the feces. All mammalian species secrete riboflavin, in its free form, into milk.

Sources   Riboflavin is widely distributed in plant and animal tissues. Milk and eggs are primary sources in the human diet. In tissues that respire (e.g., liver, kidney) riboflavin occurs as a phosphoric acid ester. Cereals contain little riboflavin except immediately after germination or if they have been enriched. Green vegetables, such as broccoli and asparagus, have a high concentration of riboflavin per unit of dry matter.

Riboflavin is stable to heat in acid solution, but is heat labile in alkaline solutions. The compound is sensitive to light; blue or violet rays destroy riboflavin.

Deficiency symptoms   A deficiency of riboflavin in the diet affects mainly ectodermal tissues, producing lesions of the skin, eye, and nervous systems. In chicks the most characteristic symptom is paralysis of the feet and legs, commonly referred to as "curled toe paralysis." A riboflavin deficiency in swine causes stiff and crooked legs, accompanied by skin eruptions. Cataracts due to pigmentation and capillary invasion of the cornea are known to occur in rats and pigs on a riboflavin-deficient diet.

In the human, skin changes (cheilosis, seborrhea) are known to be the result of a suboptimal riboflavin intake. A normochromic, normocytic anemia and ocular lesions have also been reported to occur in humans suffering from a riboflavin deficiency.

A serious deficiency of the vitamin in any young animal will inhibit growth and eventually result in death.

Riboflavin requirements   All animals and many microorganisms require riboflavin. The latter are able to synthesize it, and adult ruminants are able to obtain the vitamin from microbial synthesis in the rumen. Such species therefore do not require a dietary source of riboflavin. However, intestinal synthesis in man and caecal synthesis in the horse are not sufficient to meet the needs of those species.

Like thiamin, riboflavin is so closely associated with energy transfer that the amount of the vitamin required by animals is proportional to their intake of energy. An adult man generally needs 0.6 mg per 1,000 kcal. There is no evidence that alterations in the ratio of dietary carbohydrate to fat change human requirements for riboflavin. Similarly, the intake of protein does not affect human requirements for riboflavin. However, because flavoproteins are extremely unstable, a prolonged negative nitrogen balance will result in large losses of riboflavin in the urine.

Niacin

People have suffered from pellagra for centuries, but not until 1912 did nutritionists realize that it could be prevented by dietary means. The work of R. H. Chittenden (1917) and of J. Goldberger[*] (1926) demonstrated similarities between pellagra in man and blacktongue in dogs. At the University of Wisconsin researchers showed in 1937[†] that niacin is capable of curing blacktongue; soon afterward they also demonstrated the effectiveness of this compound against pellagra. The amide of niacin is the physiologically active compound. The vitamin is also known as nicotinic acid, or nicotinamide, and is actually the vitamin earlier called vitamin B_5.

---

[*]Goldberger, J., and Lillie, R. D., *U.S. Pub. Health Repts.* **41**(1926):1025; Chittenden, R. H., and Underhill, F. P., *Am. J. Physiol.* **44**(1917):13.

[†]Elvehjem, C. A., Madden, R. J., Strong, F. M., and Woolley, D. W., *J. Am. Chem. Soc.* **59**(1937):1767.

Box 13.2 Joseph Goldberger—a pioneer in public health nutrition

Joseph Goldberger (1874–1929) is known especially for his investigation of the causes of pellagra, although this work was but one aspect of a brilliant career in public health. His career began with a medical commission in the U.S. Public Health Service in 1899 and ended with his untimely death from cancer in 1929. He devoted the last fifteen years of his life almost entirely to the study of pellagra. However, before 1914 he was involved with research on yellow fever in Mexico and Puerto Rico, typhoid fever in the District of Columbia, dengue in Texas, typhus in Mexico City, and diphtheria in Detroit. This experience with communicable diseases was to prove invaluable in his study of pellagra.

Goldberger tackled the problem of determining what causes pellagra in the same systematic fashion that characterized his other work. On his first trip to Mississippi he noted that 68 of the 211 children in an orphanage he visited suffered from pellagra, but none of the employees in the institution had ever contracted the disease. This fact made Goldberger doubt the prevailing theory that pellagra is a communicable disease. The fact that he had contracted yellow fever, typhus, and dengue during his study of those diseases must have forcefully impressed this early observation on his mind.

Goldberger was an extremely observant individual and quickly became convinced that pellagra is a nutritional disorder. He noted that the young children in the orphanage who got milk regularly and the older children who were able to supplement their diets outside the orphanage seldom developed pellagra. On the other hand, nearly half of the children in the middle age group had pellagra. Because of these observations, three orphanages in Mississippi and Georgia participated in a study of the benefits of improving the children's diets through the addition of milk and meats. Within a few weeks all children suffering from pellagra recovered and no new cases occurred. To confirm that the disease results from deficiencies in the diet, Goldberger enlisted the cooperation of prison volunteers (the Governor of Mississippi promised to pardon those who participated) in an experiment designed to study the effect of subsisting on a diet characteristic of that consumed in villages where pellagra was a problem. Five of the eleven men who completed the study developed pellagra.

In spite of the evidence obtained in these well-designed studies, most medical practitioners refused to reject the long-held theory that pellagra is infectious. Presumably to open the eyes of his professional colleagues, Goldberger attempted to transmit the disease to himself, his wife, and a few of his close friends; all attempts failed.

Goldberger made one other important contribution to the study of pellagra: the use of the dog as an experimental animal. He had noted that, in the villages where humans suffered from pellagra, a large percentage of the mongrels suffered from blacktongue. It is perhaps fitting that Elvehjem was working with dogs when he discovered that niacin prevents pellagra.

For further information, see *J. Nutr.* **55**(1955):3.

Physiological function   Niacin is a component of two coenzymes active in the transfer of energy: nicotinamide adenine dinucleotide (NAD) and nicotinamide adenine dinucleotide phosphate (NADP). These coenzymes function as electron acceptors that accept electrons from specific substrates. These coenzymes containing niacin act in conjunction with flavoprotein enzymes in cell respiration. Thus, the functions of niacin and riboflavin are closely related; both vitamins are involved in the release of energy from carbohydrates, fats, and proteins through their association with the interdependent electron-accepting coenzymes NAD and NADP, plus FMN and FAD.

The importance of the niacin coenzymes is obvious when it is realized that they participate in at least 40 separate reactions involving electron transfers in the body. The following are a few of the different types of enzymatic reactions requiring NAD and NADP as coenzymes:

1. NAD-linked dehydrogenase reactions
   pyruvate $\rightarrow$ lactate
   vitamin A aldehyde $\rightarrow$ vitamin A alcohol
   malate $\rightarrow$ oxaloacetate
2. Conversion of aldehyde to acid
   glyceraldehyde-3-PO_4 $\rightarrow$ 1,3-diphosphoglycerate
3. NAD-linked oxidative deamination of amino acids
   glutamate $\rightarrow$ α-ketogluterate
4. Biological synthesis reactions such as synthesis of fatty acids (NAD), cholesterol (NADP), and steroid hormones from cholesterol
5. Reduction of NAD in three reactions in the tricarboxylic acid cycle (see Figure 13.1)

The two niacin-containing coenzymes are highly specific to many of these enzymatic reactions. For example, NADP is involved in the pentose shunt pathway whereas NAD is the coenzyme required for glycolysis. Similarly, in fatty acid synthesis via the malonyl CoA pathway NADP is involved, while in fatty acid degradation by the β-oxidation mechanism NAD is the coenzyme.

Metabolism   Nicotinamide and nicotinic acid are derivatives of pyridine, which fact predicts their presence in the coenzymes NAD and NADP. Because niacin is absorbed unchanged from the intestine, a lowered intake will be reflected by a decrease in the concentration of NAD and NADP in the striated muscles, but the amount of the vitamin in the blood will not be altered appreciably. Animals such as rats, pigs, dogs, and humans excrete methylated metabolites in the urine, whereas herbivores apparently excrete large amounts of niacin unchanged. Birds excrete the vitamin as dinicotinyl ornithine. Neither the acid nor the amide of the vitamin is stored in any appreciable amounts in animal tissues. The vitamin is secreted into milk and eggs.

By 1947 it had been established that the amino acid tryptophan is a precursor for the synthesis of niacin in the body. There is evidence that this synthesis takes place both in the intestine and in certain tissues within the body.

Under conditions of 100% molar efficiency, 1.7 mg of tryptophan should furnish 1 mg of niacin. In practice, however, about 60 mg of tryptophan are required to produce 1 mg of niacin in man. Ratios closer to 50:1 have been observed in chicks, rats, and pigs. The domestic cat and most insect species cannot convert tryptophan to niacin.

Although corn contains an appreciable amount of niacin, its biological availability is low because most of it occurs in a bound form. The vitamin can be released by treating the cereal with a mild alkali. Corn protein is also low in tryptophan. These two facts explain why people who consume a diet composed predominantly of corn are susceptible to pellagra. Pellagra might be considered as a dual deficiency of niacin and tryptophan.

Sources   Niacin occurs in nature mainly in its amide form; as such it is universally distributed in all living tissues. With the exception of corn, cereal grains and their by-products are good sources of niacin. Animal by-products, organ meats, peanuts, and leafy forages contain relatively large amounts of the vitamin. Although milk and eggs contain little niacin, they have a high vitamin equivalent because of their abundance of tryptophan.

Niacin, one of the most stable vitamins, is resistant to heat, light, oxidation, acid, and alkali. It is soluble in hot water; the amide is more soluble than the acid. Because of its stability, little niacin is destroyed during the preparation and processing of foods.

Deficiency symptoms   Although pellagra is usually complicated by shortages of other B vitamins, symptoms that may be attributed specifically to a deficiency of niacin include dermatitis, diarrhea, and dementia. Loss of appetite and weight, vomiting, and anemia are also commonly associated with a deficiency of this vitamin. Leg disorders (slipped tendon or perosis in birds, enlarged hocks in swine) are frequently observed in animals whose diets contain too little niacin.

In pellagra, the lack of NAD or NADP must be responsible in some way for inflammations of the skin and gastrointestinal tract because no biological function other than its participation in the two coenzymes has been discovered for niacin. The failure to find any direct association between function and clinical symptoms is not surprising considering the large number of reactions in which NAD or NADP participate as coenzymes.

Niacin requirements   All species require niacin, but as with thiamin and riboflavin, ruminants have no dietary requirements because of bacterial synthesis in the rumen. Horses, rats, and newborn calves apparently have little or no requirement for the vitamin if adequate amounts of tryptophan are available in their diets.

Although consumption of tryptophan can lower an animal's dietary requirement for niacin, this vitamin, like thiamin and riboflavin, is required in proportion to the intake of available energy. Most animals need the equivalent of 6.6 mg of niacin per 1,000 kcal. If its diet contains too little protein and/or an excess of tryptophan-deficient cereal, an animal will probably not ingest enough niacin.

Vitamin B_6

A specific dermatitis of paws and nose that occurred in rats on a thiamin- and riboflavin-supplemented diet was found by P. György in 1934* to be cured by a factor he called vitamin B_6. Shortly thereafter, this factor was synthesized in both the United States and Germany; the American researchers called it *pyridoxine* whereas the German biochemists gave it the name *adermin*. Following this, the aldehyde and amine derivatives of pyridoxine (pyridoxal and pyridoxamine, respectively) were isolated and found to have biological activity. Because of the multiple nature of this vitamin, the original term vitamin B_6 has again become its approved name.

Physiological function   Pyridoxal phosphate is the coenzyme form of vitamin B_6. It functions in conjunction with all the enzyme systems known to depend on vitamin B_6. These enzymes are concerned primarily in protein metabolism. For example, pyridoxal phosphate serves as a coenzyme in nearly all reactions involved in the nonoxidative degradation of amino acids, which include transaminations, deaminations, decarboxylations, and desulfhydrations. The coenzyme appears to require inorganic ions (e.g., Cu^{++}, Fe^{+++}, Al^{+++}) to activate most of these reactions.

Pyridoxal phosphate is also required for the normal metabolism of tryptophan. In the absence of vitamin B_6 the breakdown of this amino acid to niacin is blocked with a resulting accumulation and excretion of xanthurenic acid.

For a long time nutritionists believed that vitamin B_6 participates in the metabolism of unsaturated fatty acids, particularly in the conversion of linoleic acid to arachidonic acid. It now appears that the vitamin has an indirect effect on the metabolism of fatty acids; the exact mode of action remains unknown.

In the metabolism of carbohydrates, vitamin B_6 is involved in the release of glycogen from muscle and liver. This is because pyridoxal phosphate is a

---

*György, P., *Nature* **133**(1934):498.

coenzyme of phosphorylase. Low levels of glucose in the blood and sensitivity to insulin occur as a consequence of a vitamin B_6 deficiency, indicating that the vitamin is essential to carbohydrate metabolism.

Vitamin B_6 is not as crucial to the oxidative cycle as thiamin, riboflavin, and niacin. Vitamin B_6 affects oxidation through its role in the metabolism of amino acids.

Metabolism   Vitamin B_6 bound to protein is not easily absorbed, but the vitamin in the free form is absorbed rapidly from the intestine. It is secreted into milk and excreted primarily via the urine.

Sources   Vitamin B_6 is widely and quite uniformly distributed in both plant and animal tissues, with meat, liver, vegetables, and the outer coating of cereal grains being especially good sources. In plants, vitamin B_6 occurs chiefly as pyridoxine, an alcohol which, because it is bound to proteins, is not readily absorbable. In animal tissues, vitamin B_6 is present mainly as bound pyridoxamine; animal tissue also contains small quantities of pyridoxal and pyridoxine (about half of the pyridoxine in the body is in the enzyme phosphorylase which is active in muscle).

Vitamin B_6 is stable to heat in acid solution and relatively stable in alkaline solutions. It is quite unstable to light.

Deficiency symptoms   Acrodynia, the specific dermatitis observed in rats on a vitamin B_6 deficient diet, is not observed in other species. However, impaired growth occurs in all young animals suffering from a deficiency of vitamin B_6. Convulsions occur in pigs, rats, and chicks; and in pups and pigs the symptoms of deficiency include a microcytic, hypochromic anemia, with excessive iron deposits in the spleen.

Human infants on a diet deficient in vitamin B_6 suffer from hyperirritability and convulsions; adults develop the same type of anemia as that found in pups and pigs. Skin diseases such as glossitis, cheilosis, and stomatitis afflict people who consume the antagonist deoxypyridoxine. These symptoms differ from those resulting from a riboflavin or niacin deficiency.

Vitamin B_6 requirements   Vitamin B_6 is required by most animal species, including ruminants. Bacterial synthesis in the rumen meets the requirements of adult ruminants. Because of the wide distribution of this vitamin, it is seldom deficient in a diet consisting of natural foodstuffs.

The requirement for vitamin B_6 varies with the protein content of the diet. Although the vitamin is involved to some extent in carbohydrate metabolism (and possibly also in fat metabolism), there is no firm basis upon which to relate requirements to caloric intake. A daily allowance of 1.5 mg to 2.0 mg per day has been established for adult humans.

Pantothenic acid

Pantothenic acid was first isolated from bios in 1933 by R. J. Williams and his associates;* soon afterward researchers showed that this substance prevented a specific dermatitis in chicks, and the graying of hair in rats.

Physiological function   As far as is known at the present time, pantothenic acid is a component of only one coenzyme, coenzyme A. As a constituent of the coenzyme, the vitamin participates in all acylation reactions. The most important acyl radical is acetyl, a 2-carbon fragment holding a key position in the oxidation cycle. As will be recalled, carbohydrates, fats, and some proteins are converted to acetyl coenzyme A before they are oxidized in the tricarboxylic acid cycle. *Coenzyme A is required in any reaction in which an acetyl group is formed or is transferred from one substance to another.*

In addition to acetyl, other acyl radicals require coenzyme A. It is required whenever succinyl, benzoyl, or fatty acyl radicals are formed or transferred. Specifically, coenzyme A is required for the following important reactions:

1. Oxidative decarboxylation of pyruvic acid → acetyl-CoA.

2. Oxidative decarboxylation of α-ketoglutaric acid → succinyl-CoA.

3. Acetylation of choline.

4. Synthesis of amino-levulinic acid, which is an intermediate in the formation of porphyrin, a component part of the hemoglobin molecule.

5. Catabolism of fatty acids by the β-oxidation pathway.

6. Synthesis of fats—i.e., the reverse of the breakdown of fatty acids.

7. Synthesis of steroids, which is a crucial function because of the known relationship between pantothenic acid and the adrenal cortex. Adrenal degeneration in rats on diets deficient in pantothenic acid can be prevented by corticosterone.

Metabolism   Pantothenic acid is absorbed from the small intestine and excreted chiefly via the urine. It is stored to some extent in the liver and kidneys. Traces of pantothenic acid are found in the blood.

Sources   This member of the vitamin B complex occurs in many foods of plant and animal origin, mostly in the bound form. Organ meats (liver, kidney, brain, and heart), whole-grain cereals, and legumes are the best-known

---

*Williams, R. J., Truesdail, J. H., Weinstock, H. H., Jr., Rohrmann, E., Lyman, C. M., and McBurney, C. H., *J. Am. Chem. Soc.* **60**(1938):2719.

sources of pantothenic acid; extremely high concentrations are found in royal jelly and fish ovaries before spawning. Some green, leafy vegetables, such as broccoli, are also good sources. Free pantothenic acid is unstable in acid or alkaline solutions and is destroyed by dry heat. It is relatively stable in moist heat at a neutral pH. Only the D isomer of crystalline pantothenic acid is usable by animals.

Deficiency symptoms   Chicks, rats, dogs, pigs, and turkeys show diverse symptoms of pantothenic-acid deficiency, including retardation of growth, skin and hair lesions, gastrointestinal troubles, and lesions of the nervous system and adrenal gland.

Growth is too complicated a biochemical process to be controlled by a single vitamin, even one like pantothenic acid which plays a major role in metabolism. A deficiency of pantothenic acid causes an anemia in some species that may account for the sudden death which often follows the retardation of growth.

In rats, pantothenic-acid deficiency will prevent normal pigmentation of *skin* and *hair*. Adrenalectomy not only reverses the effect of the vitamin deficiency, but also appears to accelerate a return to normal pigmentation. In chicks, lack of pantothenic acid retards the development of feathers and causes a dermatitis in the area of the eyes, mouth, vent, and feet. Premature graying results from a deficiency of this vitamin in piebald rats, dogs, and foxes, but not in humans.

Pantothenic-acid deficient chicks develop spinal cord lesions, and mice fed an insufficient amount of the vitamin develop curvature of the spine and a twitch of the hind legs. Pigs fed a ration deficient in this vitamin develop an abnormal gait called "goose stepping." These symptoms suggest a relationship between pantothenic acid and *nerve function*. A deficiency of this vitamin might interfere with the acetylation of choline; because acetyl choline plays a vital role in nerve function, a hindrance of acetylation could produce the symptoms described above.

Gastrointestinal ulcers occur in rats and pigs on a diet deficient in pantothenic acid. Dogs may exhibit severe vomiting. It is possible that these symptoms are produced by lesions of the nervous system also caused by an interference in the acetylation of choline.

Dogs, mice, and pigs usually have normal adrenal glands when examined at the time of death from pantothenic-acid deficiency. The adrenal glands of rats, on the other hand, show hemorrhages and *necrosis of the adrenal cortex*. These symptoms can be explained as follows: pantothenic acid is required for the synthesis of cortical hormones, and if synthesis is impeded, the hormone ACTH is produced in ever-increasing amounts; its action on the already depleted glands may cause hemorrhages and necrosis.

Thus, it is possible to understand how such a large variety of symptoms can be produced by a deficiency of pantothenic acid when we consider the many fundamental biochemical reactions which are mediated by coenzyme A, the metabolically functional form of pantothenic acid.

Humans do not normally suffer from a deficiency of this vitamin. However, when volunteers were given a pantothenic acid antagonist together with a diet low in the vitamin, they reported a wide variety of symptoms including irritability, burning feet, gastrointestinal upsets, sensitivity to insulin, muscle cramps, and a decrease in muscle coordination.

Pantothenic acid requirements   Chicks, rats, pigs, dogs, and most other vertebrates require pantothenic acid. It is synthesized in the rumen of cattle, sheep, and goats, and to an appreciable extent in the intestine of rabbits, horses, and humans. Pantothenic acid is so widely distributed in natural foods that dietary deficiencies seldom arise. It is estimated that humans require less than 5.0 mg of the vitamin daily.

Biotin

Biotin, a member of the vitamin B complex, is now known to be identical to the original "biotin" required for the growth of yeast; to "coenzyme R" required for the growth of the legume nodule organism Rhizobium; and to the factor known as vitamin H in such foods as liver and kidney, which was found to be protective against "egg white injury." (Egg white injury occurs when avidin, a protein of raw egg white, combines with dietary biotin and renders it unavailable to the body.)

Physiological function   Biotin functions primarily as a coenzyme for enzymatic reactions involving the addition of carbon dioxide to other units (i.e., CO_2 fixation). All of the holoenzymes that catalyze such reactions are transcarboxylases, (e.g., acetyl CoA carboxylase, propionyl CoA carboxylase, pyruvate carboxylase), and they contain biotin as their prosthetic group. In this way, biotin plays a key role in gluconeogenesis, an important process in all animals, especially in ruminants.

Biotin is involved in both the synthesis and oxidation of fatty acids, and is required for the synthesis of dicarboxylic acids. Biotin appears to be active as well in deaminations (at least of aspartic acid, serine, and threonine), carbamylations, tryptophan metabolism (required for the synthesis of niacin), purine and protein synthesis (formation of transfer RNA), oxidative phosphorylation, and carbohydrate metabolism (utilization of glucose). The role of biotin in most of these actions is unclear; it has been suggested that the vitamin acts indirectly so that many of its effects are not tied to biotin enzymes per se.

Metabolism   Biotin is easily absorbed from the small intestine in either the free or the bound form. As with other B vitamins, excretion is mainly via the urine. Biotin, like pantothenic acid, is stored primarily in the liver and kidneys. Only traces of the vitamin are secreted into milk.

Sources   Biotin is found in many plant and animal tissues; in plant foods it occurs mainly in the free form whereas in animal food sources it occurs principally in a bound form, usually attached to an amino acid. One of the more common complexes containing biotin is biotinyl lysine, sometimes called biocytin. Liver, kidney, egg yolk, and yeast are the richest sources of biotin, although appreciable amounts are also found in cauliflower, nuts, and legumes.
    Biotin is soluble in water and alcohol, and is chemically very stable.

Deficiency symptoms   Biotin deficiency does not occur naturally, but can be produced by feeding raw egg white or a biotin-free diet in conjunction with a sulfa drug, the latter to prevent intestinal synthesis.
    Symptoms of biotin deficiency common to all species are retarded growth, dermatitis, loss of hair, and disturbances of the nervous system. Administering biotin to chicks prevents perosis, a condition also prevented by the administration of manganese, choline, folic acid, and niacin. In rats and dogs, lack of biotin produces an ascending paralysis accompanied by a cessation of growth and a spectacled eye condition. Dermatitis and spasticity of the hind legs afflict pigs who consume insufficient biotin. Biotin deficiency symptoms in humans include a fine, scaly dermatitis, loss of appetite, nausea, muscle pains, and high levels of blood cholesterol.

Biotin requirements   Although most animal species require biotin, they seldom require a dietary source of the vitamin. Biotin is synthesized not only by ruminants, but also in the intestine of such species as the rat, dog, chick, and human. It has been shown that humans and rats often excrete via the feces and urine considerably more biotin than they have ingested.

Folacin (folic acid)

Investigators originally assigned a variety of names to this vitamin, including the Wills factor, factor U, vitamin M, yeast Norit eluate factor, vitamin B^c, L-casei factor, and SLR factor. As the chemical nature of all these compounds became known, it was realized that their effectiveness was due to the presence of *pteroylglutamic acid* (PGA). Because this substance could be extracted from green leafy vegetables such as spinach, it was designated as *folic acid* (in 1941). In standardized terminology, the name folic acid (folate) applies only to pteroylmonoglutamic acid, the form of the vitamin from which active coenzymes are derived. The term *folacin* applies to the broader group of substances giving rise to folate in the body.

Folate in foods is a combination of a pteridine nucleus, *para*-aminobenzoic acid (PABA), and one to seven molecules of glutamic acid. To be of use in the body, folate must undergo reactions in which all but one of the glutamic acid molecules split off, thereby yielding PGA.

$$\underbrace{\text{Pteridine nucleus} + \text{PABA} + \text{Glutamic acid}}_{\text{PGA}} \Big/ + \text{Glutamic acid} + \text{Glutamic acid}$$

Folate can be reduced in the presence of ascorbic acid and NAD to yield tetrahydropteroylglutamic acid (H_4PteGlu), a compound also designated as tetrahydrofolic acid and tetrahydrofolacin. It is chemically very unstable, and unites easily with a single carbon unit to form 5-formyltetrahydropteroylglutamic acid (5-CHO-H_4PteGlu). This latter compound, also known as the citrovorum factor or folinic acid, is much more stable than H_4PteGlu and is considered to be the biologically active form of the vitamin. The synthetic form of 5-CHO-H_4PteGlu is called leucovorin.

$$\text{Folate} \xrightarrow[\text{NADPH}]{\text{Ascorbic acid}} \text{Tetrahydropteroylglutamic acid (}H_4\text{PteGlu)}$$

$$+$$

$$\text{Single carbon unit}$$

$$\downarrow$$

5-Formyltetrahydropteroylglutamic acid (5-CHO-H_4PteGlu)
(i.e., citrovorum factor or folinic acid)

Because 5-CHO-H_4PteGlu occurs preformed in the liver, either in the active form or conjugated with extra glutamic acid molecules, it appears that the body stores folacin in this organ as the citrovorum factor.

Physiological function   Folacin functions in a number of biological reactions effecting the transfer of single carbon units, such as methyl groups, from one compound to another. Many reactions are known in which the vitamin serves as an intermediary accepting and passing on single carbon units. For example,

1. Homocystine + Single carbon unit → Methionine

2. Glycine + Single carbon unit → Serine

3. Ethanolamine + Single carbon unit → Choline

4. Single carbon units are involved in the synthesis of (a) such purines as adenine and guanine; (b) the pyrimidine thymine and the amino acid histidine. The megaloblastic anemia that results from folate deficiency may result from a failure to synthesize the purines noted above.

In addition, folacin is involved in the oxidation of phenylalanine to tyrosine, in the oxidation and decarboxylation of tyrosine, in the formation of the porphyrin group of hemoglobin, and in the metabolism of histidine.

Folacin and vitamin B_{12} (discussed later) are interrelated; both apparently function in the metabolism or synthesis of the compounds making up nucleic acids. In addition, both appear to participate in the metabolism of methionine.

Metabolism   Folic acid often occurs conjugated with additional glutamic acid groups. These conjugated forms are active for those species containing folic acid conjugase enzymes that split the conjugated molecule.

The vitamin is absorbed through the upper part of the intestinal tract; ascorbic acid and some antibiotics facilitate its absorption. The glutamic acid molecules of conjugated folates are split off by enzymes in the brush border of the intestine.

Sources   Folacin is widely distributed in plant and animal tissues, being found in relatively large amounts in liver, kidney, yeast, mushrooms, lemons, bananas, strawberries, and vegetables such as asparagus, broccoli, lima beans, and spinach. Milk contains only a small amount of the vitamin.

Folacin is slightly soluble in water, unstable in acid solution, and stable to heat at a neutral pH. Cooking, canning, and exposure to light all reduce the amount of the vitamin available in foods.

Deficiency symptoms   Folacin deficiency symptoms, which can be produced in many species, include a retardation of growth accompanied by a macrocytic, hyperchromic anemia called megaloblastic anemia. In chicks, a deficiency of folacin also induces poor feathering.

Folacin is used to treat the human conditions of sprue and the megaloblastic anemias which occur in pregnancy and infancy. Folacin is effective in curing the anemia of pernicious anemia, but the accompanying neurological changes can be successfully treated only with vitamin B_{12}.

Folacin requirements   Most higher animals require folacin, but the only domestic animals normally requiring a dietary source of the vitamin are poultry. Ruminants synthesize folacin in the rumen, and sufficient intestinal synthesis apparently takes place in nonruminant species other than poultry to meet requirements.

Vitamin B$_{12}$ (cobalamin)

Nutritionists knew that the liver contains an anti-pernicious-anemia factor long before researchers discovered that vitamin B$_{12}$, also known as cobalamin, is this factor. Vitamin B$_{12}$ also turned out to be the substance present in proteins of animal origin, the animal protein factor (APF), that is responsible for stimulating growth in various animal species, and whose identity was sought for many years.

The term vitamin B$_{12}$ is used to designate all the chemically related compounds known to have vitamin activity. These compounds include cyanocobalamin, hydroxocobalamin, nitritocobalamin, and thiocyanate cobalamin. Of these, cyanocobalamin is the most active. All cobalamin compounds contain cobalt as an integral part of their molecules.

Physiological function   The exact metabolic function of vitamin B$_{12}$ is still not completely understood. It is known to be required for normal growth and blood formation as well as for the maintenance of nerve tissue, but the precise role of the vitamin in these processes has yet to be determined. At least five different vitamin B$_{12}$ coenzymes have been identified; the conversion of vitamin to coenzyme requires such nutrients as niacin, riboflavin, and manganese.

There is a close relationship between the physiological roles of vitamin B$_{12}$ and folacin. Both are involved with the metabolism of single carbon units. Whereas folacin participates in the *transfer* of single carbon units from one compound to the other, vitamin B$_{12}$ probably is required for the *synthesis* of single carbon units. Hence vitamin B$_{12}$ takes part in most of the reactions that have already been described for folacin. In addition, vitamin B$_{12}$ catalyzes the production of folacin from conjugated folates and aids in the formation of folacin coenzymes.

The role of vitamin B$_{12}$ in the synthesis of nucleic acids (i.e., the synthesis of thymine and the formation of deoxyribose from ribose) explains the development of macrocytic megaloblastic anemia in its absence. It has been suggested that vitamin B$_{12}$ may help to sustain nerve function through its involvement in carbohydrate metabolism (it is known that vitamin B$_{12}$ maintains glutathione in its biologically active reduced state).

Vitamin B$_{12}$ appears to function in at least one area of fat metabolism: the isomerization of methylmalonyl CoA to succinyl CoA requires a vitamin B$_{12}$

coenzyme. This reaction is extremely important in the overall process of gluconeogenesis, especially in ruminants.

Metabolism The rate of absorption of cobalamin is extremely slow. Pernicious anemia results from a complete failure to absorb the vitamin, a condition caused by gastric abnormality. The vitamin is stored in the liver. Mammals transmit vitamin B_{12} to their young via the placenta, and poultry secrete it into their developing eggs. Like other B vitamins, cobalamin's chief excretory pathway is via the urine.

Sources Vitamin B_{12} is found primarily in animal tissues, with liver being the most common and plentiful source. However, cobalamin is also found in kidney, milk and meat, and in animal feeds such as fishmeal and meatmeal. Fermentation products such as dried brewer's yeast contain vitamin B_{12} as well.

The vitamin is a dark red crystal that derives its color from the cobalt contained in the cobalamin molecule. Cobalamin is fairly soluble in water and alcohol and stable to acid and oxidation, but it is destroyed in solutions of a high pH. About 30 percent of the cobalamin in foods is destroyed by cooking.

Deficiency symptoms In humans, a deficiency of vitamin B_{12} occurs as a consequence of faulty absorption of the vitamin and results in pernicious anemia, a condition characterized by a megaloblastic type of erythropoiesis. Because the failure is in the mechanism of absorption, only injections of vitamin B_{12} can alleviate efficiently the effects of this type of anemia.

In animal species other than humans a deficiency of this vitamin manifests itself chiefly in a depression of growth rate. No anemia has been noted in nonhuman species.

A cobalamin deficiency in poultry rations results in poor egg hatchability and myoatrophy of the leg in chick embryos. In the growing chick, in addition to the retardation of growth, insufficient cobalamin can cause kidney damage and perosis. In young rats, vitamin B_{12} deficiency results in various abnormalities in the brain, eyes, and bone; a high mortality after weaning is also a common result of deficiency.

Vitamin B_{12} requirements Vitamin B_{12} is a metabolic requirement for all higher animals and many microorganisms. Ruminants synthesize the vitamin if sufficient cobalt is present in their ration (see Chapter 18, p. 262). Intestinal synthesis takes place in species such as humans, rats, and pigs; the extent of synthesis influences dietary requirement.

A diet containing 3 μg to 5 μg per day satisfies the needs of most humans.

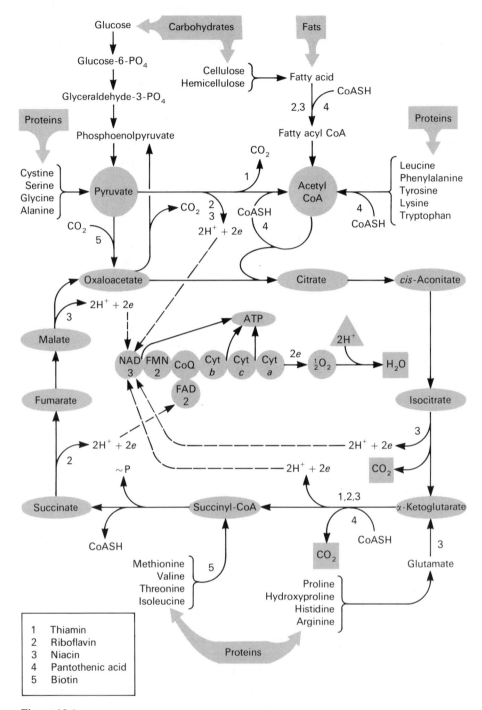

Figure 13.1
The "oxidation" of carbohydrates, fats, and proteins, showing position of certain coenzymes.

The B vitamins in the metabolic machinery

In the foregoing discussion of the various members of the vitamin B complex we have emphasized the role of many of these vitamins in the release and transfer of energy. Figure 13.1 provides a graphic representation of the coenzymatic activities of five of the B vitamins active in the metabolism of carbohydrates, proteins, and fats, showing some of the reactions in which they take part.

Suggested readings

Cooper, J. R. "The Role of Thiamine in Nervous Tissue: The Mechanism of Action of Pyrithiamine," *Biochimica et Biophysica Acta* **156**(1968):368.

Gubler, C. J. "Studies on the Physiological Functions of Thiamine. 1. The Effects of Thiamine Deficiency and Thiamine Antagonists on the Oxidation of α-keto Acids by Rat Tissues," *Journal of Biological Chemistry* **236**(1961):3112.

György, P. "Developments Leading to the Metabolic Role of Vitamin B$_6$," *American Journal of Clinical Nutrition* **24**(1971):1250.

Smith, E. L. "Vitamin B$_{12}$," *Plant Foods for Human Nutrition* **2**(1970):67.

Stadtman, T. C. "Vitamin B$_{12}$," *Science* **171**(1971):859.

Williams, R. J., Eakin, R. E., Beerstecher, E., Jr., and Shive, W. *The Biochemistry of the B Vitamins*. Reinhold Publishing Corp., New York (1950).

Wolf, H. "Hormonal Alteration of Efficiency of Conversion of Tryptophan to Urinary Metabolites of Niacin in Man," *American Journal of Clinical Nutrition* **24**(1971):792.

Chapter 14
The fat-soluble vitamins

Vitamin A

Vitamin A was the first vitamin to be identified. As long ago as 1816, xerophthalmia, a disease of the lacrimal apparatus of the eyes, was described and ascribed to the lack of a nutrient in food. Little progress was made in identifying the missing substance until nearly a hundred years later when researchers implicated a dietary insufficiency of vitamin A in the condition.

Vitamin A does not occur as such in plant tissues but rather as its precursor, carotene. Carotene, or provitamin A, can be converted by the body into the active vitamin. Thus, carotene is the chief dietary source of vitamin A for herbivores.

Chemistry of vitamin A and carotene Vitamin A and carotene are made up of repeating units of isoprene, arranged in such a way that β-carotene is in fact two molecules of vitamin A. However, the conversion of β-carotene in the intestinal mucosa, and to a lesser extent in other tissues such as the liver, yields only *one* molecule of vitamin A.

Vitamin A may exist as an alcohol (retinol), an aldehyde (retinal or retinene), or an acid (retinoic acid). The alcohol and aldehyde forms of the vitamin are readily interconverted in the body by an enzyme system in which NAD acts as a coenzyme. The aldehyde can be oxidized to the acid, but this reaction is apparently irreversible in the body. The inability of the body to

Table 14.1
Relative biopotencies of some isomers
of vitamin A

Vitamin A isomer	Relative biopotency (%)
All-*trans*	100
13-*cis*	75
11-*cis*	24
9,13-di-*cis*	24
9-*cis*	21
11,13-di-*cis*	15

convert the acid back to the alcohol or aldehyde explains why retinoic acid is effective against many of the symptoms of vitamin A deficiency, but is ineffective against night blindness and reproductive failure.

$$\text{Retinol} \underset{+ \text{NAD}}{\overset{\substack{\text{Alcohol} \\ \text{dehydrogenase}}}{\rightleftharpoons}} \text{Retinal} \longrightarrow \text{Retinoic acid}$$

In contrast to most other vitamins, vitamin A exists in a multiplicity of forms. Not only are there a number of biologically active derivatives of the vitamin A molecule itself, but also many naturally occurring active carotenoids. Furthermore, each of these vitamin A derivatives and carotenoids can exist in a variety of isomeric forms. Each of the many sources of vitamin A has a different potential for biological activity.

Table 14.1 summarizes the relative biopotencies of a few of the isomers of vitamin A. Table 14.2 gives the relative biopotencies of a few important carotenoids and two of their isomers.

Table 14.2
Relative biopotencies of some important carotenoids
and two of their isomers

Carotenoid	Relative biopotency (%)	
	All-trans *isomer*	Mono-cis *isomer*
β-carotene	100	38
α-carotene	53	13
γ-carotene	42	19
Cryptoxanthin	57	27

Physiological function   The principal role of vitamin A in the body appears to be as a regulator of the metabolism of cell structure. An animal deprived of vitamin A stops growing and eventually dies. Because a deficiency first affects epithelial cells, this vitamin probably has a specific function in the metabolism of such cells. However, at the present time its general role in cell metabolism cannot be explained in terms of specific chemical reactions.

Vitamin A plays a vital role in the regeneration of visual purple (rhodopsin) in the eye. Thus it is instrumental in preventing night blindness. The reactions constituting the regenerative process were investigated by G. Wald[*] at Harvard University, who clarified what, to that time, was an extremely complicated picture. The proportion of the total vitamin A requirement of the body involved in these reactions is small, but discovery of the reactions themselves provided the first insight into the metabolism of this vitamin.

Less well understood are the biochemical pathways through which vitamin A participates in (a) growth, (b) the maintenance of the integrity of epithelial cells, (c) the release of proteolytic enzymes from lysosomes, and (d) the synthesis of cortiocosterone from cholesterol resulting in a decrease in the body's capacity to synthesize glycogen.

Vitamin A and vision   In the retina of the eye there are structures called rods, which are concerned with vision in dim light, and cones, which are concerned with vision in bright light and are responsible for color vision. The characteristic pigments of rods and cones are the conjugated carotenoid proteins known respectively as rhodopsin and iodopsin. According to Wald they differ only in their opsin, or protein, moieties. The carotenoid common to rhodopsin and iodopsin is a *cis* isomer of retinal.

Rhodopsin, which is essential to night vision, is a bright red pigment that bleaches on exposure to light, becoming the yellow compound retinal (or retinene) through the loss of the protein opsin. Upon reduction, retinal yields retinol, which is colorless (Figure 14.1).

In the dark, rhodopsin can be regenerated. Through the action of alcohol dehydrogenase and NAD, the 11-*cis* isomer of retinol oxidizes to the corresponding isomer of retinal. Then in the absence of light, the 11-*cis*-retinal combines with the ε-amino group of a specific lysine residue in opsin to form rhodopsin or visual purple.

Some vitamin A is lost in the rhodopsin–vitamin A visual cycle, and consequently a deficiency of the vitamin eventually results in a lessened ability to see in dim light. This condition, commonly known as night blindness, is the earliest symptom of vitamin A deficiency in humans.

---

[*]Wald, G., *Nature* **139**(1937):1017.

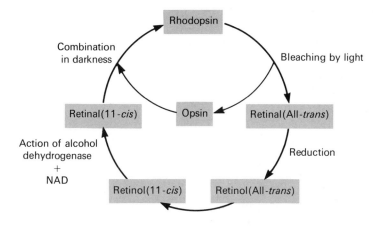

Figure 14.1
The rhodopsin–vitamin A cycle.

Metabolism of vitamin A and carotene Both vitamin A and carotene are absorbed from the small intestine, but a number of factors affect their absorption. Any condition that hinders the absorption of fat—such as biliary obstruction, fibrosis of the pancreas, or faulty chylomicron formation—will impede the absorption of the provitamin or vitamin. A low-fat diet can impair the ability of nonruminant animals to absorb carotene; in some species the dietary presence of conjugated bile acids with one free hydroxyl group enhances absorption. Low-protein diets reduce the ability to absorb vitamin A and its esters.

The ability to absorb dietary carotenoids varies from species to species. For example, humans, birds, and ruminants can absorb both vitamin A and the carotenoids whereas pigs and rats can absorb only vitamin A. Pigs and rats, however, have the ability to convert carotene to vitamin A in the intestinal mucosa.

Perhaps differences between species in the ability to convert carotene to vitamin A arise from the presence or absence in the blood of specific proteins that can form complexes with carotene to permit its absorption. Carotenoids are made water soluble (and thus soluble in blood) by reactions in the cell walls of the intestinal mucosa that result in the formation of protein complexes.

In 1948 J. Glover et al.[*] suggested that retinene is an intermediate in the conversion of β-carotene to vitamin A, and in 1954 Glover and Redfearn[†] postulated that the initial attack on β-carotene occurs at one end of the molecule and proceeds by progressive oxidation until retinene is formed.

[*]Glover, J., Goodwin, T. W., and Morton, R. A., *Biochem. J.* **43**(1948):109.
[†]Glover, J., and Redfearn, E. R., *Biochem. J.* **58**(1954):xv.

The retinene retinal can then be reduced to vitamin A retinol by alcohol dehydrogenase.

This theory for the conversion of carotene to vitamin A bears a strong resemblance to the rhodopsin–vitamin A visual processes. In both cases a carotenoid protein is degraded through retinene to vitamin A. It seems possible that the synthesis of rhodopsin from vitamin A in the retina is a model for a general class of reactions in which vitamin A is attached to other molecules to form complexes upon which the cellular activities of the vitamin depend.

We can summarize what is known about the absorption and transport of vitamin A per se as follows. Vitamin A usually occurs in sources of food as a retinyl ester, which is hydrolyzed in the lumen of the small intestine. The resulting retinol passes through the cell walls of the mucosa; inside the cells it is re-esterified preferentially with palmitic acid. Retinyl palmitate is incorporated into the chylomicrons thereby increasing its solubility in water; it is released into the lymphatic system and transported in the blood stream as part of the chylomicrons and is stored in the liver.

Stored retinyl ester is hydrolyzed in the liver by hydrolase enzymes and transported, as the free alcohol (retinol) bound to retinal-binding protein, via the bloodstream to tissues that need the vitamin for their metabolism.

Carotenes and other provitamin forms of vitamin A are transported in the body fluids as components of lipoproteins.

Sources   Vitamin A is found only in animal tissues in which the provitamin forms have been metabolized into the vitamin. Liver, the organ in which vitamin A is stored, is the richest source of vitamin A; the vitamin is also found in egg yolk and milk products. Plant materials contain only the precursors of vitamin A so that plant foods only supply the vitamin in direct proportion to the amount of carotene or other carotenoids they contain. Cryptoxanthin, a yellow pigment in corn, has some provitamin potential, but lycopene and xanthophyll, yellow pigments found respectively in tomatoes and corn, have no value as sources of vitamin A.

Vitamin A is very stable to heat, light, acid, and alkali; hence the various methods of preparing foods destroy very little of the vitamin. Drying plant materials in the sun causes some loss of vitamin A, as does prolonged storage of material dehydrated by this process. The carotenes are easily destroyed by oxygen and light.

Deficiency symptoms

1.   Deficiency of vitamin A interferes with *growth* because this vitamin takes part in the building of new cells. Vitamin A is also active in the normal development of bones as the agent that controls the activity of the osteoclasts and osteoblasts of the epithelial cartilage. One of the best-known lesions due to a deficiency of vitamin A in cattle under field conditions is a disorganized

growth of the bone. Malformation of the skull bones of young cattle can cause a constriction of the optic nerve, resulting in blindness. The same type of malformation can damage the auditory nerve, resulting in deafness.

2.   Vitamin A deficiency leads to a keratinization of the epithelial cells of the body; these cells then lose their cilia and suffer a progressive decrease in their ability to secrete mucus. The reduction in the capacity to secrete mucus is attributable to the fact that vitamin A is required for the synthesis of mucopolysaccharide, a normal constituent of mucus.

Keratinized tissue in the respiratory tract of animals deficient in vitamin A increases the severity of their colds and sinus trouble, perhaps because the affected epithelial tissues have a low resistance to infective organisms. In the alimentary tract, keratinization sometimes leads to diarrhea; and in the genito-urinary tract it probably accounts for a high incidence of kidney and bladder stones because it interferes with the elimination of urine. The keratinization of the epithelial tissues in the reproductive tract is thought to be directly responsible for the interference with reproduction associated with avitaminosis A. It is known that a deficiency of vitamin A practically eliminates spermatogenesis in the male and causes fetal resorption in the female.

3.   As we have already noted, insufficient vitamin A in the diet interferes with the regeneration of visual purple in the eye (see Figure 14.1), causing night blindness. A deficiency of vitamin A also affects the cornea of the eye, causing a condition known as Bitot's spots in its initial stages and xerophthalmia in the advanced state.

4.   There is good evidence that vitamin A is required for the release of proteolytic enzymes from the lysosomes responsible for breaking down the protein structure in bone; this breakdown must precede the synthesis of new bone structure. Hence, either a deficiency or a surplus of vitamin A results in an abnormal bone structure caused by an imbalance between the breakdown and the synthesis of bone.

5.   At least one skin condition in humans has been attributed to a dietary shortage of vitamin A—folliculosis. It occurs when eruptions at the base of the hair follicle produce a localized keratinization. The result is dry, rough skin, a condition seen most frequently around the shoulders.

Hypervitaminosis A   The earliest recorded cases of acute vitamin A toxicity were among Arctic explorers who ingested excessive amounts of the vitamin by eating the liver of polar bears. However, there have been several reports of modern-day vitamin A toxicity as a result of excessive administration of the vitamin to young children for various reasons. Hypervitaminosis A is characterized by a wide variety of symptoms, including fatigue or lethargy, abdominal discomfort, bone and/or joint pain, insomnia, restlessness, loss of hair, brittle bones, and severe headaches.

Many of the symptoms of hypervitaminosis A are quite similar to those of a deficiency of the vitamin. This may be because both result in a derangement of the lysosomes, the cell organelles that contain many of the hydrolytic enzymes.

Vitamin A requirements All mammals require vitamin A, but the requirements of many species can be met by the provitamin carotene rather than the vitamin itself. Although synthesis of carotene does occur in some animals (as in the caecum of sheep, for example), it does not help satisfy the animal's requirements because the synthesized carotene is destroyed farther down the alimentary tract. In fact, there is no known species in which synthesis provides a significant portion of the vitamin A requirement.

Body weight determines the actual vitamin A requirement of mammals. The amounts recommended as necessary to satisfy requirements vary not only from species to species but also from country to country. Differences in the quantities of vitamin A recommended arise from different assumptions about the proportion of vitamin A and carotene in a typical diet, and different interpretations of the efficiency of conversion of carotene to vitamin A.

There is evidence that an animal's requirement for vitamin A increases during the last trimester of pregnancy, during lactation, under other physiological stress, and in response to impaired intestinal absorption.

In determining how to enable an animal to meet its vitamin A requirements, it is important to know that 1.0 international unit (IU) of vitamin A is supplied by:

> 0.30 μg of all-*trans* vitamin A alcohol;
> 0.344 μg of all-*trans* vitamin A acetate;
> 0.55 μg of all-*trans* vitamin A palmitate.

It is also necessary to consider each species' capacity for converting carotene to vitamin A. Rats can convert 0.6 μg of β-carotene to 1.0 IU of vitamin A. However, as shown in Table 14.3, other species are less efficient at converting carotene.

The calculation of the ratio of 1.8 μg β-carotene to 1.0 IU vitamin A for humans is based on the assumptions that only one-third of dietary β-carotene is available for use by the human body and the body can only convert one-half of the usable carotene to vitamin A. Hence humans can only use one-sixth of the β-carotene they ingest.

Vitamin A requirements are influenced by the amount of protein in the diet. For example, inadequate protein intake decreases the efficiency of absorption of retinol as well as its transport in the blood and its metabolism; protein deficiency also depresses the rate of intestinal conversion of β-carotene to vitamin A. For these reasons, vitamin A deficiency frequently accompanies kwashiorkor.

Table 14.3
Amounts of all-*trans* β-carotene
equivalent to 1.0 IU of vitamin A
in various animal species

Species	Amount of β-carotene (μg)
Rat	0.6
Chicken	1.0
Swine	1.8
Cattle	3.0
Sheep	1.8–2.4
Horse	3.6
Dog	1.0
Human*	1.8

*The current trend is to express vitamin A requirements and potency in terms of retinol equivalents. See NAS-NRC(US), *Recommended Dietary Allowances* (8th ed.), National Academy of Sciences–National Research Council, Washington, D.C. (1974).

Vitamin D

The original antirachitic factor has become known as vitamin D. Although some ten sterol derivatives have been shown to have vitamin D activity, only two are important dietary sources of the vitamin. Ergosterol, a plant sterol, upon ultraviolet irradiation yields ergocalciferol or vitamin D_2; the irradiation of 7-dehydrocholesterol, a sterol found in the skin of animals including humans, yields cholecalciferol or vitamin D_3. Thus ergosterol and 7-dehydrocholesterol are vitamin D's chief provitamins.

Vitamin D is known as the sunshine vitamin because the ultraviolet radiation in sunlight serves as a source of the radiant energy necessary to convert the sterols of plant or animal tissues into biologically active vitamin D. Vitamin D_2 and vitamin D_3 have the same antirachitic effect in rats, dogs, pigs, ruminants, and humans, but D_2 is less active in poultry than D_3.

Physiological function Vitamin D has an important function in calcium and phosphorus metabolism; it is required for the normal calcification of growing bone. The role of the vitamin in adult animals is much less significant except during reproduction and lactation. The exact mechanisms by which vitamin D carries out its various physiological functions are not yet clear.

It has been known for many years that vitamin D enhances the absorption of calcium across the intestinal mucosa. The absorption of calcium involves an active, cation-based transport system in which phosphate is transferred secondarily to calcium. During absorption, calcium moves against a concentration gradient in the intestinal wall.

When administered to rachitic animals, vitamin D facilitates the absorption of calcium, but it takes several hours for the vitamin to achieve its effect

---

Box 14.1   Harry Steenbock and vitamin D

The most important experiment conducted by Harry Steenbock during a long and illustrious career was reported in 1923. He demonstrated that it is possible to produce indirectly the antirachitic and growth-promoting effect accomplished through the direct irradiation of an experimental animal (shown by Huldschinsky in 1919) by irradiating the food the animal eats. In other words, he showed that a food previously lacking in antirachitic vitamin acquired the potential for vitamin D activity from irradiation with ultraviolet light.

The problems Steenbock encountered in patenting his technique for irradiation were complicated, time-consuming, and personally frustrating. However, his efforts resulted eventually in the establishment in 1925 of the Wisconsin Alumni Research Foundation to which the first patent was assigned in 1928. Since that time the University of Wisconsin has benefited in countless ways from the income generated by Steenbock's discovery combined with his unselfish foresight in assigning patent rights.

Harry Steenbock (1886–1967) was born on a farm in Wisconsin of parents of German origin. Following his early schooling in rural Wisconsin, he received a B.S. degree in agriculture in 1908, an M.S. degree in 1910, and a Ph.D. degree in 1916, all from the University of Wisconsin. During his early student years, he was strongly influenced by Professor E. B. Hart (who gave him his first job as an assistant in the Department of Agricultural Chemistry at an annual salary of $720) and to a lesser extent by Dr. E. V. McCollum.

Steenbock's professional productivity really began in 1911 and lasted over half a century during which time he published more than 250 scientific papers. His research on vitamin D is legendary. Although less well known, his work on vitamin A and nutritional anemia was also important. Steenbock was the first to associate the yellow pigments in foods with vitamin A, but it was another investigator (T. Moore in England) who identified carotene as provitamin A. Steenbock collaborated on studies that led to the discovery of the independent role of copper in the curing of nutritional anemia by dietary supplements of iron. He also studied the nutritional value and biochemistry of cereals, and the nutritional effects of lipids and vitamin E.

For further information, see *J. Nutr.* **103**(1973):1235.

and its action can be blocked by agents, such as actinomycin D, that inhibit the synthesis of messenger RNA. Actinomycin D, however, is only effective if given within three hours after administering vitamin D. Furthermore, it has been shown that vitamin D induces the formation of a calcium-binding protein in the mucosa; the protein is thought to take part in the active transport of calcium. All of these findings suggest that vitamin D acts as an initiator of enzyme synthesis in the intestinal mucosa.

At the University of Wisconsin, a compound known as 25-hydroxycholecalciferol (25-HCC) was described in 1968.[*] This compound, which is produced by hydroxylating vitamin D_3 in the liver, is not only more effective than D_3 in stimulating the intestinal transport of calcium and bone resorption, but also achieves these responses more rapidly. At that time it was suggested that 25-HCC represents the metabolically active form of D_3.

More recently, it has been shown that 25-HCC is converted in the kidney to 1,25-dihydroxycholecalciferol (1,25-DHCC). The latter has been isolated in pure form and completely identified by Holick et al.[†] and is known to be much more potent (by weight) than 25-HCC in initiating both intestinal transport of calcium and the mobilization of bone minerals. However, 25-HCC is present in plasma at much higher concentrations than 1,25-DHCC and remains the most effective form of the vitamin in the cure of rickets.

Vitamin D may help regulate the disposition of calcium and phosphorus as an insoluble complex in the organic bone matrix. The details of how calcification is accomplished are not clear. However, it has been suggested that two enzymes, phosphorylase and alkaline phosphatase, are essential to the process. Vitamin D may play its role in bone calcification by helping to maintain normal levels of alkaline phosphatase in the blood.

In addition to its role in the intestinal absorption and bone resorption of calcium and phosphorus, vitamin D is somehow involved in the resorption of phosphate and amino acids from the kidney tubules, the maintenance of normal and constant amounts of calcium in the blood, and the maintenance of normal amounts of citrate in body fluids and in bones.

Metabolism   This vitamin, like vitamin A, is absorbed from the small intestine; and being fat soluble, its absorption is enhanced by any condition that increases the absorption of fat. In contrast to vitamin A, the body has little ability to store vitamin D, although some is stored in the liver, kidneys, adrenal glands, and bone. Vitamin D is excreted through the bile and the intestinal wall.

---

[*]Blunt, J. W., DeLuca, H. F., and Schnoes, H. K., *Biochemistry* 7(1968):3317.

[†]Holick, M. F., Schnoes, H. K., and DeLuca, H. F., *Proc. Nat. Acad. Sci. U.S.* **68**(1971):803.

There is a metabolic interrelationship between vitamin D, hydrocortisone, and the parathyroid hormone. For example, hydrocortisone tends to depress the level of calcium in the blood and decrease the permeability of the intestinal membrane to calcium; hence it appears to be a vitamin D antagonist. Vitamin D regulates the action of the parathyroid hormone, which in turn stimulates the mobilization of calcium from bone. Vitamin D also enhances the resorption of phosphates from the kidney whereas the parathyroid hormone has the opposite effect.

Sources   Because the irradiation of specific sterols contained in plant and animal tissues results in the formation of vitamin D, the amount of the vitamin present in plant foods depends upon the degree of exposure of the plant material to ultraviolet light following harvesting. Cod-liver oil was one of the original sources of vitamin D for both humans and animals. Other foods of animal origin, such as eggs and milk, contain the vitamin, but the amount present depends upon the season in which they are produced and the diet of the animal serving as the source of the vitamin. It is possible to increase the vitamin D content of milk through dietary additions of the vitamin, but it is much simpler to fortify the milk directly.

Although they are produced by ultraviolet irradiation, both vitamins D_2 and D_3 are unstable to continued irradiation. They are not easily oxidized and are only influenced by temperatures in excess of 140°C. The vitamins D are relatively unstable in acidic media but are stable in alkaline solutions even at high temperatures.

Deficiency symptoms   Rickets is a disease that manifests itself as a disturbance in bone metabolism, but the trouble originates in the blood that nourishes the growing bone. In rickets there is a decrease in the amount of phosphorus or calcium (or both) in the blood, and an increase in the amount of plasma alkaline phosphatase. There is also an increase in the pH of the intestinal contents and feces. The actual deformity of the bone arises from the body's failure to deposit calcium and/or phosphorus.

When we think of rickets we usually picture a child with *bowed legs* and other skeletal deformities. In bone formation, the actual calcification of the bones is preceded by the formation of cartilage. In severe cases of rickets, the formation of cartilage proceeds normally but calcification, the deposition of calcium and phosphorus salts, does not keep pace; hence the condition is characterized by cartilagenous bones. Deformities develop when the poorly calcified bones are called upon to perform the function for which normal bones are designed—i.e., the support of soft tissues. Bowing of the legs occurs because the long bones are unable to support the weight of the body.

Growth of the long bones occurs primarily in the epiphyseal region through the synthesis of new cartilage; if the cartilage fails to calcify, the epiphyses become irregularly widened from the pressure of the body's weight. The major manifestation of this enlargement is *knock-knees*.

In addition, the retarded mineralization of other bones in the body together with the gravitational and mechanical stresses associated with supporting the body in an upright position result in deformities of the ribs described as *pigeon breast* and *rachitic rosary*. Pressure on poorly calcified ribs produces a concave chest (pigeon breast), which causes a crowding of the chest cavity and an irregular spacing and swelling of the ribs, giving an appearance of beading (rachitic rosary).

The primary defect in rickets is not faulty calcification but rather the result of insufficient calcium and phosphorus in the serum which prevents calcification. In healthy individuals, the level of blood calcium is strictly maintained at a minimum of 7 mg per 100 ml by the mobilization of calcium from the bone matrix. In the rachitic individual, however, the level of serum calcium and then of serum phosphorus falls because of a lack of mineralized bone. The mobilization of bone matrix during a dietary deficiency of calcium or phosphorus results in an adult form of rickets known as osteomalacia. This condition, sometimes prevalent among pregnant and lactating women, and frequently seen in the aged, is actually a partial decalcification of normal bone which eventually produces brittleness.

Vitamin D is undoubtedly required for the calcification of teeth, but dental caries do not necessarily accompany rickets.

Hypervitaminosis D   Among humans, there is probably more reason to be concerned about vitamin D toxicity than vitamin D deficiency. The symptoms of hypervitaminosis D are the reverse of those observed in rickets. A marked hypercalcemia brings on loss of appetite, nausea, and a loss of weight. Bones are extremely dense to x-ray, and calcareous deposits are found in the joints and soft tissues such as the kidneys and arteries.

The amount of dietary vitamin D that precipitates hypercalcemia varies from one individual to another. Adults receiving 100,000 IU of vitamin D daily will develop symptoms in a matter of weeks. In infants, daily intakes of 10,000 to 30,000 IU are usually toxic. The concurrent administration of large quantities of vitamin A with potentially toxic levels of vitamin D will reduce the toxicity of the latter.

It is also noteworthy that high-potency preparations of vitamin D_2 are used as rat poisons.

Vitamin D requirements   The calcium and phosphorus content of the diet determines, to a certain extent, the vitamin D requirement. For example, if the amount of either of these inorganic elements or the ratio between them is suboptimal, the requirement for vitamin D increases. Different species require different forms and amounts of vitamin D. As already indicated, chicks and poults can efficiently utilize only vitamin D_3, whereas vitamins D_2 and D_3 are about equally active for most other species. Chicks have a higher requirement per unit of body weight than rats or pigs, and poults have an even higher requirement than chicks. The vitamin D requirement of the human child resembles that of the bird more than that of other mammals.

Because ultraviolet light can convert the provitamin in the skin and fat into the vitamin, the length of time that animals spend in the sunshine affects their dietary requirements. Darkly pigmented and hairy skins are not as easily irradiated as are fair and smooth skins. Irradiation is ineffective through glass, but it can take place in the shade on sunny days. Smoke, dust, and high humidity also decrease irradiation.

Thus, many factors—including calcium and phosphorus intake, character of skin and/or its color, environment, and living habits—influence an animal's requirement for vitamin D, making a fixed requirement difficult to assess.

Before the chemical nature of vitamin D was known, its potency, like that of vitamin A, was expressed in terms of international units (IU). One international unit of vitamin D was equivalent to 0.025 μg of cholecalciferol (D_3); in other words, 1 μg of vitamin D_3 was equivalent to 40 IU. The current trend is to express vitamin D requirements and potency in micrograms of cholecalciferol.

Vitamin E

Vitamin E was known as the "antisterility" vitamin for many years. The early work on this vitamin was carried out with rats, and in this species a dramatic improvement in fertility was observed when vitamin E was added to a diet deficient in the substance. However, this relation between vitamin E and fertility does not necessarily hold for all species. In fact, in humans and ruminants, sterility has never been linked with a deficiency of vitamin E.

Like vitamin D, vitamin E occurs in multiple forms. It consists, chemically, of tocopherols, with the alpha, beta, gamma, delta, epsilon, zeta, and eta isomers all occurring naturally and possessing characteristic biological activity. The alpha form, however, is much more active than the others, at least in its known vitamin function in the body.

Physiological function   Vitamin E was recognized as a dietary essential in 1922; since then, continuing research has clarified the vital role of vitamin E in all body cells, where it seems to be primarily associated with membrane structure. Muscular, vascular, adipose, neural, and skeletal tissues are all affected in one way or another by vitamin E. Because the vitamin is so versatile, it is not surprising that other compounds can assume specific parts of its functions. The following roles have been attributed to the tocopherols:

1.   Antioxidants in animal and plant tissues: The tocopherols are strong antioxidants capable of preventing the oxidative destruction of fats. Vitamins A and C are also protected in the presence of these compounds. The antioxidative action of tocopherols takes place not only in body cells but also in the animal's digestive tract as well as in the plant sources of tocopherols.

For years nutritionists assumed that the deleterious effects produced by polyunsaturated fatty acids in the diets of vitamin-E-deficient animals resulted from *in vivo* oxidation of these fatty acids. The resulting peroxides were believed to damage cellular structures, thereby causing the symptoms of vitamin E deficiency. Although there is little direct evidence that fatty acids actually undergo peroxidation *in vivo*, this lack of evidence does not eliminate the probability that unsaturated fatty acids increase the intracellular requirement for vitamin E.

Furthermore, fat added to the diet will destroy the vitamin E in both the diet and the digestive tract, if oxidative rancidity occurs. Hence, the quantitative relationship between vitamin E and dietary fat is of practical importance.

2.   Agents essential to cellular respiration: The action of α-tocopherol appears to be necessary in cellular respiration primarily in such tissues as heart and skeletal muscles. In this capacity the tocopherol may act as a cofactor in the cytochrome–reductase portion of the NAD oxidase and the succinate oxidase systems. Researchers have demonstrated that vitamin E restricts the specific activity of cytochrome c reductase.

3.   Regulators in the synthesis of body compounds: The tocopherols appear to be involved in the biosynthesis of DNA, probably by regulating the incorporation of pyrimidines into the nucleic acid structure. It has also been suggested that vitamin E acts as a cofactor in the synthesis of vitamin C, and that, in some fashion, it stimulates the synthesis of coenzyme Q.

It is of interest to note that the *in vitro* antioxidative powers of the tocopherols are the reverse of the biological potencies in the body. The *in vivo* potency of vitamin E decreases from the alpha to the delta isomers ($\alpha > \beta > \gamma > \delta$), whereas the *in vitro* antioxidant powers of the isomers are the reverse.

Metabolism   Vitamin E is absorbed in the small intestine in the presence of bile, α-tocopherol being the most efficiently absorbable form. Some species of animals are able to store considerable amounts of the vitamin in such diverse tissues and organs as fat, muscle, adrenal glands, heart, and liver. As with other fat-soluble vitamins, its path of excretion is via the feces. Tocopherols pass through the placental membranes and also into the mammary gland, and thus the diet of female mammals influences the store of the young at birth and the amount the young subsequently obtain from the mother's milk.

Sources   Several forms of tocopherol of varying biological activity occur throughout the plant kingdom, particularly in green plants, but all homologues do not occur together. Alpha-tocopherol is the most widely distributed isomer; it is the sole tocoperhol in the green parts of plants. The other tocopherols are found together with the alpha form in the seeds of plants, and particularly in the oils extracted from these seeds. In general, the amount of tocopherol in these oils parallels their content of polyunsaturated fatty acids. A small amount of vitamin E is found in such animal products as liver, eggs, fish, and butter.

Naturally occurring α-tocopherol is the d-epimer, and it has been shown that d-α-tocopherol has 1.2 times the biological potency of the dl-form. This is of significance because vitamin E can be prepared synthetically, but all of the synthetic vitamin is the dl-form.

The heating of cooking oils destroys practically all of their vitamin E potency. Compared to the oils, fruits and vegetables are poor sources of tocopherol, but they lose very little of their potential for vitamin activity during normal cooking procedures.

Deficiency symptoms   The most outstanding characteristic of vitamin E deficiency is the great variety of tissue alterations seen in different species. Changes have been shown to occur in the reproductive, nervous, and circulatory systems, in the muscles, liver, alimentary tract, and fat depots. Some species manifest only a single symptom, whereas others react with a wide range of pathologies. All are preventable with α-tocopherol. Table 14.4 lists some of the commonly seen symptoms of vitamin E deficiency and the species manifesting them.

Table 14.4
Some of the symptoms of vitamin E deficiency in different species

Symptoms of deficiency	Species showing symptoms
Infertility	Rats, guinea pigs, mice, hamsters, rabbits, pigs, dogs, chicks, monkeys
Brown pigment in uterus	Rats
Brown pigment in adipose tissue	Rats, mice, hamsters, mink
Skeletal muscular dystrophy	Adult rabbits and hamsters, weanling rats, lambs, pigs, guinea pigs, calves
Exudative diathesis	Chicks, rats, pigs
Encephalomalacia	Chicks
Liver necrosis	Rats, mice, chicks, pigs
Cardiac muscle abnormalities	Rabbits, rats, monkeys, cattle, lambs, poultry
Dental depigmentation	Rats, hamsters

Many dietary factors seem to contribute to the development of these vitamin-E-deficiency symptoms. Total fat, unsaturated fats, cod-liver oil, amount of protein, choline, cystine, inositol, cholesterol, vitamin A, and minerals all have, at one time or another, been considered capable of causing or aggravating one or another of the deficiency symptoms listed in Table 14.4.

Vitamin E deficiency is seldom seen in humans. There have been reports, however, of remarkable positive responses to orally administered tocopheryl acetate in premature infants suffering from *scleroma neonatorum*, a condition characterized by edema, skin lesions, and blood abnormalities. Furthermore, individuals suffering from protein deficiency diseases such as kwashiorkor have very little tocopherol in their serum; the fragility of their red blood cells is greater than normal and they frequently suffer from an accompanying anemia.

Interrelating substances   It is well established that some of the biochemical functions of the tocopherols can be carried out in full or in part by a variety of chemically unrelated substances. For example, selenium is more efficient in alleviating some of the disorders that investigators originally thought responded only to vitamin E therapy (exudative diathesis, liver necrosis, muscle dystrophy), but selenium has little or no effect on other disorders cured by vitamin E (encephalomalacia, brown pigment in uterus). The amino acids cystine and methionine delay the onset of muscular dystrophy in chicks fed a vitamin-E-deficient diet.

Antioxidants also prevent the appearance of some of the symptoms of vitamin E deficiency. For example, antioxidants such as ethoxyquin (EHQ) give some protection against encephalomalacia and exudative diathesis in chicks, and against muscular dystrophy and brown pigment in the uterus in rats. Another chemical antioxidant, N-N' diphenyl-*p*-phenylene (DPPD), can fulfill an even wider range of vitamin E functions.

Researchers are still elucidating the interaction between vitamins A and E. Vitamin E probably aids in the absorption or utilization of vitamin A and the carotenes. Excessive ingestion of vitamin A or carotene appears to increase the requirement for vitamin E, whereas excessive vitamin E in the diet in relation to vitamin A seems to deplete vitamin A reserves.

Vitamin E requirements   An animal's quantitative requirement for vitamin E appears to be related to metabolic size (e.g., $wt_{kg}^{.75}$). Except under conditions of stress, animals seldom need a supplementary dietary source of tocopherol if they consume a mixed diet. This is because of the wide distribution of vitamin E in plant tissues.

Vitamin E requirements are usually expressed in international units (IU). One international unit of vitamin E is equivalent to 1 mg of dl-α-tocopheryl acetate, and 1 mg of naturally occurring d-α-tocopherol is equivalent to 1.49 IU.

The recommended intake of vitamin E for humans varies from 10 to 15 IU per day. Humans require more of the vitamin if their diet contains polyunsaturated fatty acids. The requirements of farm animals depend upon the amount of polyunsaturated fatty acids, selenium, cystine and methionine, and vitamin A in the ration. Agriculturalists used to add 10 to 20 IU of vitamin E per kilogram of swine and poultry ration. Since 1974, when the United States Food and Drug Authority approved selenium as a feed additive, the amount of supplementary vitamin E in feed has been reduced to 5 to 10 IU/kg.

Box 14.2   Vitamin E for humans

The following is a summary of an official statement of the Food and Nutrition Board of the National Academy of Sciences–National Research Council (1973) on "Supplementation of Human Diets with Vitamin E."

"Misleading claims that vitamin E supplementation of the ordinary diet will cure or prevent such human ailments as sterility, lack of virility, abnormal termination of pregnancy, heart disease, muscular weakness, cancer, ulcers, skin disorders, and burns, are not backed by sound experimentation or clinical observations. Some of these claims are based upon deficiency symptoms observed in other species. Careful studies over a period of many years attempting to relate these symptoms to vitamin E deficiency in human beings have been unproductive.

"The wide distribution of vitamin E in vegetable oils, cereal grains, and animal fats makes a deficiency in humans very unlikely. Premature infants or individuals with impaired absorption of fats may require supplemental vitamin E, but they should, in any event, be under the care of a physician."

More recently, A. L. Tappel at the Davis campus of the University of California has claimed that vitamin E fulfills two additional major functions. The first is that this vitamin slows the aging process in animal cells. Tappel asserts that within the fat components of animal tissues, aging is taking place as the result of an on-going series of destructive chemical reactions and vitamin E is the natural inhibitor of these destructive processes. The second claim is that vitamin E plays a role in the fight against air pollution. This assertion was made on the basis of some evidence from experiments with rats indicating that the vitamin can protect lung tissue from the noxious effects of smog.

We would like to emphasize that, as of 1976, neither of these claims had been clearly substantiated by other researchers.

Vitamin K

Vitamin K has been known since 1934, when, in Denmark, H. Dam and F. Schönheyder* concluded that the hemorrhagic condition of chicks fed an ether-extracted diet was caused by an avitaminosis; they called the new factor that relieved the symptoms of deficiency vitamin K. The deficiency also occurs in humans, rats, mice, and rabbits, but only if the mechanism of fat absorption is defective. Vitamin K, which belongs to a group of chemical compounds known as the quinones, is multiple in nature. Vitamin K_1, which occurs only in green plants, is also known as phylloquinone; vitamin K_2, which comprises a group of menaquinones, occurs as the result of synthesis by microorganisms.

Several synthetic compounds have been prepared that possess vitamin K activity, the best known of which is menadione (2-methyl, 1,4-naphthoquinone). Menadione is even more active than vitamin K_1. Naturally occurring vitamin K is fat soluble, but some of the synthetic compounds are soluble in water.

Physiological function   In higher animals vitamin K regulates the plasma content of proteins required for blood coagulation—i.e., of prothrombin (Factor II), proconvertin (Factor VII), plasma thromboplastin component (Factor IX), and Stuarts factor (Factor X). However, there is no agreement as to whether the vitamin controls the production of these four compounds or whether they are all derived from a parent molecule.

An appreciation of the processes involved in clot (fibrin) formation is fundamental to an understanding of the action of vitamin K in the body. Although clotting is a complex process, it may for our purposes be summarized by the "cascade" sequence illustrated in Figure 14.2.

---

*Dam, H., and Schönheyder, F., *Biochem. J.* **28**(1934):1355.

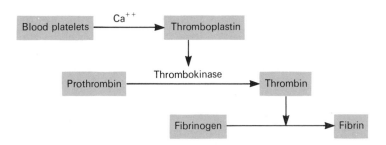

Figure 14.2
The role of prothrombin in the blood clotting process.

If we accept the theory that vitamin K controls the synthesis in the liver of one or more of the protein compounds (prothrombin, proconvertin, etc.) required for blood coagulation, the question remains: how is clotting accomplished? One theory that received early acceptance is that the vitamin functions at the RNA translation stage in protein synthesis. This possibility is represented schematically in Figure 14.3.

In this series of reactions, it is proposed that vitamin K is required to mediate the entry and attachment of specific soluble RNA (sRNA) molecules, each bearing its own particular amino acid, to ribosomal RNA. When properly aligned, the amino acids are joined in peptide linkage; the protein and sRNA units detach from each other, and the process can begin again. The proteins that require vitamin K for their synthesis are presumably those required for blood coagulation.

The most recent suggestion is that there is a specific precursor (protein) to prothrombin, and under the influence of vitamin K this precursor is converted to prothrombin by the carboxylation of the glutamic acid residues in the amino terminal of the protein.

Although there is some indication that vitamin K participates in electron transport and oxidative phosphorylation in microorganisms, there is no evidence that it fulfills these functions in higher animals.

Vitamin K antagonists   The discovery of vitamin K antagonists stemmed primarily from investigations into a disorder in cattle known as "sweet clover poisoning." The hemorrhagic disease occurs in herbivores if they consume sweet clover hay that has undergone spoilage during harvesting or storage. The causative agent has been identified as dicumarol, an oxidation product of coumarin.

Warfarin, a commercial product used primarily as a rat poison, is similar in structure to dicumarol, but it is an even more potent anticoagulant. It is

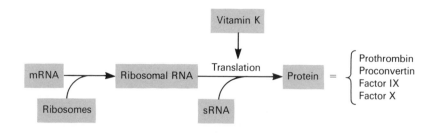

Figure 14.3
The role of vitamin K in the RNA translation stage of protein synthesis.

generally assumed that such anticoagulants compete directly with vitamin K for a receptor protein, or proteins, in the parenchymal cells of the liver.

Because they decrease the ability of blood to clot, coumarin anticoagulants are medically useful in treating some forms of atherosclerosis, thrombosis, and phlebitis.

Metabolism   The absorption, excretion, and secretion of vitamin K are similar to those of vitamin E. However, there is little storage of this vitamin in the body, except in the liver.

Sources   Alfalfa is an especially rich source of vitamin K, which occurs in lesser quantities in other foods of plant origin, including dark leafy vegetables, tubers, grain seeds, and fruits.

Vitamin K is destroyed by light, acid, alkali, and different oxidizing agents; it is stable to reducing agents and heat.

Deficiency symptoms   Fowl appear to be the type of animal most susceptible to vitamin K deficiency; absence of a dietary source of this vitamin leads to subcutaneous and intramuscular hemorrhages in poultry. A hemorrhagic syndrome occurs occasionally in humans but usually only if there is an impairment of biliary function. Vitamin K deficiency is sometimes found in newborn infants. The deficiency symptoms are similar to those caused by dicumarol.

Vitamin K requirements   All mammals require vitamin K to synthesize prothrombin, but because bacteria in the alimentary tract produce the vitamin, mammals do not necessarily depend upon a dietary source of vitamin K. Birds, however, have such a short intestinal tract and harbor so few microorganisms that they require a dietary source of vitamin K. Even among birds, different species have different needs. Chicks, ducklings, and goslings require dietary vitamin K, whereas pigeons and canaries are much less susceptible to a deficiency of this vitamin.

In recent years, vitamin K has become a routine addition to swine rations. Experimental work has shown that this addition is particularly valuable when high-moisture grains are used.

Humans normally do not require a dietary source of the vitamin, but some diseases increase the apparent need for vitamin K. Thus, vitamin K has proved of therapeutic value as a preoperative and postoperative measure to prevent the risk of bleeding; in treating cases where absorption is impaired, as in obstructive jaundice; and in treating hemorrhagic diseases of the newborn.

Suggested readings

Bieri, J. G. "Vitamin E," *Nutrition Reviews* **33**(1975):161.

Capen, C. C., Cole, C. R., and Hibbs, J. W. "Influence of Vitamin D on Calcium Metabolism and the Parathyroid Glands of Cattle," *Federation Proceedings* **27**(1968):142.

DeLuca, H. F. "Vitamin D: The Vitamin and the Hormone," *Federation Proceedings* **33**(1974):2211.

DeLuca, H. F., and Suttie, J. W. *The Fat-Soluble Vitamins*. University of Wisconsin Press, Madison (1970).

Draper, H. H., and Csallany, A. "Metabolism and Function of Vitamin E," *Federation Proceedings* **28**(1969):1690.

Haussler, M. R. "Vitamin D: Mode of Action and Biochemical Applications," *Nutrition Reviews* **32**(1974):257.

Kelleher, J., and Losowsky, M. S. "The Absorption of α-tocopherol in Man," *British Journal of Nutrition* **24**(1970):1033.

Olson, J. A. "Metabolism and Function of Vitamin A," *Federation Proceedings* **28**(1969):1670.

Olson, R. E. "The Mode of Action of Vitamin K," *Nutrition Reviews* **28**(1970):171.

Owen, E. C. "Some Aspects of the Metabolism of Vitamin A and Carotene," *World Review of Nutrition and Dietetics* **5**(1965):132.

Roels, O. A. "Vitamin A Physiology," *Journal of the American Medical Association* **214**(1970):1097.

Suttie, J. W. "Vitamin K and Prothrombin Synthesis," *Nutrition Reviews* **31**(1973):105.

Ullrey, D. E. "Biological Availability of Fat-Soluble Vitamins: Vitamin A and Carotene," *Journal of Animal Science* **35**(1972):648.

Wald, J. "Molecular Basis of Visual Excitation," *Science* **162**(1968):230.

Chapter 15
Other vitamins or vitamin-like compounds

Vitamin C

Scurvy was already a well-known disease when North America was discovered. Sailors who spent months on the sea almost invariably developed scurvy unless citrus fruits were included in their diet. It was not until the twentieth century, however, that vitamin C was discovered to be the antiscorbutic factor present in citrus fruits. A dietary deficiency of vitamin C will cause scurvy only in humans, guinea pigs, monkeys, red-vented bulbul birds, and Indian fruit-eating bats. These species are genetically deficient in the enzyme L-gulonolactone oxidase. Other animals are capable of synthesizing the vitamin from glucose via glucuronic acid and gulonic acid lactone.

Vitamin C was the first vitamin to be synthesized in the laboratory. Because it is a derivative of hexose, it can be classified as a carbohydrate. It occurs in two forms, both of which are biologically active. These forms are ascorbic acid (the reduced form) and dehydroascorbic acid (the oxidized form). These components are readily and reversibly oxidized and reduced, but if the "dehydro" form is oxidized further to diketogulonic acid, a reaction that is not reversible, the compound loses its potential for biological activity.

Ascorbic acid $\rightleftharpoons$ Dehydroascorbic acid $\longrightarrow$ Diketogulonic acid
(biologically   (biologically   (biologically
active)   active)   inactive)

Physiological functions   In spite of the relatively early laboratory synthesis of vitamin C, we still know very little about its specific functions in the body. Its outstanding chemical property is its reversible oxidation and reduction capacity, and therefore it most likely functions in some way as a transporter of hydrogen in cellular respiration. For example, ascorbic acid in the oxidized form is capable of picking up hydrogens from gluthathione and passing them on to molecular oxygen. However, a reaction such as this has yet to be fitted into the currently accepted scheme of intermediary metabolism. A role for vitamin C in tissue respiration would explain the

---

Box 15.1   James Lind and scurvy

The lifetime of James Lind (1716–1794) spanned a large part of the era of empire expansion, when adventurers and explorers undertook long sea voyages to claim new lands. Scurvy was the principal health problem encountered by the seamen of that period.

Through his experiments and writings on scurvy, James Lind was largely responsible for eliminating this scourge of sailors. Lind was born in Edinburgh, Scotland, and at the age of fifteen was apprenticed to a local physician. Upon completion of his medical apprenticeship in 1739, he joined the British navy as a surgeon's mate.

While on board the *Salisbury*, Lind carried out his now famous experiment on twelve patients suffering from advanced scurvy. He divided the patients into 6 groups of 2 men each, and gave only one pair of subjects two oranges and one lemon daily. The condition of these two patients improved rapidly and dramatically; the improvement was obvious in as little as six days from the commencement of treatment. Not only did Lind demonstrate the value of citrus juices in the treatment of scurvy, he also described a method whereby they could be preserved for long voyages through concentration by evaporation.

Because of these discoveries and of his recognition that a variety of "stress factors" encountered during sea voyages (e.g., exposure to cold and wetness, inadequate nutrition in addition to insufficient vitamin C) accentuate the severity of scurvy, Lind has often been referred to as one of the fathers of modern preventive medicine.

Despite Lind's position in the Royal Navy and the conclusiveness of his experimental results, it was not until 1795 (one year after his death) that orders were given to make the issue of lemon juice compulsory on all British naval ships.

For further information, see *J. Nutr.* **50**(1953):3.

increased survival time induced by administering vitamin C to rats suffering from hemorrhage or deprived of oxygen.

The main physiological defect in scurvy is the failure of collagen to form in the fibroblasts of connective tissue. Collagen is a structural protein that binds cells together; it contains large amounts of proline and hydroxyproline. The enzyme *collagen proline hydroxylase* effects the conversion of proline to hydroxyproline in the body; ascorbic acid and oxygen are required for the conversion. The importance of ascorbic acid in collagen formation explains why wound healing is impaired in scorbutic individuals: the new connective tissue that must be formed is primarily collagen.

The dentin in teeth is formed by a layer of cells known as odontoblasts. Because ascorbic acid is required for the normal development of odontoblasts, there is a defect in dentin formation if ascorbic acid is not available during the critical period of tooth formation.

Ascorbic acid is also necessary in the metabolism of tyrosine. A deficiency of the vitamin will result in the build-up and excretion of an intermediary product, *p*-hydroxyphenylpyruvate. The role of ascorbic acid in the metabolism of tyrosine, along with its function in the formation of tetrahydropteroylglutamic acid (HP_4teGlu), emphasizes the interdependence of folacin and ascorbic acid. This interdependence also explains, in part, the fact that anemia invariably accompanies scurvy.

Vitamin C enhances the absorption of iron from the gut, presumably by maintaining iron in the reduced, and hence more absorbable, form. Furthermore, ascorbic acid activates certain iron-containing enzymes.

Investigators have suggested a number of other functions for ascorbic acid, but because the evidence for most of these functions is not conclusive, researchers have not yet been able to elucidate the biochemical activity of the vitamin.

1. Ascorbic acid may participate in the metabolism of steroids, particularly in the synthesis of steroid hormones by the adrenal cortex.

2. Ascorbic acid may play a role in the metabolism of lipids because blood cholesterol levels appear to fall with the administration of ascorbic acid and rise during a deficiency of the vitamin.

3. During exposure to low temperatures, animals may benefit from large doses of ascorbic acid.

4. Limited evidence exists that animal requirements for ascorbic acid increase during infection (e.g., tuberculosis).

5. Ascorbic acid is needed for the conversion of tryptophan to serotonin.

6. Administering the reduced form of vitamin C reduces an animal's requirements for thiamin, riboflavin, pantothenic acid, folacin, vitamin A, and vitamin E.

Metabolism   Ascorbic acid is absorbed from the small intestine and excreted via the urine. The level of vitamin C in the plasma reflects very closely the intake. There is practically no storage of this vitamin in the body, but tissues functioning at a high metabolic rate have been observed to have a high ascorbic acid content. Vitamin C is secreted in the milk of lactating animals.

Sources   Vitamin C is found almost exclusively in foods of plant origin (and in kidney). Citrus fruits and leafy vegetables are the usual sources, although an appreciable amount of ascorbic acid is also found in green peppers, strawberries, and tomatoes. Human milk contains three to four times as much vitamin C as cow's milk. Cow's milk is a poor source of vitamin C for the human infant.

Ascorbic acid is highly soluble in water and slightly soluble in alcohol. It is quite stable in the dry crystalline state, but is easily oxidized in solution. The instability in solution increases as the pH of the solution increases.

Box 15.2   Vitamin C and the common cold

Publication of the book *Vitamin C and the Common Cold*, written by two-time-Nobel-prize-winner Linus Pauling, resulted in the consumption of enormous quantities of ascorbic acid by people seeking to prevent and cure the common cold. The book also ushered in a tremendous debate among advocates of Pauling's philosophy, and nutritionists, clinicians, and pharmacologists who challenged the efficacy of ascorbic acid in this context and who expressed concern over the safety of doses of 1 to 5 gm daily for prophylaxis, and as much as 15 gm daily for treatment of a cold. The fact that there was little scientific evidence to confirm either the usefulness or the hazards of large daily doses of ascorbic acid did not deter either side in the debate.

It is interesting that the major negative response to Pauling's recommendations came from nutritionists. The fact that ascorbic acid is a required nutrient seemed to many of them "to put the ball squarely in their court." Most nutritionists who took exception to the hypothesis that ascorbic acid is effective against the common cold overlooked the fact that the daily intakes recommended by Pauling were 30 to 300 times higher than the amount considered adequate to meet the normal dietary need for ascorbic acid, which placed the debate in the court of the pharmacologists, rather than the nutritionists. Some nutritionists even questioned Pauling's competency to comment on health and nutrition in spite of his contribution to the explanation of sickle cell anemia.

Any method of food processing that applies heat or increases the surface area of the food exposed to air or water will destroy most of the vitamin. Prolonged storage also reduces the ascorbic acid content of foods.

Deficiency symptoms   The classical symptoms of scurvy are hemorrhages throughout the body (due to the increased fragility of the capillaries), swollen and bleeding gums, and anemia. During the chronic or developing stages of a vitamin C deficiency a decline in weight is noted, along with sore and swollen joints, bones that fracture easily, and difficulty in wound healing. In fever and in tuberculosis there is a depletion of whatever reserves of ascorbic acid the body may have had.

Vitamin C requirements   Only humans, the other primates, and guinea pigs require a dietary source of vitamin C. Feeding ascorbic acid to cows does not increase the amount of vitamin in the milk because ascorbic acid is destroyed in the rumen. The basis for the vitamin C requirement of humans

The book's chief virtue is that it questions some of the fundamental concepts of nutrition that are based on the minimal intakes required to prevent deficiency symptoms. It has also generated a flurry of research into the efficacy of ascorbic acid in preventing and curing the common cold and into the possible hazards of taking megadoses of ascorbic acid year round. Despite a large number of double-blind studies (in which neither the physician nor the patient knew which subjects received the ascorbic acid and which received the placebo), the question of whether vitamin C is effective in reducing the severity of the common cold remains largely unanswered.

The reported undesirable side effects of large amounts of ascorbic acid are insignificant or rare, and although they may be troublesome, they are of little consequence to health. However, the possibility of an increased requirement for vitamin C in infants born of mothers who took large doses of ascorbic acid during pregnancy and the possibility that ascorbic acid destroys vitamin B_{12} both suggest that users of large doses of vitamin C should observe the same precautions normally applied to the use of other drugs. Users should be aware that toxicity may exist and that the risk of undesirable side effects may be greater in certain physiological states (e.g., pregnancy). Whether the benefits of a slight reduction in the severity of a cold outweigh the potential hazards of megadoses of ascorbic acid is a question even the most authoritative experts in the field avoid.

is indefinite. A man weighs about 70 times as much as a guinea pig, whereas his probable vitamin C requirement is only 20 times as great. The optimal requirements are still uncertain, and different dietary standards often differ in their recommended allowances.

Although vitamin C was the first vitamin to be synthesized, less is known for certain about it than about many of the more recently identified vitamins.

Choline

Choline does not really qualify as a vitamin because it is actually a structural component of fat and nerve tissue, and is not known to participate in any enzyme system. However, because of its biological function and its distribution in foods it is often considered in a discussion of vitamins.

Choline has been known for many years because of its relationship to the phospholipids and to acetylcholine. The phospholipids, lecithin and sphingomyelin, are the principal bound forms of choline, and although acetylcholine is physiologically important in the transmission of nerve impulses, quantitatively it forms but a small part of the total choline in the body. Nutritionists have long recognized the role of phospholipids in the body, but they have more recently determined the significance of choline as a specific dietary requirement. Choline is present in all foods that contain fat.

Physiological functions   As a component of phospholipids, choline is essential in the building and maintenance of cell structure; and as a component of acetylcholine it is active in the transmission of nerve impulses. Choline also plays an essential role in fat metabolism in the liver by making possible the transport of excessive fat as lecithin. For this reason, choline is referred to as a "lipotropic factor."

Along with other compounds, choline is a source of biologically labile methyl groups. These methyl groups are always attached to a sulfur or a nitrogen atom that has acquired an additional covalent bond and a positive charge. Methionine is an example of a sulfur-containing compound that acts as a methyl donor; choline and betaine are nitrogen-containing compounds that serve in this capacity.

Metabolism   Methionine, as well as choline, is a lipotropic factor. This is because the labile methyl groups provided by methionine can combine with ethanolamine to form choline. Conversely, the methyl groups from choline can combine with homocysteine to form methionine. This phenomenon is known as transmethylation.

In addition to its interrelationship with methionine, choline is associated with biotin and folacin; a deficiency of any one of the three will cause perosis in chicks. Choline, vitamin B_{12}, and folacin are also interrelated; all engage in specific aspects of the chemistry of methyl groups.

Deficiency symptoms   A nonspecific symptom of choline deficiency in all species is the retardation of growth. More specific symptoms are fatty livers, degenerated renal tubules, enlarged spleens, and a generalized hemorrhagic condition of the kidneys. In poultry, egg production is inhibited in adults and perosis is observed in the young.

Choline requirements   All animal species have a metabolic requirement for choline. The requirement of the guinea pig is abnormally low because this species does not possess a hepatic choline oxidase. A dietary deficiency of this "vitamin" is seldom encountered, although the tendency toward low-fat diets may dictate the inclusion of choline in the diets of some species.

The actual requirement for choline depends on the amount of methionine present in the diet because the body can synthesize choline from methionine and ethanolamine.

Methionine can completely eliminate mammalian requirements for choline but not those of young birds. For the first eight weeks of life, a chick or poult has only a limited capacity to methylate ethanolamine, and thus choline must be provided in its diet. Beyond eight weeks of age, biosynthetic mechanisms can provide sufficient choline for both chicks and poults. High levels of dietary protein tend to increase the choline requirements of birds.

Myo-inositol

Myo-inositol is another substance that cannot be classified as a true vitamin, but because it possesses functional similarities to the vitamins, we will discuss it in this category. There are nine possible stereoisomers of inositol (related chemically to glucose), but myo-inositol is the only one that is biologically active.

Myo-inositol is a constituent of the cells in practically all plant and animal tissues, and is present in these cells in relatively large amounts. In animal cells it occurs primarily as a phospholipid, which is found in highest concentration in skeletal and heart muscle and in the brain. In cereal grains, myo-inositol is present in the complex compound, phytic acid, the organic acid that ties up calcium, zinc, and iron, thereby preventing their absorption.

The physiological function of myo-inositol is still unclear, although it appears to be directly related to the function of phospholipids. The following roles have been suggested for myo-inositol.

1. It is essential for the growth of liver and bone marrow cells.

2. It retards the loss of ascorbic acid in scorbutic guinea pigs.

3. It is involved in the synthesis of RNA.

4. It serves as an intermediary product between carbohydrate and aromatic compounds.

5. Like choline, it has lipotropic properties, but more for the cholesterol- than for the fat-type of fatty livers.

In addition to myo-inositol being a growth factor for some yeasts and fungi, a deficiency will cause growth retardation and loss of hair in young mice, and loss of hair around the eyes in rats. Myo-inositol appears to be required in the diet of the mouse, rat, hamster, and chick, but there is still uncertainty about whether it is merely performing some of the functions of certain B vitamins or whether it is itself an essential metabolic requirement.

Coenzyme Q (ubiquinone)

Coenzyme Q, or ubiquinone, is a collective name for a group of lipidlike compounds that are chemically somewhat similar to vitamin E. These compounds consist of a substituted benzoquinone ring with a long isoprenoid side chain. The large number of biologically active forms of coenzyme Q have between 30 and 50 carbon atoms in the side chain (i.e., 6 to 10 isoprenoid units). The 50-carbon side chain occurs exclusively in mammalian tissues.

Coenzyme Q can be found in most living cells where it seems to be concentrated in the mitochondria. Because it is synthesized in the cell, it cannot be considered a true vitamin. The isoprenoid side chain of ubiquinone is synthesized from acetate or mevalonate, whereas phenylalanine is the precursor of the benzoquinone ring of coenzyme Q.

Because of the ease with which it can be reversibly oxidized and reduced, coenzyme Q is involved in cellular electron transport. It appears to function as an integral link in the respiratory chain in which energy is released to form such high-energy compounds as ATP. Coenzyme Q participates in the oxidation of succinate and reduced NAD, and it may be an integral component of liver aldehyde oxidase.

Ubichromenol, a compound similar to vitamin E in both biological activity and structure, can be formed from ubiquinone. Because ubichromenol has antioxidant properties *in vitro*, it is possible that the vitamin E–like effect of some of the members of the coenzyme Q group of compounds may be related to these properties.

Lipoic acid

Lipoic acid is a fat-soluble compound essential for growth in several species of microorganisms. It can be synthesized by higher animals and for this reason is not considered a vitamin.

The physiological function of lipoic acid is closely associated with that of TPP: both are required for the oxidative decarboxylation of α-keto acids (see page 163). Lipoic acid is concerned with the conversion of the initial decarboxylation product (an aldehyde) to an activated acid. The reduction of the disulfide ring in the lipoic acid molecule brings about the transfer of an acyl group. Lipoic acid thus functions both in dehydrogenation and in the transfer of acyl groups.

Because the body can synthesize the lipoic acid needed for these functions, animals and humans do not require a dietary source of the compound.

Suggested readings

Baker, E. M., Saari, J. C., and Tolbert, B. M. "Ascorbic Acid Metabolism in Man," *American Journal of Clinical Nutrition* **19**(1966):371.

Folkers, K., Smith, J. L., and Moore, H. W. "On the Significance of Biological Activities in the Coenzyme Q and Vitamin E Groups," *Federation Proceedings* **24**(1965):79.

Hodges, R. E., Hood, J., Canham, J. E., Sauberlich, H. E., and Baker, E. M. "Clinical Manifestations of Ascorbic Acid Deficiency in Man," *American Journal of Clinical Nutrition* **23**(1971):432.

Kinsman, R. A., and Hood, J. "Some Behavioral Aspects of Ascorbic Acid Deficiency," *American Journal of Clinical Nutrition* **23**(1971):455.

Olson, R. E. "Anabolism of the Coenzyme Q Family and Their Biological Activities," *Federation Proceedings* **24**(1965):85.

Section IV
THE NUTRITIONALLY IMPORTANT MINERAL ELEMENTS

We come now to the inorganic elements essential to the structure and/or operation of the metabolic machine. Like the vitamins, they can function as structural entities in various parts of the body or as cofactors that activate enzyme systems. Mineral elements, in addition, have general functions that depend on their unique physical or physiochemical properties.

In fulfilling their nonspecific functions, the mineral elements frequently operate in balanced pairs or in small groups; for example, they work in combination to maintain the acid-base balance of body fluid, to regulate the behavior of body gels, and to control the movement by osmosis of body fluids. The collective action of the mineral elements is unique among the nutrients.

The skeleton is composed largely of inorganic material, but the units of the skeleton are vital to both the physiology and the structure of the body: they serve as sites of temporary storage for such regulatory nutrients as calcium, phosphorus, magnesium—nutrients that must be continuously present in critical concentration in the blood or other fluids—as well as being rigid members of a frame that gives the body its shape and motility.

We know less about the roles of those elements needed in trace amounts than about the activities of the other nutritionally important mineral elements, but we are certain that some of these "trace" elements are integral parts of such complicated and essential molecules as hemoglobin and cyanocobalamin. We also know that phosphorus, an essential component of bone, is in fact the very core of the energy transmission system of the metabolic machine (see Section II), and its partner, calcium, activates the ATPase enzyme.

Finally, some inorganic elements are nutrient or toxin depending on circumstances, and others that are toxic may be present in some edible materials and thus accidentally ingested. To understand the nutritional significance of the inorganic nutrient elements and their toxic relatives, it is necessary to consider them individually. This we shall do in the next four chapters.

Chapter 16
Inorganic elements—general

The periodic system lists 104 elements. With the exception of the organically bound elements having a molecular weight of 16 and less (i.e., hydrogen, carbon, nitrogen, and oxygen), all of the elements could be considered in a discussion of the metabolism of the inorganic elements. However, of the 104 elements only a few occur in measurable amounts in the body, and even fewer are known to be of vital importance to the organism.

In discussing the metabolism of the inorganic elements we shall consider only those which occur in measurable amounts in the body. There are less than 40 elements that fall into this category, and most of them have been shown to be either useful or harmful to the organism. We shall deal chiefly with the so-called essential minerals.

Essential mineral elements

An inorganic element is considered to be essential to the body if it meets all of the following criteria.

1. It must be present in fairly constant concentration in the healthy tissues of all living animals, with little variation from one animal to another.

2. Deficiency in the otherwise nutritionally adequate diets of various animal species must result in the development of reproducible structural and/or physiological abnormalities; the diets must contain all other known dietary essentials in adequate amounts and proper proportions, and must be free from toxic properties.

3. Addition of the element to such selectively deficient diets must either prevent or reverse the development of the abnormalities.

4. The abnormalities induced by deficiency must be accompanied by specific biochemical changes that are prevented or reversed when the deficiency is removed.

Each of the elements listed in Table 16.1 has been found to meet these requirements, and therefore is considered essential.

Table 16.1
The essential mineral elements

Macroelements		Trace or microelements	
Principal cations	Principal anions		
Calcium	Phosphorus	Manganese	Cobalt
Magnesium	Chlorine	Iron	Molybdenum
Sodium	Sulfur	Copper	Selenium
Potassium		Iodine	Chromium
		Zinc	Tin
		Fluorine	Nickel
		Vanadium	Silicon

The essentiality of the principal cations and anions is indicated by the elemental composition of the body (see Table 16.2). Ninety-six percent of the body weight consists of the four organically bound elements. The principal cations and anions together account for 3.45% of the body weight, the remainder being composed of trace elements.

The number of essential minerals is believed to be the same for all species, with one exception: cobalt is a necessary dietary inclusion only in the rations of herbivorous animals. This fact raises the question: Do higher organisms actually require cobalt or do they only require it to supply the microflora in the digestive tract who use it as a building unit in their synthesis of vitamin B_{12}?

Table 16.2
Elemental composition of the body of most animals *(by weight)*

Element	Percentage of body weight		Approx. no. of grams in a 70-kg man
Oxygen	65.0		45,500
Carbon	18.0		12,600
Hydrogen	10.0	96	7,000
Nitrogen	3.0		2,100
Calcium	1.5		1,050
Phosphorus	1.0		700
Potassium	0.35		245
Sulfur	0.25	3.45	175
Sodium	0.15		105
Chlorine	0.15		105
Magnesium	0.05		35
Iron	0.004		3
Manganese	0.0003		0.2
Copper	0.0002		0.1
Iodine	0.00004		0.03

SOURCE OF DATA: Hawk, P. B., Oser, B. L., and Summerson, W. H., *Practical Physiological Chemistry* (13th ed.), The Blakiston Co., New York (1947).

Possibly essential mineral elements

The Australian authority on mineral metabolism, E. J. Underwood, has proposed that a limited group of trace elements be categorized as "possibly essential minerals."* As is implied, some evidence has been produced suggesting that the elements falling into this category are required, but this evidence is not sufficient to demonstrate that the elements meet all of the requirements for essentiality. This category is a temporary one; as more information becomes available it should eventually disappear, because the "possibly essential" elements will be classified finally as either essential or nonessential. At present the following elements fall into the category of possibly essential minerals:

> Arsenic   Cadmium
> Barium   Strontium
> Bromine

*Underwood, E. J., *Trace Elements in Human and Animal Nutrition* (3rd ed.), Academic Press, New York (1971).

Potentially toxic mineral elements

Practically any element can be toxic to the body if an animal consumes it in large enough quantities, or for sufficiently long periods. However, the following trace elements are toxic in relatively small quantities, and occur naturally either in foods, in the water supply, or in the air:

(a)	(b)	(c)
Copper	Arsenic	Lead
Molybdenum	Cadmium	Mercury
Selenium		
Fluorine		
Silicon		

It is of interest to note here that the "toxic" minerals in group (a) have already been categorized as "essential," whereas those in group (b) have been categorized as "possibly essential." We must recognize therefore that the same element can be either essential or toxic to the organism, depending on the amount ingested.

Nonessential mineral elements

There are a number of inorganic elements present in measurable amounts in the animal body for which no metabolic role has been found. At present such elements fall into the nonessential category, and it is generally believed that their "normal" presence in the body is incidental to their presence in plant tissues consumed by the animal. The following are the most abundant and important of these nonessential elements:

Aluminum	Germanium	Rubidium
Antimony	Gold	Silver
Bismuth	Lead	Titanium
Boron	Mercury	

Among these are lead and mercury, both highly toxic, and both sometimes accidentally ingested.

The determination of minerals in food

The common method of determining the total inorganic content of a food is very rough. It consists merely of measuring the total ash remaining after combustion of the organic matter. There are two basic reasons why this figure is of little value either for expressing mineral requirements or for indicating the useful mineral content of foods.

In the first place, the body has specific requirements for certain inorganic elements. That is, under defined conditions the body requires specific amounts of elements such as calcium, phosphorus, iron, in order to function normally. Statement of a requirement of 2% ash in the diet is without nutritional meaning; it might be fulfilled by the inclusion of 2% of silicon.

Secondly, ash may not be a true measure of total *inorganic* matter present. For example, if excessive amounts of base-forming minerals are present in a food, organic carbon may be bound as a carbonate and may be determined as such, making it impossible to ascertain whether the mineral was present originally in organic or inorganic combination. Furthermore, some inorganic elements such as sodium, chlorine, and sulfur may be lost during combustion.

Many nutritionists now think that the most important reason for determining the total ash in a given food is to permit calculation of the nitrogen-free extract by difference, as described in the proximate analysis of foodstuffs in Chapter 2.

General functions of minerals

Each of the essential mineral elements serves the body in one or more of *four* different ways:

1. As a constituent of skeletal structures.

2. In maintaining the colloidal state of body matter, and regulating some of the physical properties of colloidal systems (viscosity, diffusion, osmotic pressure).

3. In regulating acid-base equilibrium.

4. As a component or an activator of enzymes and/or other biological units or systems.

Some essential minerals serve the body in only one of these ways; others may serve in all four capacities. As we discuss these elements individually we shall indicate which of the functions each one performs, and thus establish the fundamental reason for its inclusion in a diet or ration.

Skeletal structures. Minerals are crucial constituents of skeletal structures such as bones and teeth. Calcium and phosphorus together account for a high percentage of the inorganic compounds in these structures, and when present in normal amounts give the required rigidity and strength to them. (We shall deal in some detail with bone formation and bone metabolism in Chapter 17.)

Colloidal systems   The animal organism is composed mainly of colloidal systems, the most important of which is protoplasm itself. To understand how minerals act in the maintenance of this state it may be well to review some facts of physical chemistry.

A colloidal system is one in which particles, called the *disperse phase,* are distributed throughout a solvent, called the *dispersion medium.* The differentiation between a true solution and a colloidal solution is made according to particle size. That is, the molecules (or ions) of a true solution are not visible, whereas the particles of a colloidal solution are visible under an ultramicroscope. The disperse phase of a colloidal solution is more or less stable, the stability of the colloidal particles or droplets usually being secured by an outer layer of oriented molecules that gives each particle an electrical charge.

The *interfacial tension* of the surface layer of particles in a colloidal solution is decreased by NaCl but increased by $CaCl_2$. This means that NaCl decreases both the size and the stability of the particles, whereas $CaCl_2$ increases them. Protoplasm and other colloidal solutions can solidify without the separation of water, forming *gels.* This ability to solidify is increased through the action of calcium ions, and counteracted by both sodium and potassium ions.

Thus, *viscosity,* which depends on the state of solidification of a gel, is influenced by the concentration of Ca, Na, and K ions. *Diffusion,* being dependent on particle size, is also regulated by minerals. Osmotic pressure measures the tendency for a solvent (normally water in living organisms) to move through a membrane from a dilute solution into a more concentrated one. Osmotic pressure is inversely proportional to the molecular weight of the solute. Inorganic elements, because they form ions and molecules of low molecular weight, affect osmotic pressure more than an equal weight of large organic molecules. It is through their effect on *osmotic pressure* that the mineral elements become the main regulators of the exchange of water and solutes through the cell walls.

By controlling the flow of water and solutes, minerals play a key role in intestinal absorption and the exchange of water between the blood and both the intercellular and the intracellular fluids. The exchange of sodium and potassium ions across cell membranes is also responsible for the transmission of nerve impulses. Finally, such minerals as calcium, magnesium, sodium, and potassium function in muscle contraction.

Acid-base balance   Inorganic elements help to regulate the acid-base equilibrium in the body. To maintain health—that is, the normal operation of the organism—the pH of the blood and other body fluids must be held within a narrow range. For example, the pH of the blood of a healthy man is 7.4 ± 0.1, and the extremes between which life is possible are 7.0 and 7.8.

The potential acidity or alkalinity of the foods ingested by animals, however, covers a wide range and depends on the minerals present. Certain foods, such as vegetables or fruits, leave on combustion an ash in which the basic elements (Na, K, Ca, Fe, and Mg) predominate; they are therefore known as base-forming foods. Other foods, such as cereals, meat, and fish, leave an ash in which the acid-forming elements (Cl, P, and S) predominate, and these are known as acid-forming foods. Although sulfur is present in foods mainly in neutral form in the sulfur-containing amino acids (methionine, cystine, cysteine), it is nevertheless oxidized in the body to sulfuric acid, and thus is an acid-forming mineral. Therefore, foods containing a large amount of protein are generally acid-forming. Contrary to popular belief, citrus fruits are not acid-forming. They do contain citric acid and acid potassium citrate, but the citrate radicals are completely metabolized in the body, leaving only potassium. Many "acid" fruits therefore are really base-forming foods.

Components or activators of body compounds   Some inorganic elements are known to be components of enzymes or enzyme systems. For example, there are the well-known iron- and copper-containing enzymes, cytochrome oxidase and tyrosinase, respectively. Certain minerals are required for the activiation of enzymes or enzyme systems. Calcium, magnesium, and manganese are of particular significance as enzyme activators.

Other biologically important compounds contain minerals as an inherent part of their structure. For example, the thyroxine and hemoglobin molecules contain iodine and iron, respectively. More will be said about the relationship between the various inorganic elements and enzymes, hormones, and other biological units in the later chapters of this section.

To summarize how the essential minerals function in the body, we can say that they serve either as building units of the skeleton or as regulators of body processes. In the latter capacity they may exert a direct influence on the physiochemical equilibrium of the body and/or they may serve as active units in enzyme or other biologically important systems.

Suggested readings

McCall, J. T., Goldstein, N. P., and Smith, L. H. "Implications of Trace Metals in Human Diseases," *Federation Proceedings* **30**(1971):1011.

Mertz, W. "Some Aspects of Nutritional Trace Element Research," *Federation Proceedings* **29**(1970):1482.

O'Dell, B. L. "Trace Elements in Embryonic Development," *Federation Proceedings* **27**(1968):199.

Underwood, E. J. *Trace Elements in Human and Animal Nutrition* (3rd ed.). Academic Press, New Work (1971).

Wacker, W. E. C. "Metalloenzymes," *Federation Proceedings* **29**(1970):1462.

Chapter 17
Essential macroelements

Calcium and phosphorus

The nutritional role of calcium is closely related to that of phosphorus. We shall therefore consider the two elements together. In addition, because most species utilize calcium and phosphorus in conjunction with vitamin D, we shall describe the function of the vitamin in the metabolism of the minerals.

Calcium and phosphorus together account for over 70% of the total ash in the body. They are the chief elements of the skeleton; 99% of the calcium and about 80% of the phosphorus found in the body are located in the bones and teeth. Because most of the calcium and phosphorus in the body is found in the skeleton, we shall consider briefly the composition, formation, and metabolism of bone.

Composition of bone   The water and fat content of bone is highly variable, and for this reason the composition of bone is often expressed on a dry, fat-free basis. For example, it is known that with advancing age there is a progressive dehydration of the body. This dehydration applies equally to bone. Thus, the fetal bone contains more water than the bone of the very young, and this dehydration of bone progresses into old age. The condition of an animal affects the fat content of its bones. Because deposition of adipose fat occurs in the bone marrow, an obese individual has significantly more fat in the bone than does his lean counterpart. The protein and ash content of bone can also vary, but the prerequisites of variation are relatively drastic conditional changes. The commonly accepted makeup of "normal" bone is shown in Table 17.1.

Table 17.1
The composition of "normal" bone

Component	Fresh basis (%)	Dry, fat-free basis (%)
Water	45	—
Fat	10	—
Protein	20	45
Ash	25	55

The inorganic material of bone consists chiefly of calcium, phosphate, and carbonate, with small amounts of magnesium, sodium, strontium, lead, citrate, fluoride, hydroxide, and sulfate. The more abundant of these substances are present in approximately the following proportions in the bone ash.

$Ca_3(PO_4)_2$ 84% $Mg_3(PO_4)_2$ 1%

$CaCO_3$ 10% $MgCO_3$ 1%

$Ca_3(Citrate)_2$ 2% Na_2HPO_4 2%

The specific inorganic composition of bone is not constant, but despite the wide variations that have been detected chemically, x-ray diffraction studies have revealed only one crystal structure. This is known as the *apatite lattice*. The hexagonal crystals in the lattice are small and consequently offer a large surface that can absorb compounds other than constituents of the crystal lattice itself. The most acceptable theory is that the crystal structure of bone salts is a hydroxy apatite

$$Ca_{10}(PO_4)_6(OH)_2$$

in which fluorine or carbonate can replace the OH, the rest of the components being held by surface forces. In addition, magnesium can replace the calcium without significantly changing the x-ray diffraction pattern.

Regardless of the exact chemical compounds with which we are dealing, the elementary composition of bone is quite constant under normal conditions. In particular, the ratio of calcium to phosphorus by weight does not deviate appreciably from 2:1.

Morphologically, bones of the skeleton are of two kinds. Vertebrae, skull, mandibles, and ribs, referred to as *soft bones,* are rich in areas (spongiosa) from which bone salts are easily and readily withdrawn. On the other hand, the *long bones,* though containing within their shafts relatively spongy areas called trabeculae, consist mainly of cortical bone, a more dense formation which offers greater resistance to mobilization than do regions rich in spongiosa. The trabeculae are presumably temporary mineral depots from which the elements are drawn to maintain the blood levels between dietary intakes. The substance of the soft bones forms a reserve that is mobilized extensively in such conditions as lactation. The shafts of the long bones are probably the last to be sacrificed to meet "operating" needs in the face of a persistent restriction of dietary intake.

Bone formation   The process of bone formation differs somewhat from one bone to another. In general, however, all bone formation is essentially a deposition of mineral elements onto an organic matrix. The exact mechanism of calcification is still not fully understood, but it is probably that dicalcium phosphate ($CaHPO_4$) is central to the process. It is postulated that the events of bone formation, approximately in order of occurrence, are as follows:

1. Dicalcium phosphate aggregates, presumably into submicroscopic particles.

2. Three molecules of dicalcium phosphate condense to form one molecule of tricalcium phosphate, leaving one molecule of phosphoric acid.

3. Tricalcium phosphate is unstable, but such ions as carbonate, fluorine, or hydroxyl quickly attach to it to complete the crystal structure characteristic of the apatite minerals.

4. Further additions to and substitutions in the molecule continue over a long period of time, increasing the stability of the mineral and decreasing its solubility.

The tentative mechanism of calcification is shown in Figure 17.1.

This theory of bone formation explains why bone salt once formed is less soluble than the salts formed in the process of its deposition, and why ready solution of bone salt from bone is negligible, even in the presence of low-ion products in the plasma, unless some mobilizing mechanism comes into action.

Bone metabolism   Evidence from many sources indicates that there is an active metabolism in bone. The labile fraction of bone is reportedly in equilibrium with the plasma, and the stable fraction is in equilibrium with the labile portion.

The rapidity of calcium and phosphorus turnover in the bone is often not appreciated. The exchange of calcium and phosphorus between the bones and the soft tissues proceeds continuously, with about 20% of these elements being exchanged between the two types of tissues annually.

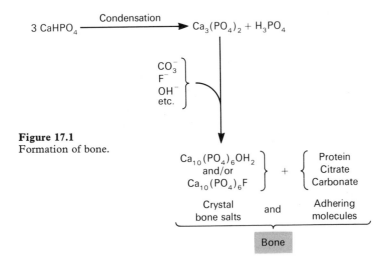

Figure 17.1
Formation of bone.

If the dietary intake of calcium does not meet the requirements of the body, an organism can draw upon its bone reserves, which are stored in the soft bones and in the trabeculae of the long bones.

An organism utilizes bone calcium during periods of stress (i.e., during formation of milk or of fetal bones) through the resorption of entire bone rather than through simple decalcification; both the inorganic and organic components disappear during the process. The exact mechanism for mobilizing calcium from the bone is not completely understood, but it is known to be controlled by the parathyroid hormone (parathormone), and affected by vitamin D. The phosphorus which is released simultaneously with the calcium does not appear to be used to meet the nutritional requirements for phosphorus because it is promptly excreted via the urine.

Osteoporosis   A condition found primarily among middle-aged women, osteoporosis is characterized by a diminution in the absolute amount of bone in the skeleton; the composition of the remaining bone is normal. It is believed that the rate of bone formation in osteoporosis is normal but that bone resorption takes place at an increased rate. The increase in resorption may result from an attempt to maintain the normal level of calcium in the blood despite an inadequate intake of calcium or an abnormally large requirement for calcium caused by faulty absorption. Osteoporosis also results in an inability to reduce the amount of calcium excreted in the urine even when dietary intake is low.

Treatment of the condition by dietary means has proven successful. A diet that contains both a large amount of calcium and sufficient vitamin D can stop bone resorption.

A high incidence of bone fractures accompanies osteoporosis, and the fractures take considerably longer to heal than those in patients with normal bone.

Osteomalacia   In contrast to osteoporosis, osteomalacia is a condition in which the mineral content of the bone is depleted while the absolute amount of bone in the skeleton remains normal. Osteomalacia is found in mature vertebrates exhibiting a continued negative mineral balance. Such a condition may be the result of a suboptimal intake of calcium and phosphorus, a faulty absorption of these elements, an overactive parathyroid, or the special demands for mineral elements created during pregnancy or lactation.

In osteomalacia the bones are gradually weakened. Such bones break easily, and fractures are common in humans as well as in farm animals suffering from the disease. The posterior paralysis of pregnant sows is frequently the result of fracture of a vertebra and a consequent pinching of the spinal cord.

Rickets   Rickets, which occurs only in growing animals, is the result of a subnormal calcification caused by a lack of adequate calcium and/or phosphorus in the diet, a decrease in the ability to absorb these inorganic elements, or a suboptimal intake of vitamin D. The primary trouble in rickets lies in the composition of the blood or the fluid bathing the bone, which is characterized by a low level of calcium and/or phosphorus. Rickets due to a deficiency of calcium is the more prevalent.

Rickets causes an enlargement of the joints and a beading of the ribs from which lameness and stiffness develop. The strains on the bones can cause the misshapen bones seen in chicken breasts, bowed legs in humans, and arching backs in calves.

All growing animals are subject to rickets, and in all cases cures may be effected by dietary measures.

Calcium in soft tissues   Calcium is an essential constituent of all living cells, and the 1% of total body calcium not in the bones and teeth is widely distributed throughout the soft tissues. The greatest concentration, however, is found in the blood; all of the larger animals have 10 mg of calcium per 100 ml of serum.

Part of the calcium in the serum exists as a colloidal calcium-protein salt. This fraction is called nondiffusible calcium, because the colloidal particles are too large to pass through the pores of an organic membrane.

However, about 60% of the calcium in the serum occurs in inorganic bondage as phosphate or bicarbonate. This fraction is called diffusible calcium, and it is of particular significance in nutrition because it is more readily ionized and therefore more available than the colloidal form.

The vital minimum level of calcium in the serum is regulated by the parathyroid hormone, and not by dietary calcium intake. As need arises, parathormone maintains the minimal level of calcium in the serum by mobilizing calcium from the bones.

In addition to increasing the amount of calcium released from bone, parathormone simultaneously stimulates the kidney to resorb more of this calcium and enhances the absorption of calcium from the intestinal tract. When the demand for calcium decreases to normal (e.g., following birth or lactation), the activity of the parathyroid returns to normal as well.

During hypercalcemia, the parathyroid stimulates the thyroid gland to secrete increased quantities of calcitonin. The effect of calcitonin is the opposite of that of parathormone; it serves to decrease the level of calcium in the blood. The central role of the parathyroid gland in maintaining desirable levels of calcium in the blood is obvious.

In addition to initiating the process of blood clotting and activating several important enzymes (see pp. 237–238), the calcium present in soft tissues carries out a number of regulatory functions in the body.

1. In the cell membrane, calcium is closely bound to lecithin where it controls the permeability of the cell membrane and thus regulates the uptake of nutrients by the cell.

2. Calcium stimulates muscle contraction; an excessive amount of calcium in the blood can cause a state of tonic contractions known as calcium rigor, whereas abnormally low levels may result in a state of spasmodic contractions known as tetany.

3. Calcium plays a role in regulating the transmission of nerve impulses from one cell to another through its control over the formation of acetylcholine.

4. Calcium may be an essential component of the physiological mechanism involved in the absorption of vitamin B_{12} from the intestinal tract and the absorption of the vitamin on the cell membrane.

Phosphorus in soft tissues   The 20 percent of the body's phosphorus not in the bones and teeth is, like calcium, widely distributed throughout the soft tissues. There are 35 mg–45 mg of phosphorus per 100 ml of blood. Whereas calcium is concentrated in blood serum, most of the phosphorus is found in the red blood cells in various combinations.

In every 100 ml of blood plasma there are 3 mg–5 mg of inorganic phosphorus. This is the fraction with which we are most concerned when considering an animal's nutritional requirement for phosphorus. The so-called normal level of inorganic phosphorus in blood plasma, however, is subject to rather wide fluctuations not related to dietary intake. Therefore, plasma phosphorus level is useful as a guide to dietary sufficiency only if observed over a long period.

In addition to its function within the osseous tissues, the phosphorus abundantly available in the soft tissues of the body fulfils important functions in several life processes. For example:

1. Phosphorus plays a primary role in carbohydrate metabolism through the formation of hexosephosphates, adenosine phosphates, and creatine phosphate.

2. Phosphorus is active in fat metabolism through the intermediary formation of lecithins.

3. Phosphorus is a constituent of the phospholipids which are present in all tissues, and which are especially abundant in nerve tissues.

4. Phosphorus is present in the nucleoproteins of the chromatin material of cells, and in phosphoproteins such as casein.

5. Phosphates help to regulate the acid-base balance (i.e., neutrality) of the body. For example, the phosphate ion is found in the urine in two forms—the acid phosphate or monobasic ion ($H_2PO_4^-$), and the dibasic ion ($HPO_4^=$); the ratio of these two ions determines in large measure the pH of the urine, because they constitute the major buffer system present.

Absorption of calcium and phosphorus   The efficiency of absorption of these elements is difficult to determine because they are partly re-excreted into the large intestine as endogenous calcium and phosphorus. Apparent digestibility figures are therefore meaningless. The nutritionist is interested in the net absorption (i.e., the amount of these elements that is not excreted via the feces or urine). Net absorption is determined in balance experiments.

The proportion of calcium or phosphorus that appears in the feces as compared to that in the urine depends mainly on the amounts of each in the food. For example, if the dietary calcium intake is high, the percentage of the total excretion taking place via the kidneys will be low, and vice versa.

The absorption of calcium takes place principally in the proximal part of the small intestine, whereas phosphorus is absorbed mainly in the lower part of this organ. The amount of calcium and phosphorus absorbed is difficult to assess because it can be affected by a number of factors.

SOURCE OR FORM IN WHICH INGESTED   In general, the usual inorganic sources of calcium and phosphorus are better utilized than the organic sources of these elements.

In certain foods, such as cereal grains and proteins of vegetable source, 50%–80% of the phosphorus occurs in the form of phytin, which is usually the calcium-magnesium salt of phytic acid (the hexaphosphate ester of inositol). This organic form of phosphorus must be hydrolyzed to inositol and phosphoric acid before it can be utilized. Such hydrolysis is accomplished in the rumen and ruminants are therefore able to utilize this form of phosphorus quite readily. However, in species such as the pig and the chicken, only about 30% of the phosphorus in phytin is considered to be biologically available.

Phytin can be split by the enzyme phytase, which has been identified in several cereal grains. The presence of this enzyme may explain why calcium, magnesium, and phosphorus are more available in leavened than in unleavened breads. Phytase has also been identified in the intestinal mucosa of a number of animal species, including the human; however, there is disagreement about the physiological role of intestinal phytase in making calcium and phosphorus biologically available.

Foods containing oxalic acid may interfere with the absorption of dietary calcium through the formation of insoluble calcium oxalate. Only a few foods are high in oxalic acid. Among them are

Spinach	0.89%	Poke	0.48%
Swiss chard	0.66%	Purslane	0.91%
Beet tops	0.91%	Rhubarb	0.50%

Calcium ingested with diets extremely high in fats may combine to form insoluble calcium soaps. However, because calcium is absorbed in the proximal part of the small intestine, most of the calcium is usually absorbed before the neutral fats are hydrolyzed to their component fatty acids.

Certain other inorganic elements such as iron, aluminum, magnesium, beryllium, and strontium may interfere with phosphorus absorption by forming insoluble phosphates.

THE pH OF INTESTINAL FLUIDS   As already noted, calcium and phosphorus are absorbed at different points in the small intestine; the normal pH of intestinal fluids varies from 6.5 at the duodenum to 7.5 or 8.0 at the ileocaecal valve.

Calcium absorption is facilitated by high gastric acidities and hence by acid-forming foods in general. Dietary lactose also improves the absorbability of calcium. For many years nutritionists thought that this effect is produced by the relatively slow digestion of this disaccharide, leading to its fermentation to lactic acid in the lower intestinal tract. Scientists no longer accept this hypothesis; they now think that the formation of a specific soluble sugar-calcium complex is responsible for the increased absorption.

It is noteworthy that in rickets the reaction of the intestinal contents, as well as of the feces, is usually more alkaline than usual. Rickets does not necessarily follow the occurrence of an alkaline intestinal reaction, however, because rickets has occurred in both acidic and alkaline conditions.

THE RATIO OF CALCIUM TO PHOSPHORUS   If a diet contains an excess of calcium over phosphorus—that is, more calcium than can be absorbed in the first part of the small intestine—free calcium will be present at the points where phosphorus is absorbed. This excess calcium will combine with the phosphorus to form insoluble tricalcium phosphate, and thus interfere with the absorption of phosphorus.

An excess of dietary phosphorus over calcium will in the same way decrease the absorption of both calcium and phosphorus. Therefore the ratio of dietary calcium to phosphorus affects the absorption of both of these elements: an excess of either one impedes absorption. However, the normal

---

Box 17.1   Parturient paresis (milk fever)

One of the most common disturbances associated with lactation in dairy cows is parturient paresis, or milk fever. The disease occurs at the time of parturition and the onset of lactation. It is a metabolic disorder that is characterized by a generalized paralysis, collapse of the circulatory system, and a gradual loss of consciousness. If left untreated the condition frequently results in death. One of the main features of parturient paresis is a sharp decrease in the amount of calcium and inorganic phosphorus in the plasma. The hypocalcemia can vary from mild (7.5 mg/100 ml) to severe (5.0 mg–6.0 mg/100 ml); normal concentrations of calcium in the plasma range from 8.5 mg–11.4 mg/100 ml. The decline in plasma calcium and inorganic phosphorus is more pronounced with advancing age and number of lactations. Milk fever seldom occurs before the third parturition and is most common in high-producing cows.

Parturient paresis represents a failure of the homeostatic mechanisms governing calcium metabolism to adjust to the challenge of the sudden secretion of 13 g–18 g of calcium daily in colostrum or milk, compared to prior fetal needs of only 5 g per day. Although there is a slight decline in the level of calcium in the plasma of a mastectomized cow at parturition, lactation is the main cause of hypocalcemia in parturient cows. Parturient paresis can be successfully treated by the intraveneous infusion of calcium (usually as calcium borogluconate), but treatment is costly and inconvenient. In addition it has been estimated that milk fever can shorten the productive life of a dairy cow by as much as 3.4 years. Thus emphasis has been placed on prevention.

Investigators have reported that the prepartal and immediate postpartal intake of specific nutrients can determine the incidence of parturient paresis. Although there is some correlation between the level of calcium and phosphorus in the prepartal ration and the development of the condition, the relationship does not depend solely on the ratio of Ca:P in the ration. The hypothesis that a

variations that may be encountered in dietary calcium : phosphorus ratios do not have a significant effect on absorption.

DIETARY VITAMIN D   Vitamin D helps to prevent rickets by enhancing the absorption of calcium. The possible mechanism whereby the vitamin functions in this regard (i.e., as an inducer of enzyme synthesis is the intestinal mucosa) has already been outlined in Chapter 14.

OTHER FACTORS   Other less specific factors have also been suggested as being influential in calcium absorption. For example, as the need for calcium

---

prepartum ration low in calcium and high in phosphorus provides protection is based on the theory that such a diet stimulates the secretion of parathormone which in turn initiates the mobilization of bone calcium pre- and immediately postpartum. However, recent findings do not support the "parathyroid insufficiency theory" although the precise relationship of parathormone and other hormones (e.g., epinephrine, ACTH, glucocorticoids, and calcitonin) to calcium homeostasis and the development of parturient paresis is not well understood.

The fact that vitamin D is important in the intestinal absorption of calcium and the mobilization of calcium in bone induced researchers in 1955 to test the effect of feeding dairy cows massive doses of vitamin D (20 to 30 million IU) for a short period prior to parturition. Because of the risk of toxicity from massive doses of vitamin D, agriculturalists have recently begun to use the vitamin D metabolite 25-hydroxycholecalciferol (25-HCC). The discovery that vitamin D must be metabolically activated to carry out its characteristic physiological functions and that 25-HCC acts more rapidly and is metabolized more rapidly than the vitamin resulted in the use of the compound in the prevention and treatment of parturient paresis. Any toxicity produced by the metabolite is readily alleviated by simply stopping treatment. Early experiments were very encouraging, but the results of field studies have been inconclusive. Therefore, although administration of 25-HCC is effective in reducing the incidence of parturient paresis, widespread acceptance of this treatment awaits further testing.

Parturient paresis is a complex disorder that requires a thorough understanding not only of the nutrition and management of dairy cattle, but also of physiology, biochemistry, and endocrinology.

For further information, see *J. Dairy Sci.* **57**(1974):933.

increases during pregnancy and lactation, or during prolonged periods of abnormally low calcium intake, the rate of absorption of the element appears ·to increase. Ingesting a large amount of protein also enhances the absorption of calcium, but because a high-protein diet increases the amount of calcium excreted in the urine, the net effect is a negative calcium balance. Emotional stress, increased gastrointestinal motility, a decrease in the mobility of the body, and aging all appear to decrease the rate of absorption of calcium.

Calcium and phosphorus requirements   Because of the large number of different factors that affect the absorption of calcium and phosphorus, it is difficult to determine accurate and fixed values for the requirements of these elements. In addition, individuals can adjust to a wide range of calcium and phosphorus intakes, in part because the body can adapt to a low intake even though in so doing it diminishes its reserves against periods of stress.

Nevertheless, the following factors have a direct bearing on calcium and phosphorus requirements.

THE RATIO OF CALCIUM TO PHOSPHORUS   From the ratio of calcium to phosphorus in the bone, which is 1.95:1, it is possible to estimate the optimal calcium-to-phosphorus ratio in the diet. For most species the satisfactory range lies between 1:1 and 2:1. Ratios within this range have been found satisfactory for normal calcification of bone and for reproduction.

INTAKE OF VITAMIN D   The ratio of calcium to phosphorus means little unless the amount of vitamin D in the diet is adequate. Rickets can occur not only in animals on a high-calcium–low-phosphorus diet or in those on a low-calcium–high-phosphorus diet, but also in individuals who ingest the normal proportion of calcium and phosphorus without ingesting sufficient vitamin D.

RATE OF GROWTH OF ANIMAL   Experimental studies of calcium and phosphorus requirements often overlook the effect of total food intake on the rate of increase in body weight. Vitamin deficiency symptoms have been shown to occur sooner on deficient diets if food intake is ample. Similarly, calcification of bones is impaired to a greater extent on a rachitongenic diet if food intake is liberal.

Requirements for calcium and phosphorus therefore depend in part on rate of growth and the amount of food ingested. For example, mineral levels sufficient for a daily gain of 0.5 kilogram in hogs may be entirely inadequate for hogs gaining at the rate of 1.0 kilogram per day.

PHYSIOLOGICAL STATE   Infants and adults have a similar absolute requirement for calcium and phosphorus (expressible in mg/day). Growing children, adolescents, and pregnant and lactating females all require more than this amount of these minerals. The daily intake of elderly people should be at least equivalent to that of younger adults; however, because many older people decrease their intake of food, they should consider supplementing the calcium and phosphorus in their diets.

Sources of calcium and phosphate   Foods vary widely in the amount and proportion of calcium and phosphorus they contain (see Table 17.2).

These data reveal the following facts. All cereals are low in total calcium; the outer coating of cereal grains contains most of both their calcium and

Table 17.2
Composition of various foods according to the percentage of calcium and phosphorus and the proportion of calcium to phosphorus they contain (*on a dry basis*)

Food	Ca	P	Ca:P ratio
Barley	0.09	0.47	0.19
Maize	0.04	0.31	0.13
Oats	0.10	0.39	0.26
Rice, brown	0.03	0.22	0.14
Wheat: whole	0.05	0.41	0.12
bran	0.16	1.32	0.12
flour (80% extraction)	0.02	0.19	0.10
Soybean meal (44% protein)	0.36	0.75	0.48
Alfalfa: whole plant	1.72	0.31	5.55
leaves	2.38	0.29	8.21
stems	0.89	0.22	4.04
Asparagus	0.26	0.75	0.35
Spinach	1.00	0.55	1.82
Beans: green, snap	0.56	0.44	1.27
white	0.16	0.48	0.33
Cow's milk: whole	0.91	0.71	1.28
skim	1.38	1.02	1.28
Eggs, less shell	0.19	0.83	0.23
Beef, round	0.04	0.61	0.07
Salmon, canned	0.79	1.05	0.75
Tuna, canned	0.01	0.62	0.02
Oranges, peeled fruit	0.29	0.14	2.07
Peaches	0.08	0.17	0.47

their phosphorus. In the vegetative parts of plants the leaves carry most of the calcium. Leguminous plants are richer in calcium than nonleguminous plants. Milk is an excellent source of both calcium and phosphorus, and skim milk is a better source than whole milk. Eggs are low in calcium but rich in phosphorus. Meats are poor sources of calcium.

The values in Table 17.2 (and in other such tables) are averages; actual mineral content is subject to rather wide variations from sample to sample. For example, the calcium and phosphorus of plant materials, other than seeds, varies with the mineral content of the soil in which they are grown; and the proportion of leaf to stem is also significant. In foods of animal or marine origin, such as fish meal or meat meal, the proportion of bone to flesh materially affects the amount of calcium.

If a diet is low in calcium or phosphorus, these elements are added usually in the form of inorganic salts. In animal rations the calcium and phosphorus supplements commonly used are equivalent, per unit of element contained. The average composition of a few of these products is shown in Table 17.3.

Table 17.3
Percentage of calcium and phosphorus in a few common supplementary sources of these elements (*on a dry basis*)

Product	Calcium	Phosphorus
Raw bone meal	27.3	13.0
Steamed bone meal	30.5	14.3
Dicalcium phosphate	23.1	18.7
Rock phosphate	32.0	18.0
Defluorinated phosphates	33.1	18.0
Ground limestone	33.8	—
Oyster shells	38.0	—

Depraved appetite in cattle   A deficiency of phosphorus in the ration of cattle can produce "pica," or "depraved appetite," which is one of the first effects of phosphorus deficiency. The animals thus affected chew bones, wood, hair, rocks, etc., have a rough hair coat, and become emaciated.

A possible secondary effect of bone chewing is death from botulism from bones infected with *Clostridium botulinum*. Other infections due to the consumption of putrid material in an effort to satisfy the depraved appetite are the "loin disease" of cattle in Texas, and "lamsiekte" of sheep and cattle in South Africa.

Pica is not specifically indicative of a phosphorus deficiency. It can also be produced by deficiencies of copper, cobalt, or even iron. Indeed, it can be unrelated to diet. However, if calves are not affected but the cows are, a phosphorus deficiency is the likely cause.

Calcium–thrombin relationship Calcium is essential to the process of blood clotting through its relationship to thrombin. Thrombin is the complex that clots fibrinogen. Thromboplastin catalyzes the conversion of prothrombin, anormal constituent of the blood, to thrombin. Calcium stimulates the release of thromboplastin from the blood platelets. Thus calcium is needed to initiate a series of reactions that culminates in the formation of a blood clot (see Figure 17.2).

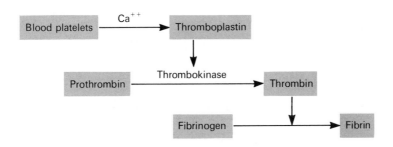

Figure 17.2
Role of calcium in blood clotting.

Calcium–enzyme relationships An important function of calcium, often obscured by its role in the formation of skeletal tissue, is as an activator of several important enzymes.

ESTERASES Pancreatic lipase. The lipase in pancreatic juice is the most important fat-splitting enzyme in the digestive tract. It hydrolyzes the neutral fats in the food into fatty acids and β-monoglyceride. Calcium activates this enzyme:

$$\text{Tripalmitin} + 2H_2O \xrightarrow{\substack{\text{Pancreatic} \\ \text{lipase}}} 2 \text{ Palmitic acid} + \beta\text{-monoglyceride}$$

ACID PHOSPHATASE After phosphorylation, glucose becomes available for glycogen formation, reconversion to glucose, breakdown to lactic acid anaerobically, or complete oxidation aerobically. Reconversion to glucose is controlled by the enzyme phosphatase, which catalyzes the hydrolysis of glucose-6-phosphate to glucose and inorganic phosphate. Calcium activates this enzyme:

$$\text{Glucose-6-phosphate} \xrightarrow{\substack{\text{Acid} \\ \text{phosphatase}}} \text{Glucose} + \text{Phosphate}$$

CHOLINESTERASE   Brain tissue contains an enzyme, choline acetylase, which promotes the synthesis of acetylcholine from choline and acetic acid. Acetylcholine plays an important role in the chemical transmission of nervous impulses.

$$\text{Choline} + \text{Acetic acid} \xrightarrow{\text{Choline acetylase}} \text{Acetylcholine}$$

Physiological control over the excessive accumulation of acetylcholine constantly being produced by normal nerve impulses appears to be accomplished by the enzyme cholinesterase, which catalyzes the hydrolysis of acetylcholine into the relatively inert compounds, choline and acetic acid:

$$\text{Acetylcholine} \xrightarrow{\text{Cholinesterase}} \text{Choline} + \text{Acetic acid}$$

Calcium diminishes the amount of acetylcholine formed, apparently by activating the enzyme cholinesterase; it is possible, however, that calcium acts conversely by inhibiting the enzyme choline acetylase. Whichever is the case, the action of calcium in inhibiting the formation of acetyl choline explains one of the major functions of the mineral in the soft tissues of the body: decreasing the irritability of cells.

ATPASES   Hydrolysis of adenosine triphosphate (ATP) is effected by ATPases which split the terminal pyrophosphate linkage, yielding adenosine diphosphate and inorganic phosphate:

$$\text{ATP} \xrightarrow{\text{ATPase}} \text{ADP} + P_i$$

At least two such enzymes occur in muscle: myosin ATPase and actomyosin ATPase. The former is activated by calcium and inhibited by magnesium; the latter is activated by magnesium and inhibited by calcium.

SUCCINIC DEHYDROGENASE   In the citric acid cycle (see Chapter 11), succinic acid is oxidized to fumaric acid:

$$\text{Succinic acid} \xrightarrow{\text{Succinic dehydrogenase}} \text{Fumaric acid} + 2H$$

This reaction is accomplished by the enzyme succinic dehydrogenase which is activated by calcium.

Phosphorus–enzyme relationship   Unlike calcium, phosphorus is not known to activate or inhibit any enzyme. However, phosphorus can be an integral part of an enzyme. For example, pepsin, the proteinase of gastric juice, contains phosphorus, and the yellow enzymes (Warburg's yellow enzyme, xanthine-oxidase, and others) contain phosphorus in their prosthetic group.

Magnesium

The distribution of magnesium in the animal body is similar to the distribution of phosphorus. About 60% of the body's magnesium is found in the skeleton. The remaining 40% is scattered throughout the body fluids. Next to potassium, magnesium is the most plentiful cation of the intracellular fluids. Blood serum contains 1 mg–3 mg of magnesium per 100 milliliters.

Muscle tissue contains more magnesium than calcium. In blood, where the reverse is true, the magnesium content is very constant. This is also true of the body as a whole; the concentration of magnesium remains at about 0.05% during growth, whereas the percentage of both calcium and phosphorus usually increases.

Absorption and excretion of magnesium   Magnesium is absorbed from the small intestine, and like calcium and phosphorus it may be re-excreted in considerable amounts by the intestinal mucosa lower in the tract. Hence, net absorption is the only valid estimation of its effective utilization.

Magnesium is excreted in both the feces and urine, but its major output is in the feces which normally contain 65% or more of the magnesium excreted. Excessive intakes of magnesium give rise to increased excretion of calcium in the urine, and excessive intakes of calcium result in increased excretion of magnesium in the urine.

Symptoms of magnesium deficiency   Like calcium, magnesium depresses nervous irritability, but to an even greater extent. Diets extremely low in magnesium will cause the level of magnesium in the serum to drop as low as 0.5 mg per 100 ml, and the following sequence of conditions will occur if the dietary insufficiency is not rectified:

1. Vasodilation, resulting in a reduction in blood pressure (manifested outwardly by a flushing of the skin).

2. Hyperirritability.

3. Tetany, followed by death.

In spite of the marked drop in the amount of magnesium in the serum of individuals suffering from a dietary deficiency, the levels of calcium and phosphorus in the blood remain normal. Because a low level of calcium in the serum also produces tetany, the condition caused by insufficient magnesium in the serum is distinguished from the usual tetany as "magnesium-tetany." Magnesium-tetany has been found both in children and in calves fed milk alone for extended periods or fed milk plus a magnesium-deficient supplement.

A disease of cattle called "grass-tetany" or "grass staggers" is associated with a magnesium deficiency. The condition has been noted primarily in dairy cattle shortly after calving and subsisting on good pasture. Nervousness, muscle twitching, and, finally, convulsions occur; and fatalities are usually high. In grass-tetany the calcium content, as well as the magnesium content, of the blood serum is low.

Magnesium and calcium interrelationships   The intravenous injection of magnesium causes large urinary losses of calcium. Therefore the question arises whether a high dietary intake of magnesium will have a deleterious effect on calcium assimilation. Recent studies have indicated that when magnesium is *ingested* instead of *injected* it does not enter in excessive amounts into the bloodstream because of selective absorption. In fact, in experiments with pigs, chickens, and rats it has been shown that dolomitic limestone is a satisfactory source of calcium for bone formation, despite its high magnesium content.

The relationship of magnesium and calcium in bone formation is emphasized by the fact that magnesium can be substituted for calcium in the apatite structure without significantly changing the x-ray diffraction pattern.

Sources of magnesium   Most leafy vegetables and cereal grains are rich sources of magnesium, whereas milk and animal products are much poorer sources. Table 17.4 illustrates this divergence in the magnesium content of various foods.

Table 17.4
Magnesium content of
some foods (*in mg/100 g*)

Food	Magnesium
Beef, lean	24
Eggs	11
Milk, cow's	12
Milk, human	4
Peas	140
Spinach	97
Corn	121
Wheat	165
Soybeans	210

Magnesium–enzyme relationships Magnesium activates many enzyme systems, particularly those concerned in carbohydrate metabolism. Magnesium is also capable of inactivating certain enzymes, and is known to be a component of at least one enzyme.

KINASES The enzymes that catalyze the transfer of the terminal phosphate of ATP to sugar or other acceptors are named by adding the suffix "kinase" to the name of the particular acceptor (e.g., hexokinase for the enzyme that phosphorylates hexoses). Most kinases require magnesium for their activation.

MUTASES The suffix "mutase" designates those transphosphorylations that occur at a low energy level, and in which the end result appears to be a molecular rearrangement (e.g., phosphoglucomutase). Mutases also appear to require magnesium for their activation.

ATPASES As already noted, at least two such enzymes occur in muscle: myosin ATPase and actomyosin ATPase. The former is activated by calcium and inhibited by magnesium; the latter is activated by magnesium and inhibited by calcium.

CHOLINESTERASE We have mentioned previously that calcium activates the enzyme cholinesterase. Magnesium has been found to be capable of activating this enzyme as well. Thus, the role of calcium and magnesium in reducing cell irritability appears to be associated with their common influence on acetylcholine.

ALKALINE PHOSPHATASE Alkaline phosphatase is found in ossifying cartilage and bone, in the kidneys, and in intestinal mucosa. In cartilage and bone and in the kidneys it can act as an esterase by hydrolyzing hexose phosphates and glycerophosphate. In the intestinal mucosa alkaline phosphatase acts as a nuclease. In either case, magnesium has been shown to activate alkaline phosphatases.

ENOLASE In the chain of reactions that produces pyruvic acid from glucose, an enzyme, enolase, plays a significant role. Enolase is a hydrase which dehydrates 2-phosphoglyceric acid to phosphopyruvic acid; it must be activated by magnesium to function normally.

ISOCITRIC DEHYDROGENASE In one stage of the citric acid cycle (see Chapter 11), isocitric acid is oxidized to α-ketoglutaric acid.

$$\text{Isocitric acid} \xrightarrow{\text{Isocitric dehydrogenase}} \alpha\text{-ketoglutaric acid} + 2H$$

This reaction is catalyzed by the enzyme isocitric dehydrogenase, which can be activated by magnesium.

ARGINASE Metalloproteins are protein enzymes that contain inorganic elements as components of their molecules. The metalloprotein arginase is responsible for the splitting of the amino acid arginine to ornithine and urea. The inorganic element contained in the arginase molecule is magnesium.

OTHER ENZYMES Magnesium can also activate other less well-known enzymes such as deoxyribonuclease, leucine aminopeptidase, and glutaminase; it inhibits the enzyme ribonuclease.

Sodium, potassium, and chlorine

Sodium, potassium, and chlorine occur almost entirely in the fluids and soft tissues of the body, sodium and chlorine being found chiefly in the body fluids, and potassium occurring mainly in the cells. They serve a vital function in controlling osmotic pressures and acid-base equilibrium. They also play important roles in water metabolism.

All three elements are closely related metabolically. Both sodium and potassium ions occur in the body mainly in close association with the chloride ion, and therefore a sodium or potassium deficiency is rarely found in the absence of a chlorine deficiency.

Sodium The adult human body contains about 100 g of sodium, over half of which is distributed in the extracellular fluids (i.e., plasma, interstitial fluids). The remainder of the body's sodium is found in the skeleton. Within the cells, sodium is present in relatively low concentration, being replaced largely by the cations potassium and magnesium. Generally, attempts to alter the sodium content of the blood by reducing the intake of the mineral have been ineffective; body growth ceases, but the composition of the blood does not change.

Sodium is rapidly absorbed from the small intestine, but apparently some absorption also takes place from the stomach. Practically all of the ingested sodium (85%–90%) is excreted via the urine as chlorides and phosphates. The ratio of potassium to sodium in the urine is generally about 3:5.

Experiments with rats have shown that a sodium deficiency will adversely affect appetite, normal increase in weight, storage of energy, and the synthesis of both fat and protein.

The major functions of the sodium ion in the animal body appear to be connected with the regulation of osmotic pressure and the maintenance of acid-base balance. In addition, the sodium ion has an effect on irritable tissues such as muscle, which does not appear to be related to osmotic forces, and which is counteracted by the presence of the calcium ion in the proportion of about 1 or 2 calcium ions to 100 sodium ions. This, at least in part, is the basis for restricting dietary salt in cases of hypertension and cardiac disease.

Sodium plays a specific role in the absorption of carbohydrate; the sodium ion promotes the absorption of glucose against a concentration gradient (see Chapter 7).

Most animal tissues contain a large amount of sodium whereas plant foods are deficient. Although low in sodium, plants are usually high in potassium, and the ingestion of plant material causes an increase in the amount of sodium excreted via the urine.

There are no known sodium–enzyme relationships that are of significance in the animal body.

Potassium   Potassium, like sodium, is present in tissues only as the potassium ion. The adult human body contains about 250 g of potassium, almost entirely within the cells rather than in the extracellular fluids. In fact, potassium is the most plentiful cation of the intracellular fluids.

Potassium is absorbed primarily from the small intestine, and excreted in the urine.

Growth in rats may be retarded by restricting the daily intake of potassium. In humans a deficiency of potassium causes weakness and muscular paralysis accompanied by a fall in the level of potassium in the plasma. In other animals hypertrophy of the heart and kidneys has been noted.

By regulating intracellular osmotic pressures and acid-base balance, potassium apparently fulfills, in the cells, the same general functions sodium carries out in the extracellular fluids of the body. The potassium ion has a stimulating effect on muscular irritability, which, like that of sodium, tends to oppose the effect of the calcium ion. Nevertheless, under conditions created by the severe dietary restriction of salt, calcium appears to be important in supporting the minimal essential potassium content of body tissues.

Via mechanisms that are not clear at this time, the potassium ion takes part in the metabolism of both carbohydrates and proteins. For example, both the formation of glycogen and the breakdown of glucose require potassium. Protein synthesis also requires this ion.

The amount of potassium in the body correlates with lean body mass. This knowledge forms the basis for calculating lean body mass *in vivo* by determing how much radioactive potassium 40 is present in the body; because the ratio of potassium 40 to total body potassium is constant, it is possible to calculate the total potassium content and use that figure to estimate lean body mass.

The abundance of potassium in both plant and animal foods precludes the danger of a deficiency of this element in a mixed diet.

POTASSIUM ENZYME RELATIONSHIP   Pyruvic acid kinase is one of the kinase enzymes that requires magnesium for its activation. However, it appears that it requires potassium as well, which means that it takes two inorganic elements to activate this enzyme.

Chlorine   Like sodium and potassium, chlorine is found in biological material exclusively in ionic form. The adult human body contains approximately 100 g of chlorine; most of it is found in the extracellular fluids of the body, but it is present to some extent in red blood cells and to a lesser extent in the cells of other tissues.

This element is absorbed chiefly from the small intestine. Chlorine present in excessive amounts in the diet is excreted via the urine. Excreted chlorine is usually accompanied by excess sodium or potassium, unless the body has a need to conserve base, in which case the ammonium ion accompanies the chloride ion.

Chlorine is essential to the regulation of osmotic pressure, constituting about two-thirds of the total anions of blood plasma and making up a similar fraction of the other extracellular fluids of the body. Although a close relationship exists between chlorine and sodium in certain physiological processes, the chloride ion has functions that are peculiar to it, and that are essentially independent of the functions of the sodium ion.

For example, chlorine is the chief anion of gastric juice, being present in approximately the same concentration as in the blood. In gastric juice it is accompanied by the hydrogen rather than the sodium ion, as in plasma and other extracellular fluids of the body. Another specific function of the chloride ion is in the "chloride-shift" in the blood during the transport of carbon dioxide; the bicarbonate (HCO_3) content of the blood plasma is significantly increased by exchange with plasma chloride, the latter entering the red blood cells.

No chlorine–enzyme relationships have been definitely established, although chlorine may have some bearing on the activity of salivary amylase.

Salt (NaCl)   Salt, being a condiment, is frequently consumed in great excess of body requirements. The ability of the body to adapt itself to wide ranges of salt intake is shown by the fact that the human kidney can excrete as little as 1 g or as much as 40 g of salt per day, depending on intake. With normal kidneys and adequate water intake, the body can tolerate a large intake of salt, but in animals previously salt starved, large and sudden intakes of salt may prove toxic. Sodium toxicity appears to be more common if excess sodium is accompanied by a deficiency of potassium. Excessive salt intakes result in water retention in the body, causing edema.

A continuous excessively low intake of salt can have adverse effects on health, indicated by loss of appetite and weight, and concentration of blood with resulting retention of nitrogenous waste products. A deficiency of salt is found more often in herbivora than in other animals because forages and grains are relatively low in salt content. A deficiency can occur in humans as a consequence of losses through excessive sweating. In sweat, both NaCl and KCl are lost as well as water. It is not sufficient to replace the liquid losses in sweating with pure water—the salt losses also have to be replaced. However, after the body becomes acclimatized to heat, the sodium content of sweat is greatly reduced, and the allowance for salt can be nearly normal.

Sulfur

The sulfur of the body occurs almost entirely in organic compounds, notably in proteins in which it is present as cystine and methionine. Of the total sulfur content of whole blood, a portion is present as the inorganic sulfate ion; another portion is in the form of various organic compounds that may be present, most of which are found in the red blood cells (e.g., insulin, glutathione); and the remainder is found in the sulfur-containing amino acids present in the blood.

The sulfate that is excreted in the urine arises principally from oxidation of the sulfur of protein within the body; a relatively small amount comes from ingested sulfates. The sulfate ion is excreted with greater difficulty than any other inorganic radical ordinarily present in normal blood. A retention of 30 times the normal blood value has been observed.

Strictly speaking, the metabolism of sulfur does not belong under the heading of inorganic element metabolism, because only an insignificant part of that ingested is in inorganic form. Inorganic sulfur is ineffective in satisfying body requirements.

Nevertheless, a small amount of inorganic sulfur in the diet of ruminants can improve their ability to utilize urea as a source of nitrogen. However, inorganic sulfur can be dangerous if ingested in large amounts. It appears that, through the action of the microflora in the digestive tract of ruminants, H_2S is produced which is easily absorbed and capable of causing disturbances.

Sulfur–enzyme relationships   Sulfur is not known to activate any enzyme. However, because enzymes are proteins, many of them contain sulfur-containing amino acids.

Sulfur in other biological units   Insulin, taurine, condroitin, heparin, fibrinogen, and glutathione, all compounds of biological significance in the body, are known to contain sulfur. The importance of the sulfur in the regulatory systems of which these compounds are a part seems to stem from the reversible oxidation of the sulfhydryl group to the disulfide group:

$$(-SH) \rightleftharpoons (-S-S-)$$

Sulfur is also a component of two B vitamins—thiamin and biotin—and of lipoic acid.

Suggested readings

Benson, J. D., Emery, R. S., and Thomas, J. W. "Effects of Previous Calcium Intakes on Adaptation to Low and High Calcium Diets in Rats," *Journal of Nutrition* **97**(1969):53.

Braithwaite, G. D., and Riazuddin, S. "The Effect of Age and Level of Dietary Calcium Intake on Calcium Metabolism in Sheep," *British Journal of Nutrition* **26**(1971):215.

Briscoe, A. M., and Ragan, C. "Effect of Magnesium on Calcium Metabolism in Man," *American Journal of Clinical Nutrition* **19**(1966):296.

Care, A. D. "Significance of the Thyroid Hormones in Calcium Homeostasis," *Federation Proceedings* **27**(1968):153.

Council on Foods and Nutrition. "Symposium on Human Calcium Requirements," *Journal of the American Medical Association* **185**(1963):122.

Forbes, R. M. "Mineral Utilization in the Rat. I. Effects of Varying Dietary Ratios of Calcium, Magnesium and Phosphorus," *Journal of Nutrition* **80**(1953):321.

Kellogg, W. W., Cadle, R. D., Allen, E. R., Lazrus, A. L., and Mantell, E. A. "The Sulfur Cycle," *Science* **175**(1972):587.

Leitch, I. "The Determination of the Calcium Requirements of Man," *Nutrition Abstracts and Reviews* **6**(1937):553; **8**(1938):1.

Newman, W. F., and Newman, M. W. *The Chemical Dynamics of Bone Mineral.* University of Chicago Press, Chicago (1958).

O'Dell, B. L. "Magnesium Requirement and Its Relation to Other Dietary Constituents," *Federation Proceedings* **19**(1960):648.

Peeler, H. T. "Biological Availability of Nutrients in Feeds: Availability of Major Mineral Ions," *Journal of Animal Science* **35**(1972):695.

Pike, R. L., and Gursky, D. S. "Further Evidence of Deleterious Effects Produced by Sodium Restriction during Pregnancy," *American Journal of Clinical Nutrition* **23**(1970):883.

Reddy, B. S. "Calcium and Magnesium Absorption: Role of Intestinal Microflora," *Federation Proceedings* **30**(j1971):1815.

Schofield, F. A., and Morrell, E. "Calcium, Phosphorus, and Magnesium," *Federation Proceedings* **19**(1960):1014.

Seelig, M. S. "The Requirement of Magnesium by the Normal Adult," *American Journal of Clinical Nutrition* **14**(1964):342.

Tadayyon, B., and Lutwak, L. "Interrelationships of Triglycerides with Calcium, Magnesium, and Phosphorus in the Rat," *Journal of Nutrition* **97**(1969):246.

Taylor, T. G. "The availability of the Calcium and Phosphorus of Plant Materials for Animals," *Proceedings of the Nutrition Society* **24**(1965):105.

Wacker, W. E. C. "Magnesium Metabolism," *Journal of the American Dietetic Association* **44**(1964):362.

Wasserman, R. H. "Calcium and Phosphorus Interactions in Nutrition and Physiology," *Federation Proceedings* **19**(1960):636.

Chapter 18
Essential trace elements

In the mid-1950s seven trace elements were known to be essential: manganese, iron, copper, iodine, zinc, cobalt, and molybdenum. By the mid-1970s this number had been doubled by the addition of fluorine, selenium, tin, chromium, vanadium, silicon, and nickel. Obviously, dramatic progress in the area of bioinorganic chemistry has replaced that associated with vitamin and amino acid metabolism that characterized the first two-thirds of the twentieth century. Progress in this field can be attributed to improved analytical procedures for trace elements and the introduction of ultraclean isolator techniques.

Manganese

Manganese is found in fairly constant amounts in both plant and animal tissues. The small amounts of manganese in the animal body, 12 mg–20 mg in a 70 kg man, are concentrated primarily in the bone, although significant amounts are also present in the liver, muscle, and skin.

In addition to interfering with normal growth, a deficiency of the element frequently affects skeletal development, resulting in shortened and often deformed limbs. As long ago as 1936, it was discovered that perosis (or slipped tendon) in poultry is the result of a lack of manganese in the ration.

Using laboratory animals and pigs as subjects, researchers have shown that manganese is essential for normal reproduction in mammals. In females, late sexual maturity, irregular ovulation, and weak young at birth are characteristic results of a low-manganese diet. In males, sterility due to testicular degeneration follows the ingestion of such diets.

No deficiency of this trace element occurs in any normal human diet.

Absorption and excretion   Relatively little is known about the precise mechanism of absorption of manganese from the gastrointestinal tract, although it is recognized that an excess of either dietary calcium or phosphorus reduces the availability of the trace elements.

The chief channel of excretion of manganese is through the liver into the bile. Excretion takes place as well via the pancreatic juice into the small intestine. The concentration of manganese in the various body tissues is quite stable under normal conditions; this has been attributed to well-controlled excretion rather than to regulated absorption.

Manganese–enzyme relationships   Manganese activates enzymes *in vitro*; this is not a specific property of manganese, however, because other bivalent ions, such as magnesium, fulfill the same role under these conditions.

The first identification of a specific physiological function for manganese was by R. M. Leach and A. M. Muenster, who demonstrated that the element takes part in the synthesis of the mucopolysaccharides of cartilage by acting as a catalyst on glucosamine–serine linkages.* Another biochemical role for manganese became evident when investigators found that pyruvate carboxylase contains the trace element and that through this enzyme, manganese functions in the transcarboxylation phase of the enzyme reaction.

A further role for manganese in carbohydrate metabolism was demonstrated when G. S. Everson and R. E. Shrader showed that the trace element functions in the utilization of glucose.†

There is also evidence of a manganese–arginase relationship; in both rats and rabbits, the activity of liver arginase is reduced as a result of manganese deficiency.

Manganese in lipid metabolism   Supplementing manganese-deficient diets with either manganese or choline reduces the amount of both liver and bone fat in rats; supplementing similarly deficient rations with just manganese reduces fat deposition and back fat in pigs. However, neither the choline–manganese interaction nor the lipotropic action of the trace element is clearly understood.

---

*Leach, R. M., Jr., and Muenster, A. M., *J. Nutrition* **78**(1962):51.

†Everson, G. J., and Shrader, R. E., *J. Nutrition* **94**(1968)89:269.

Iron

Iron is present in the body in small amounts. In an adult man there are about 4 g–5 g of iron, 70% of which is found in hemoglobin. The remaining 30% is found chiefly in the liver, to some extent in the spleen and bone marrow, in plasma where it is practically all bound to the blood protein transferrin, and as a constituent of various oxidation-reduction enzymes essential for the life of cells in general.

In hemoglobin, iron is found in the heme portion of the molecule:

$$\text{Hemoglobin} \xrightarrow{\text{Hydrolysis}} \text{Globin (96\%)} + \text{Heme (4\%)}$$

Myoglobin, an iron-containing compound in muscle, differs from hemoglobin only in the nature of the protein component of the molecule.

The iron in the liver, spleen, and bone marrow is a component of two compounds—ferritin and hemosiderin. Ferritin is a soluble iron–protein complex containing up to 20% iron; hemosiderin is an insoluble iron–protein complex that can contain up to 35% iron. Iron is drawn equally well from both of these compounds for erythropoiesis and for the placental transfer of iron to the fetus.

Absorption and excretion   Iron is absorbed primarily from the small intestine, although some may be absorbed from the stomach. Dietary iron appears to be absorbed in nutritionally significant amounts only when it is in the inorganic form, and ferrous iron is more available for absorption than ferric iron. Hence the presence of any reducing substance (e.g., ascorbic acid) augments the ability to absorb iron.

There is good evidence that the absorption of iron is influenced by the state of the body's iron stores. Dietary iron appears to pass into the epithelial cells of the intestinal lining as a chelate with such carbohydrates as fructose or sorbitol or some amino acids. The rate at which iron is released from the epithelial cells to the general circulation depends upon the state of transferrin in the plasma. If the transferrin is relatively saturated with respect to its iron-binding capacity, little iron is absorbed from the cells. However, if there is a relatively large quantity of unbound transferrin, the amount of iron released from the epithelial cells increases. Therefore, when the iron in transferrin achieves equilibrium with the iron reserves present in ferritin, absorption drops to a minimum. The body's need for iron thus affects the absorption of the element from the gastrointestinal tract.

Iron can be absorbed rapidly, appearing in the red blood cells in about four hours after ingestion. However, it takes about a week for the complete conversion of absorbed iron into hemoglobin. Once absorbed, iron is tenaciously held by the body, and only very small amounts are excreted. This means that the iron requirement of an adult is small, except for replacing blood losses.

Iron is excreted in the urine at the rate of only 1 mg–3 mg per day. Greater amounts are found in the feces, but this probably represents, for the most part, unabsorbed iron from dietary sources. Sweat is also an important excretory route.

Iron released by the normal destruction of red blood cells can be used again to form hemoglobin, almost without loss.

Consequences of iron deficiency   Anemia is the well-known result of a deficiency of iron. In anemia the number of red blood cells is reduced; in addition changes in cell size and in the hemoglobin content of the cells can occur.

There are several causes of anemia. Anemias of hereditary, pathological, and nutritional origin are known. Nutritional anemia can occur at any time of life, though it is more likely to develop during the suckling period of mammals when milk, which is extremely low in iron, is the major or only component of the diet. Normally young mammals are born with a reserve of iron sufficient to last throughout their nursing period, or at least until food other than milk is consumed. The piglet has a 3–4 day store of iron, and the human infant a 5–6 month store. Since calves, foals, and lambs begin to eat grass or hay shortly after birth, no nutritional iron problem arises.

Nutritional anemia due to iron deficiency occurs in human babies and piglets if:

1. The maternal diet during gestation is deficient in iron, causing the newborn to have an insufficient store of the element; feeding iron to the lactating female is of no use, because such treatment does not increase the iron content of the milk.

2. Premature birth occurs, which results in a smaller iron store than normal; the iron content of the fetus is increased mainly during the last trimester of pregnancy.

3. The number of newborn is abnormally high; multiple births in humans or large litters in pigs result in a reduced supply of iron to each of the young.

In both species, anemia due to iron deficiency can be prevented in sucklings by feeding or injecting iron. Because newborn pigs have an extremely small store of iron at birth and because they consume only a small quantity of dry diet before three to four weeks of age, it is usually necessary to administer iron to young pigs. Many animal breeders use iron dextran, and inject baby pigs with this compound at least during the first week of life.

An iron deficiency in sheep and cattle can cause a depraved appetite (pica) much like that due to a deficiency of phosphorus. It is characterized by diarrhea, loss of appetite for normal foods, and anemia.

Metabolic functions of iron   Iron is an essential constituent of the respiratory pigment, hemoglobin. It also plays a role in cellular oxidations, being a component of certain enzymes concerned with the transfer of electrons ($Fe^{++} \rightleftharpoons Fe^{++}$). (See iron–enzyme relationships described below.)

Sources of iron   Table 18.1 lists the total content of iron in a few foods. The iron in these foods is not equally available to all species, but in general, the iron of leafy plants is relatively inaccessible, whereas most of the iron in inorganic sources is readily available.

Table 18.1
Iron content of some foods (*in mg/100g*)

Food	Iron content
Blood	50.0
Dry yeast	35.0
Beef liver	8.0
Spinach (fresh)	3.6
Eggs	3.0
Beef muscle	2.5
White flour (nonenriched)	1.0
Milk	0.25

Animals can utilize sulfate, chloride, citrate, and fumarate salts far better than oxide and carbonate salts. In general, the greater the solubility of an iron salt the greater its potential utilization by the body.

Iron–enzyme relationships

CYTOCHROMES   Iron is a component of cytochrome oxidase, the enzyme that oxidizes reduced cytochrome c, and of cytochrome c itself.

HYDROPEROXIDASES   Hydroperoxidases is the name proposed to include both catalases and peroxidases. In general, catalases prevail in animals and peroxidases in plants, but there are many exceptions. Nevertheless, iron is a component of both the catalase and peroxidase molecules.

Catalases: The overall formula of the reaction catalyzed by catalases is

$$2H_2O_2 \xrightarrow{\text{Catalase}} 2H_2O + O_2$$

The release of oxygen gas from H_2O_2 is the spectacular feature of this reaction.

Peroxidases: The overall formula of the reaction catalyzed by peroxidases is

$$H_2O_2 + Acceptor \cdot 2H \xrightarrow{\text{Peroxidases}} 2H_2O + Acceptor$$

No oxygen is evolved; instead, an acceptor is oxidized.

XANTHINE AND ALDEHYDE OXIDASE   These enzymes contain iron in addition to molybdenum and FAD.

SUCCINIC DEHYDROGENASE   This is another of the so-called heme enzymes and hence contains iron as an integral part of its structure.

Copper

Copper and iron are sometimes considered together because of their similar properties and joint importance in the formation of hemoglobin. Like iron, copper is stored in the liver; to a lesser extent it is found as well in the brain, bone marrow, spleen, heart, and kidney. Whereas iron is an essential constituent of hemoglobin, copper is not a part of this molecule; rather its relation to the formation of hemoglobin appears to be in promoting the maturation of red blood cells and in increasing their survival time.

Because of this relationship, anemia can result from a copper deficiency as well as from an iron deficiency. If iron salts are given to prevent anemia, copper as such need seldom be given since it is normally present in sufficient amounts as an impurity of the iron salts. The requirement for copper is only between one-twentieth and one-tenth that for iron.

Like iron, copper plays a part in certain oxidation-reduction enzyme systems of the cell ($Cu^{++} \rightleftharpoons Cu^+$). This role as a component of enzyme complexes is probably of greater significance than its role in the formation of hemoglobin.

In addition to these better-known functions, copper has a role in maintaining the integrity of the myelin sheath surrounding nerve fibers; bone and connective tissue formation; the formation of the melanin pigment of skin and hair through its association with the tyrosinase molecule; keratinization of wool; reproduction; and cardiac function.

Absorption and excretion   Copper is absorbed from the upper small intestine. In the bloodstream, this element is present in almost equal amounts in the plasma and the red blood cells. Approximately 80% of plasma copper occurs as ceruloplasmin, an α_2-globulin-copper complex; the remainder is loosely bound to blood albumin. About 60% of the copper in red blood cells is present as erythrocuprein, a compound synthesized in the bone marrow.

Only about 4% of the copper ingested leaves the body via the urine. Fecal material contains unabsorbed copper, both that which has poured into the gut via bile secretions and that which has been lost directly through the intestinal wall.

Excretion rates for copper appear to be increased by high levels of cadmium, zinc, or a combination of high molybdenum and sulfate intake.

Consequences of copper deficiency   A nutritional anemia may result from a prolonged deficiency of copper. However, a number of other conditions also arise from an insufficient intake or availability of copper.

For example, *sway-back*, or *neonatal ataxia*, a condition found in certain parts of England in newborn lambs, is caused by an apparent copper deficiency in spite of the fact that the copper content of the pastures of these animals is normal. The affected pastures apparently contain some factor or factors that either limit the absorption of copper or promote its excretion. Sway-back may therefore by regarded as a conditioned copper deficiency. It can be prevented by administering a supplement of 5 mg of copper daily to pregnant ewes.

Falling disease in grazing cattle in Australia is caused by a chronic copper deficiency resulting from a low content in the herbage. The primary lesion of this condition is an atrophy of the myocardium with replacement fibrosis. Falling disease is characterized by staggering, falling, and a sudden death probably caused by acute heart failure. *Peat scours*, occurring in parts of New Zealand, is a condition that arises from the consumption of pastures that are excessively high in molybdenum and low in copper. It can be completely controlled by raising copper intakes to normal levels.

Copper deficiency in sheep results in marked changes in the fleece. The fibers become progressively less keratinized and hence less crimped, the rate of wool growth is reduced, and black wool turns white.

A deficiency of copper decreases fertility of cattle by depressing or delaying estrus. In rats, a deficiency of this element results in fetal death and resorption, whereas in poultry ingesting insufficient copper, hatchability is reduced and embryonic abnormalities can occur.

In 1961 investigators discovered that aortic rupture in chicks is caused by a copper deficiency. At about the same time, other workers described cardiovascular changes in copper-deficient pigs which resulted in ruptures of major blood vessels. In both cases, there was histological evidence of abnormalities in the elastic membranes of the aorta and of the coronary and pulmonary arteries. Since these discoveries, much effort has been devoted to elucidating the role of copper in elastin biosynthesis.*

---

*Hill, C. H., Starcher, B., and Kim, C., *Fed. Proc.* **26**(1968):129.

Copper toxicity   Although copper is essential to the normal functioning of the body, intakes of 100 mg per day by adult sheep are toxic, and intakes of 50 mg per day produce kidney trouble (i.e., tubules become blocked with hemoglobin).

Copper toxicity in sheep is accentuated if the ration is low in molybdenum. Typical symptoms of copper toxicity are found in sheep in parts of Australia where pastures contain high levels of copper but are deficient in molybdenum. The addition of molybdenum to rations high in copper counteracts possible copper poisoning. It is therefore apparent that copper and molybdenum are biologically antagonistic, and that the copper-to-molybdenum ratio in the ration is metabolically significant. Manganese and sulfate have also been implicated in the copper–molybdenum relationship.

Copper poisoning can occur in pigs ingesting rations that contain more than 250 ppm of copper. Increasing the animals' intake of zinc and iron appears to afford protection against such toxicity.

In humans, *Wilson's disease*, a rare disorder of genetic origin, results from an abnormal copper metabolism: body tissues retain an excessive amount of copper because of a failure to produce ceruloplasmin, the regulator of the levels of copper in the plasma.

Copper as a growth promotant   If 100 ppm or more of copper are included in an animal's diet, the trace element can display antibacterial properties against a broad spectrum of organisms. Consequently, copper is sometimes used (particularly in the United Kingdom) as a growth promotant in swine and poultry rations, where it functions in the same way as an antibiotic.

Copper–enzyme relationships

AMYLASES   Amylases can be easily inactivated by heavy metals, especially copper.

TYROSINASE   Tyrosinase is found in both animal and plant tissues. It oxidizes various phenolic compounds such as tyrosine, phenol, catechol, and cresol. For example:

Catechol   + O_2 $\xrightarrow{\text{Tyrosinase}}$ O-Quinone   + H_2O

Water, not hydrogen peroxide, is always formed as a result of oxidation by this enzyme, and gaseous oxygen serves as the hydrogen acceptor. Copper is an integral part of the tyrosinase molecule.

OTHER ENZYMES   Other "copper enzymes" found in the body include cytochrome oxidase, uricase, amine oxidase, and dopamine-β-hydroxylase.

Copper is also a component of the molecule of certain enzymes found in plant tissues (e.g., ascorbic acid oxidase and phenolase). It has been proposed that one or more of these copper-containing enzymes functions in plant tissues in much the same way as cytochrome oxidase does in animal tissues.

Iodine

The animal body contains 10 mg–20 mg of iodine, about 70%–80% of which is found in the thyroid gland. Iodine is also found in muscle tissue, the ovaries, and certain parts of the eye. Its chief role, however, appears to be as a component of thyroxine and tri-iodo-thyronine.

The thyroid gland is under the influence of a thyrotropic hormone from the anterior pituitary. The extent of the secretion of this pituitary hormone depends on the secretion of thyroxine. A decline in the level of thyroxine in the blood stimulates the pituitary to produce more of its thyrotropic hormone, which in turn influences the thyroid to produce more thyroxine. (See Figures 18.1 and 18.2.)

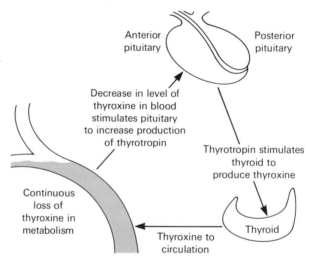

Figure 18.1
Thyrotropin from the anterior pituitary stimulates the thyroid to produce thyroxine, some of which is continuously lost in metabolism. As the level of thyroxine in the blood declines as a consequence of the metabolic loss, the pituitary is stimulated to produce sufficient thyrotropin to maintain the thyroxine equilibrium.

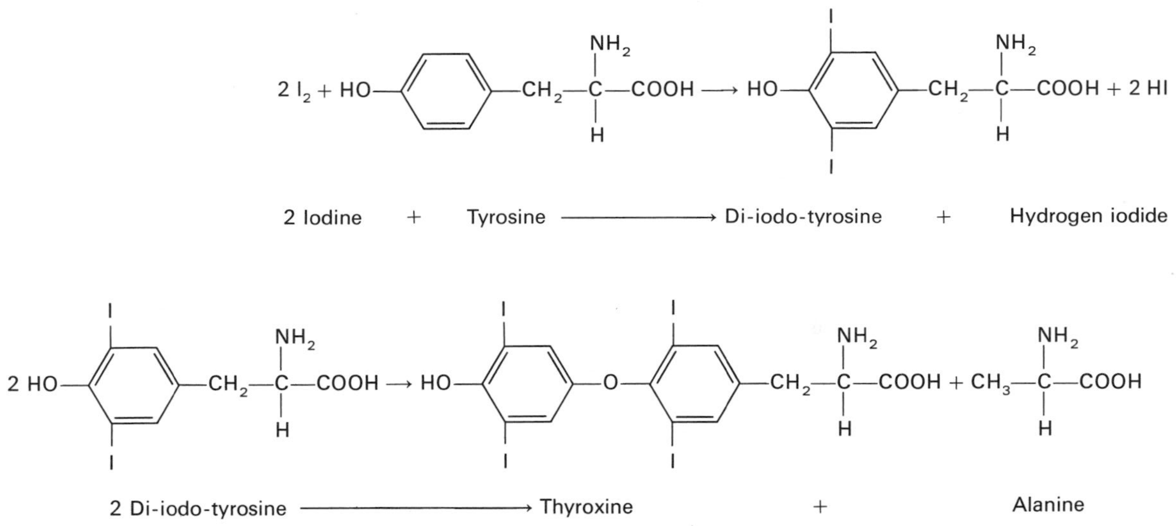

Figure 18.2
Steps in the formation of thyroxine.

Iodine is absorbed primarily in the small intestine as iodide. About 30% is preferentially picked up by the cells of the thyroid; the remainder is taken up by the kidney and excreted in the urine. A significant quantity of iodide is trapped by the salivary gland, but salivary iodide remains in the inorganic form and is normally completely reabsorbed so that there is little actual loss of the element via this route.

The iodide picked up by the thyroid is quickly oxidized to iodine which then combines with the amino acid tyrosine to form such compounds as mono-iodo-tyrosine and di-iodo-tyrosine. The iodinated tyrosine molecules unite to form either thyroxine (see Figure 18.2) or tri-iodo-thyronine (i.e., 1 molecule of mono-iodo-tyrosine plus 1 molecule of di-iodo-tyrosine). Tri-iodo-thyronine is a more active form of the hormone than thyroxine but is found in relatively small amounts in the blood.

Both thyroxine and thyronine are components of a mucoprotein, thyro-globulin, which is secreted into the jellylike substance of the anterior of the thyroid gland where it appears to slowly but steadily undergo hydrolysis; in the process it liberates the hormones which diffuse into the blood and per-form the physiological function of regulating the metabolic rate of all body processes. The overall stimulation or depression of basal metabolic rate is directly proportional to the thyroxine secreted. However, different tissues are stimulated differentially.

Among the trace elements, iodine is unique in the ease of its mammary transfer; as a result, the amount of iodine in milk is determined by dietary intake.

The element is excreted primarily via the urine, although small amounts are lost in the feces and in sweat.

Consequences of iodine deficiency   In the absence of sufficient thyroxine, the thyroid, as a consequence of the action of the thyrotropic hormone from the anterior pituitary, enlarges to what is called *goiter*. Thus goiter may indicate a dietary insufficiency of iodine, a deficiency of iodine (inhibition of uptake by thyroid) conditioned by the presence of goitrogens in the diet, or a metabolic defect in the synthesis of thyroxine, caused by certain types of goitrogens or by a constitutional disability.

Because the need for iodine, or rather thyroxine, varies with the activity of the body functions it controls, goiter usually develops in periods when metabolic rate is high, such as during puberty and pregnancy.

Goiter occurs in the newborn primarily as a result of insufficient iodine in the diet of the pregnant female. Other symptoms of deficiency include hair-lessness and thick, pulpy skin in calves and pigs and enlarged necks in calves. The thyroid hormone is essential for normal growth and reproduction in all mammals and birds. In humans, a type of dwarfism known as cretinism develops as a result of iodine deficiency; endemic goiter is frequently as-sociated with feeble-mindedness and deaf-mutism in children.

Iodine deficiency is a regional problem. Geographic areas in which the iodine content of the soil is low produce crops low in this element. Goiter is also common in areas where the drinking water contains little iodine. To prevent goiter in iodine-deficient areas, supplementary iodine is provided usually in the inorganic form as either potassium or sodium iodide.

Goitrogenic substances   Goitrogens are substances that are capable of producing goiter by interfering with the synthesis of thyroid hormone. As long ago as 1928 researchers reported that goiter developed in rabbits fed a diet consisting mainly of fresh cabbage and that the condition could be prevented by supplementing the diet with iodine. Since that time, a wide range of plants, including practically all cruciferous species, have been shown to have goitrogenic properties.

The development of the rapeseed industry in Canada and other countries has been impeded by the discovery of goitrogenic activity in *Brassica* seeds which can only be partially controlled by supplemental iodine. The goitrogen *goitrin* (5-vinyl-2-oxazolidinethione) has been shown to be the primary responsible agent, although both the 3-butenyl and 4-pentyl derivatives of isothiocyanate are also present in the seeds. However, plant breeders have succeeded in selecting lines that are almost free of these compounds.

Goitrogens are widely used in the treatment of thyrotoxicosis in humans, and have also been used in livestock and poultry rations because of their ability to promote fattening. Those used for such purposes include methyl and proply thiouracil, carbimazole, and methimazole.

When foods containing goitrogenic substances (cabbage, turnips, etc.) are consumed in normal quantities and are cooked in water, goiter is much less likely to develop because the wet cooking process eliminates the enzyme that liberates the active goitrogen from its inactive precursor.

Zinc

Most of the zinc in the body is found in the liver, muscle, male sex organs, bones, epidermal tissues, and blood, although a rapid metabolism of zinc also occurs in the pancreas, kidney, and pituitary gland. In the blood, 75% of the zinc is found in the erythrocytes, 22% in the serum, and the remaining 3% in the leucocytes.

Because many plants contain zinc and animals require a very small amount of the element, there is seldom any danger of a deficiency under normal conditions. Under certain conditions, however, a deficiency of zinc occurs in both laboratory and domestic animals, in birds, and in humans. Symptoms of a deficiency include retarded growth, reduced appetite, impaired reproductive development and function, gross lesions in epithelial tissues, and impaired bone growth.

Zinc can cure or prevent parakeratosis in pigs, a skin disease of considerable economic significance. Rations high in calcium and low in zinc predispose pigs to parakeratosis. In poultry, zinc is required for growth, feathering, and skeletal development.

Only extreme deprivation will cause symptoms of zinc deficiency in humans. Such symptoms include retarded growth and hypogonadism. Although the precise mode of action of zinc in tissue repair is not known, the element appears to play a positive role in wound healing. Recent research has revealed that zinc therapy can diminish the effects of some types of atherosclerosis. In alcoholics afflicted with cirrhosis, disorders in zinc metabolism have been observed.

The main site of zinc absorption is the duodenum, and the element is excreted primarily in the feces. Absorption is enhanced when the intake of zinc is low, and it declines when intake is high. Dietary excesses of calcium, copper, and phytic acid all inhibit zinc absorption. Cadmium appears to be a zinc antimetabolite (see Chapter 19).

Zinc–enzyme relationships

CARBONIC ANHYDRASE   A major physiological role of zinc is as an active component of the enzyme carbonic anhydrase, which is found chiefly in the red blood cells and also in the parietal cells of the stomach. Carbonic anhydrase catalyzes the following reaction.

$$CO_2 + H_2O \; \overset{\text{Carbonic}}{\underset{\text{anhydrase}}{\rightleftharpoons}} \; H_2CO_3 \rightleftharpoons HCO_3^- + H^+$$

This reaction plays an important role in the transport of respiratory carbon dioxide by the blood. The reaction may also be responsible for the fact that the stomach produces a secretion (HCl) that is about three million times more acidic than the blood.

OTHER METALLOENZYMES   Zinc is also the metallic component of a number of other metalloenzymes, including pancreatic carboxypeptidase, alkaline phosphatase, various dehydrogenases (alcohol, lactate, malate, glutamate), and tryptophan desmolase. Furthermore zinc serves as a cofactor in a number of enzyme systems, including arginase, enolase, several peptidases, oxalacetic decarboxylase, and carnosinase.

Through these various relationships with enzymes, zinc takes part in a wide range of cellular activities; it is active in the synthesis and metabolism of RNA and protein in both plants and animals.

Box 18.1 Phytate and the availability of inorganic elements

The 1955 report that it is possible to cure or prevent parakeratosis in pigs fed a diet based on corn and soybean meal by zinc supplementation ushered in an era of research not only on zinc nutrition but on how phytate and calcium affect the availability of this element. Phytate, which occurs naturally in all foods of plant origin, is generally assumed to be the hexaphosphate of inositol. In cereals, the phosphorus in phytin may constitute as much as 80% of the total phosphorus. Phytate occurs in foods in association with protein, which accounts in part for the high phytate content of soybean, sesame, and rapeseed meal.

The anionic character of phytate makes it ideal for forming complexes with mineral elements, particularly the transitional elements such as zinc, iron, and manganese. The solubility of these complexes varies with pH and calcium ion concentration. Calcium promotes the complexing of zinc to phytate; the zinc complex is the most insoluble at approximately pH 6. The effect of pH on solubility is particularly significant because pH 6 is the approximate pH of the duodenum and upper jejunum, the area of the intestinal tract where zinc and many of the heavy elements are absorbed. Neither phytate nor the zinc–phytate or calcium–zinc–phytate complexes are absorbed.

The bran fraction of grains is particularly rich in phytate. This localization of phytate in the bran of cereals undoubtedly contributes significantly to the mineral deficiencies observed among populations in Iran and other countries in the Middle East. Unleavened bread made from high-extraction flours may comprise 70% to 80% of the daily intake of energy of many Mideastern villagers. The fact that the dietary staple for many of the people in this area is unleavened bread compounds the problem because the phytase in yeast and in the flour itself hydrolyzes phytate during leavening.

Although the complexing of zinc following the regular consumption of whole wheat bread does not constitute a serious nutritional problem in the more developed countries, there are potential areas of concern with phytate even in these regions. Dried prepared cereals, consumed regularly because of their convenience, are normally eaten with milk. Milk is not a particularly rich source of zinc but when it is consumed alone, the zinc is readily available. However, when milk is added to cereal, the calcium in the milk and the phytate in the cereal act synergistically to complex the zinc, thus rendering the zinc less available. This interaction can be particularly critical in young infants.

Supplementation with adequate zinc can overcome the adverse effects of phytate. This is the usual practice followed today in livestock feeding. A similar approach may be followed in human nutrition although supplementation with other chelating agents, such as EDTA or histidine, and the use of the phytate-splitting enzymes in yeast offer other means of decreasing the adverse effect of phytate on the availability of zinc.

Zinc–hormone relationships   Nutritionists have postulated a relationship between zinc and the action of such hormones as insulin, glucagon, FSH, LH, and corticotrophin. However, a specific role for zinc in hormonal function has not yet been established.

Cobalt

Cobalt is an inorganic element that is of significance primarily in ruminant nutrition. Early evidence suggested that cobalt is needed to maintain the normal activity of the microflora of the intestinal tract. One theory was that cobalt suppresses the growth of pathogenic bacteria in the rumen. However, it has now been shown that cobalt is actually an integral part of vitamin B_{12} and is used in the synthesis of this vitamin by the rumen microflora. A deficiency of vitamin B_{12} is therefore responsible for the metabolic failure found in cobalt deficiency in ruminants.

As is true of iodine, cobalt deficiency is a regional problem. The clinical evidence of a cobalt deficiency in cattle includes long rough hair coat, scaliness of the skin, absence of estrus, abortion, low milk yield, loss of appetite, rapid loss of weight, and anemia. Loss of appetite and dramatic recovery following administration of a cobalt supplement are the principal diagnostic criteria for determining a deficiency in dairy cattle.

Large intakes of cobalt can be toxic, but there is a very wide margin between essential and harmful levels.

Molybdenum

A condition in cattle known for a long time in England as *teartness* was identified in 1938 as molybdenum poisoning. It occurs where the forage contains 0.002% or more of the element. Potentially toxic levels in soils and forages have also been found in Canada, the U.S.A., Ireland, and in New Zealand where the clinical toxicity is known as *peat scours*. Although cattle and sheep are most susceptible to high levels of molybdenum, species such as rats, rabbits, guinea pigs, pigs, and poultry can also suffer from excesses of this element.

The chief symptoms of molybdenum poisoning are extreme diarrhea, retarded growth, loss of body weight, and anemia. In addition, loss of coat color, alopecia, dermatosis, male sterility, and decreased lactation have been observed in certain species. The extent to which these various symptoms occur depends upon the amount of molybdenum ingested relative to the amount of copper and inorganic sulfate or sulfate-producing substances. The interrelationship between molybdenum, copper, and sulfate was discussed earlier in this chapter.

Xanthine oxidase is an enzyme found in animal tissues; it catalyzes reactions typified by the following:

$$\text{Xanthine} \xrightarrow{\text{Xanthine oxidase}} \text{Uric acid}$$

This enzyme catalyzes the oxidation of aliphatic and aromatic aldehydes, reduced NAD, and a number of purines (e.g., xanthine, hypoxanthine).

The first indication of an essential role for molybdenum was when this metal was shown to be a component of the xanthine oxidase molecule, and it was shown that xanthine oxidase levels in the tissues of animals are affected by the levels of dietary molybdenum. More direct evidence that molybdenum is essential in the diet of lambs, chicks, and turkey poults has been obtained through feeding highly purified diets.

There is very little evidence that molybdenum has any direct relationship to human health or disease. Claims that this element prevents or reduces the incidence of dental caries have not yet been proven conclusively.

Selenium

Selenium is one of the elements that recently has come into prominence as an essential trace element. It is now known that selenium can perform some of the functions originally attributed exclusively to vitamin E. For example, it protects rats against necrotic liver degeneration, chicks against exudative diathesis, and lambs, calves, and chicks against muscular dystrophy when these animals are fed certain vitamin E–deficient diets. The protection afforded by vitamin E against all of these conditions is variable but usually less satisfactory than that provided by selenium. On the other hand, neither the resorption sterility in rats nor the encephalomalacia in chicks that occur on vitamin E–deficient diets will respond to treatment with selenium.

Good evidence that selenium is a dietary essential independent of, or in addition to, its function as a substitute for vitamin E was provided by J. N. Thompson and M. L. Scott.[*] In their experiments, purified diets low in selenium resulted in poor growth and high mortality in chicks even when vitamin E was added; increasing the amount of tocopherol in the diet prevented mortality, but growth was inferior to that obtained when selenium but no vitamin E was included in the diet. These findings provided a clear indication that selenium does not function merely as a substitute for vitamin E. (The interrelationship between vitamin E, selenium, and the sulfur-containing amino acids has already been discussed in Chapter 14.)

---

[*]Thompson, J. N., and M. L. Scott, *J. Nutrition* **97**(1969):335; **100**(1970):797.

The exact physiological function of selenium is still far from clear. The functions that have been attributed to the element include the following: acts as nonspecific antioxidant and protects against peroxidation in tissues and membranes; participates in the biosynthesis of ubiquinone (coenzyme Q); participates in hydrogen transport along the respiratory chain; and influences the absorption and retention of vitamin E and of triglyceride.

The identification of selenium as the active site of the enzyme glutathione peroxidase tends to discount the possibility that selenium acts merely as a nonspecific antioxidant in the body.* Glutathione peroxidase contains 0.34% selenium. Selenium also appears to be a constituent of a special cytochrome in muscle and heart, and of two bacterial enzyme complexes (formic dehydrogenase and glycine reductase) which contain selenium enzymes.

Prior to the discovery of the essentiality of selenium, great emphasis had been placed upon its toxic properties. The cause of alkali disease (blind staggers), a disease of livestock which had long been known in certain regions of the world, was eventually traced to the ingestion of high levels of selenium. The symptoms of selenium poisoning occur in approximately the following order: dullness and lack of vitality, emaciation and roughness of hair coat, loss of hair, soreness of the hooves, stiffness and lameness, abdominal pain, grating of teeth, excessive salivation, gastrointestinal stasis, and paralysis of the swallowing and respiratory mechanism.

Selenium poisoning afflicts grazing animals if the forage contains 5 ppm or more of the element, or if the plants consumed by the animals are grown on soil containing more than 0.5 ppm of selenium. Within plants grown on seleniferous soil, the greatest concentration of selenium is in the leaves; less is found in the stem, and still less in the seed. In the seeds, selenium is closely bound to the protein fraction, but it can be removed from the vegetative part of plants by hot water.

High levels of selenium are thought to exert their toxic effects through the removal of sulfhydral groups essential to oxidative processes. A diet high in protein provides some protection against selenium poisoning, as does a diet high in sulfate. More dramatic, however, is the fact that a small amount of arsenic in drinking water (5 ppm) prevents selenium toxicity.

It is not clear whether selenium deficiency or selenium poisoning occur in humans. Data from epidemiological studies with children suggest that a higher-than-normal intake of selenium increases the incidence of dental caries. Researchers have also suggested but not yet proven that selenium acts as a carcinogen in rats but as a protective agent against cancer in humans.

---

*Rotruck, J. T., Pope, A. L., Ganther, H. E., Swanson, A. B., Hafeman, D. G., and Hoekstra, W. G., Science **179** (1973): 179, 588.

Fluorine

Fluorine is found in various parts of the body, but is particularly abundant in bones and teeth; it normally constitutes 0.02%–0.05% of these tissues as an integral part of the apatite molecule. This regular occurrence suggests that a small amount of fluorine is an essential dietary constituent. The fluoride ion, at appropriate levels of intake, assists in the prevention of dental caries.

The mechanism by which the element acts in this capacity is not completely understood. However, it appears that crystals of fluoroapatite can replace some of the calcium phosphate crystals of hydroxyapatite that are normally deposited during tooth formation. Fluoride may also replace some of the carbonate normally found in the tooth. These fluoride substances are apparently more resistant to the cariogenic action of acid-producing bacteria in the mouth.

Fluorine is now considered an essential trace element because, in addition to its beneficial effects on the pigmentation of incisors and in the prevention of dental caries, it enhances the growth of rats: 2.5 ppm of fluoride in the diet produce an optimal rate of growth in this species. In addition, K. Schwarz has indicated that "fluorine concentration in blood plasma is homeostatically controlled, bone and teeth serve as storage organs containing normally between 100 ppm and 7,000 ppm, the fetus contains fluorine, the placenta plays an active role in fluoride transfer, rather constant concentrations are maintained in soft tissues such as liver, heart and brain, and the element occurs in practically all foods and feeds."[*]

Absorption and excretion   Fluorine is absorbed primarily from the small intestine. A large proportion (90%) of ingested flourine is normally absorbed, although large amounts of dietary calcium, aluminum, and fat will depress its uptake. That portion of absorbed fluorine which is not taken up by bones and teeth is excreted in the urine, with the result that the level of fluoride in blood plasma is quite constant.

Toxicity   In addition to its role in preventing dental caries and in promoting normal growth, fluorine has nutritional importance because it is toxic when the amount ingested exceeds 30 ppm–40 ppm of the dry matter of the diet. In fluorosis the enamel of the teeth loses its luster, becoming chalky and mottled. The permanently growing incisors in the rat do not wear away normally and become elongated. In cattle, sheep, and hogs, on the other hand, the teeth become soft and are rapidly worn down. When taken in large quantities over a period of time, fluorine eventually interferes with growth,

---

[*]Schwarz, K., *Fed. Proc.* **33**(1974):1748.

reproduction, and lactation. It is unclear how this interference occurs, but the drastic reduction in appetite that accompanies fluorosis is considered by many to be the primary cause. Fluorine might also inhibit certain enzymes concerned with carbohydrate and lipid metabolism (e.g., glucose-6-phosphate dehydrogenase, ATPases, lipase, alkaline phosphatase). The effects of fluorine are cumulative, so that continuous intakes of small quantities can eventually produce toxic effects.

Excessive fluorine intake can be a practical problem in mineral mixtures fed to animals if fluorine is a contaminant of the phosphorus source used. Rock phosphates carrying more than 0.1% fluorine are dangerous sources of phosphorus and should be used in mineral mixtures only if they have been defluorinated.

Tin

On the basis of the findings of K. Schwarz et al.,[*] tin has been elevated to the list of essential trace minerals. Schwarz and his colleagues demonstrated that in rats maintained on purified diets in trace-element-controlled isolators, dietary supplements of 1.5 ppm–2.0 ppm of tin stimulated significant growth. The tin was provided in various forms and in amounts similar to those normally present in foods and tissues. Tin is thought to function as an oxidation-reduction catalyst.

This element is poorly absorbed and retained by humans and hence its primary excretory pathway is the feces; minimal amounts are found in the urine.

The distribution of tin in human tissues is wide but highly variable, with significant differences being related to age and geographical location. The element tends to accumulate in the lungs with age, but not in the liver, kidney, aorta, or intestine. There is apparently no placental transfer of tin, but it is available to the newborn in milk.

Vanadium

Some interesting biological functions have been suggested for vanadium over the years. For example, vanadium has been said to be involved in bone and tooth calcification and to help prevent dental caries; it has also been suggested that this element can exchange with phosphorus in apatite crystals.

Vanadium has also been shown to inhibit the synthesis of cholesterol.

---

[*]Schwarz, K., Milne, D. B., and Vinyard, E., *Biochem. Biophys. Res. Comm.* **40**(1970):22.

This inhibition appears to be accompanied by a decrease in the phospholipid and cholesterol content of plasma and a reduction in the amount of cholesterol that accumulates in the aorta. Vanadium counteracts the stimulation of cholesterol synthesis by manganese; similarly, manganese nullifies the inhibitory action of vanadium.

L. L. Hopkins and H. E. Mohr have pointed out that vanadium is an essential trace element for chicks and rats.* If either of these species consumes a diet low in vanadium, the rate of body and/or feather growth decreases, reproduction and survival of the young is impaired, iron metabolism is altered, the metabolism of hard tissue is impaired, and the level of lipid in the blood is altered. The probable requirement of these species is 50 ppb–500 ppb. It is likely that vanadium, like tin, functions as an oxidation-reduction catalyst in the organism.

In the animal body, vanadium is present primarily in the bones, teeth, and fatty tissues. The lungs may also contain appreciable amounts of the element, but this is believed to be the result of inhaling atmospheric dusts. The element appears to be poorly absorbed and is excreted mainly via the feces.

Excessive vanadium has been shown to be toxic to rats and chicks, but it is not particularly toxic to humans.

Chromium

Although a wide margin of safety exists between the amounts of chromium ordinarily consumed and those likely to be harmful to the body, the early biological interest in chromium was confined to investigating its potential toxicity for humans.

Evidence gathered more recently shows that trivalent chromium plays an important role in carbohydrate metabolism; specifically it takes part in the metabolism of glucose and the action of insulin. W. Mertz and his colleagues at the Human Nutrition Research Division of the United States Department of Agriculture in Beltsville, Maryland, showed that animals raised on a diet of torula yeast were unable to metabolize carbohydrates normally. Little improvement was noted when vitamin E, selenium, or cystine were added to the diet, but a factor present in brewer's yeast restored carbohydrate metabolism to normal. Investigators called this factor GTF (glucose tolerance factor) and subsequently demonstrated that trivalent chromium is an essential component of GTF.

It is now established that trivalent chromium acts as a cofactor with insulin at the cellular level, through the formation of a complex with membrane sites, insulin, and chromium.

---

*Hopkins, L. L., and Mohr, H. E., *Fed. Proc.* **33**(1974):1773.

The amount of chromium in body tissues is highest at birth, falls quite rapidly during the early years of life, and then levels off or declines slowly throughout the rest of life. A large number of humans lose their ability to metabolize sugar normally as they approach middle age. This leads to a condition termed *maturity onset diabetes*. Preliminary evidence from the Beltsville group suggests that dietary supplements of chromium can alleviate this condition. However, this same group of researchers stresses that chromium per se should not be considered a hypoglycemic agent, a substitute for insulin, nor a *cure* for diabetes.

Findings that the addition of chromium to low-chromium diets reduces the level of cholesterol in the serum of rats and humans suggest that chromium plays a role in the metabolism of lipids.

Chromium may also affect the metabolism of proteins. There is evidence that rats fed diets deficient in chromium and protein have an impaired capacity to incorporate certain amino acids, such as methionine, serine, etc., into the protein of their hearts.

The supplementation with chromium of diets otherwise nutritionally adequate improves the growth rate of rats; dietary supplements of chromium also increase the longevity of male (only) rats and mice. Repeated pregnancies can deplete the tissue stores of females subsisting on a chromium-deficient diet.

From relative nutritional obscurity the trace element chromium has come to the fore as an important factor in carbohydrate metabolism, with probable roles in lipid and protein metabolism as well.

Silicon

Silicon is found in all plant and animal tissues, sometimes in very large amounts; for example, the ash of wheat straw contains as much as 70% silicon oxide, and the ash of feathers is more than 70% silicon. Plants may take up silicon from the soil; the mineral can also infiltrate their cellulosic fraction. The highest concentrations of silicon in animal tissue are found in the skin and its appendages.

Silicon appears to be essential for chicks and rats; its absence from the diet impedes normal growth and skeletal development.[*] A deficiency produces abnormalities of articular cartilage and connective tissue in chicks. Silicon appears to take part in the synthesis of mucopolysaccharides and is a component of the mucopolysaccharide–protein complexes of connective tissue. In fact, it may contribute to the structural integrity of connective tissue by serving as a cross-linking agent.

The metabolism of silicon can be very extensive. Silicon is absorbed read-

---

[*]Carlisle, E. M., *Fed. Proc.* **33**(1974):1758.

ily, but it is also excreted easily, via both the feces and the urine; hence storage in the body is limited. Blood may contain up to 1 mg per 100 ml; once silicon has entered the bloodstream, it passes rapidly into the urine; even over a wide range of intake, the concentration of silicon in the blood remains relatively constant.

The silicon content of the aorta, skin, and thymus decreases significantly with age; this is probably related to the fact that the mucopolysaccharide content of body tissues also declines with aging.

Urinary silicon is normally eliminated efficiently. However, under conditions that are still poorly understood, part of it may be deposited in the kidney, bladder, or urethra to form calculi or uroliths.

Silicon was initially best recognized through its role in silicosis. This lung condition is due partly to the mechanical effect of silicon oxide dust deposited in the lungs, and due partly to the uptake of silicon particles by the lysosomes with a resulting damage to lysosomal membranes through hydrogen-bonding interactions. The amount of silicon in the blood and urine increases in silicosis.

Nickel

It has taken some time to substantiate that nickel is essential in the diets of higher animals. Early evidence that it can partially replace cobalt in the treatment of cobalt deficiency in sheep has never been confirmed. However, in a review of earlier work, F. H. Nielsen and D. A. Ollerich defend the claim that nickel is a truly essential trace element.*

They point out that a deficiency of nickel in chicks results in suboptimal liver function as evidenced by ultrastructural degeneration, reduced oxidative ability, increased lipid, and a decreased phospholipid fraction. Rats deprived of nickel also show a reduced oxidative ability in the liver and abnormalities in the polysome profile.

Nickel is biologically active *in vitro*. For example, it activates such enzymes as arginase, tyrosinase, deoxyribonuclease, acetyl coenzyme A synthetase, and phosphoglucomutase. Nickel also enhances the adhesiveness of polymorphonuclear leucocytes *in vitro*, and stabilizes RNA and DNA against thermal denaturation. However, it is still not known whether these *in vitro* phenomena relate to *in vivo* functions of nickel, although they do suggest that the element can participate in various biochemical reactions.

Nickel is widely distributed in low concentrations in body tissues. It is poorly absorbed and hence is excreted mainly in the feces. There is evidence that the body does not readily retain the element, nor does it accumulate it

---

*Nielsen, F. H., and Ollerich, D. A., *Fed. Proc.* **33**(1974):1767.

with age in any organ with the possible exception of the lungs.

Because this element is relatively nontoxic, nickel contamination is not a serious health hazard.

Suggested readings

Ammerman, C. B., and Miller, S. M. "Biological Availability of Minor Mineral Ions: A Review," *Journal of Animal Science* **35**(1972):681.

Anonymous. "Endemic Goiter," *Nutrition Reviews* **21**(1963):73.

Bing, F. C. "Assaying the Availability of Iron," *Journal of the American Dietetic Association* **60**(1972):114.

Carnes, W. H. "Role of Copper in Connective Tissue Metabolism," *Federation Proceedings* **30**(1971):995.

Handler, P., Rajagopalan, K. V., and Aleman, V. "Structure and Function of Iron-Flavoproteins," *Federation Proceedings* **23**(1964):30.

Hegsted, D. M. "The Recommended Dietary Allowances for Iron," *American Journal of Public Health* **60**(1970):653.

Krehl, W. A. "Selenium—The Maddening Mineral," *Nutrition Today* **5**(1970):26.

Leach, R. M., Jr. "Role of Manganese in Mucopolysaccharide Metabolism," *Federation Proceedings* **30**(1971):991.

Luecke, R. V. "Significance of Zinc in Nutrition," *Borden Reviews of Nutrition Research* **26**(1965):45.

Mertz, W. "Chromium Occurrence and Function in Biological Systems," *Physiological Reviews* **49**(1969):163.

Mills, C. F. "Metabolic Interrelationships in the Utilization of Trace Elements," *Proceedings of the Nutrition Society* **23**(1964):38.

Munro, H., and Drysdale, J. W. "Role of Iron in the Regulation of Ferritin Metabolism," *Federation Proceedings* **29**(1970):1469.

Prockop, D. J. "Role of Iron in the Synthesis of Collagen in Connective Tissue," *Federation Proceedings* **30**(1971):984.

Ross Conference on Pediatric Research. *Iron Nutrition in Infancy.* Ross Laboratories, Columbus, Ohio (1970).

Schroeder, H. A. "The Role of Chromium in Mammalian Nutrition," *American Journal of Clinical Nutrition* **21**(1968):230.

Schwarz, K. "Recent Dietary Trace Element Research, Exemplified by Tin, Fluorine and Silicon," *Federation Proceedings* **33**(1974):1748.

Sullivan, J. F., and Heaney, R. P. "Zinc Metabolism in Alcoholic Liver Disease," *American Journal of Clinical Nutrition* **23**(1970):170.

Underwood, E. J. *Trace Elements in Human and Animal Nutrition* (3rd ed.). Academic Press, New York (1971).

Westmoreland, N. "Connective Tissue Alterations in Zinc Deficiency," *Federation Proceedings* **30**(1971):1001.

Chapter 19
Other inorganic elements

Possibly essential minerals

The small group of inorganic elements potentially required by the body, which have as yet failed to meet all the criteria for essentiality, include at present arsenic, barium, bromine, cadmium, and strontium. Because of the rapid advances being made in bioinorganic chemistry, it is possible that by the time this chapter is being read, new information will have enabled nutritionists to categorize these trace elements as either essential or nonessential.

Arsenic Because it gained historical notoriety as a poison, the more valuable aspects of arsenic have been obscured. Solutions containing arsenic have long been used as tonics for men and animals and for the treatment of human anemias. It has also been claimed that administration of various forms of this element improves the appearance of the skin and hair of rats, mice, and horses.

In the field of animal nutrition, the role of various organic arsenicals in improving growth rate and feed efficiency has been recognized for some time. Four organic arsenic compounds have proven of value in this respect, but no definite relation between structure and growth-promoting ability has been uncovered. Therefore, the exact mode of action of these compounds is not known, although some (the arsonic acids) appear to act in much the same way as antibiotics do in stimulating growth.

Scientists have not yet clearly demonstrated that arsenic is an essential trace mineral, despite indications that it is.

Arsenic occurs in air, soil, and seawater. Although most foods consumed by humans contain less than 0.5 ppm of arsenic on a fresh basis, those of marine origin (e.g., oysters, mussels, prawns, shrimps) are very much richer in the element. In the human body, arsenic is found in greatest concentration in the skin, nails, and hair.

Absorption and subsequent retention of arsenic in the body vary with the amount and chemical form ingested. The more toxic arsenic compounds are retained in the tissues in greater amounts and are excreted more slowly than the less toxic forms. The arsenic found in most foods is readily absorbed and quickly excreted in the urine. Inorganic arsenic is well absorbed also, but is retained longer and in greater quantities in the tissues.

Barium   In spite of reports that barium stimulates plant growth and of findings that it may be essential for normal growth in rats and guinea pigs, there is still no conclusive evidence that barium is in fact an essential trace mineral for any animal species.

Barium occurs in highly variable concentrations in various soils, plants, and animal tissues. The element is poorly absorbed from most foods, and that which is absorbed is poorly retained in the body tissues. In the human, barium is found in the adrenal glands, brains, heart, kidney, liver, lungs, spleen, and muscle.

Bromine   Bromine can completely replace chloride in the growth of several halophytic algal species and can substitute for a part of the chloride requirements of chicks. Bromine also produces a small but significant growth increase in chicks fed a special synthetic diet, and in mice given a diet containing iodinated casein.

Further investigation and confirmation of data is necessary before this element can be fully accepted as a member of the essential group. Bromine is so universally present in both animal and plant tissues that naturally ocurring deficiencies in animals are unlikely.

All animal tissues except the thyroid contain 100 times as much bromine as iodine. In the thyroid the proportions are reversed. Bromine is retained for only short periods in the tissues, being excreted mainly via the urine. Bromide and chloride interchange to some degree in the body tissues, so that the administration of the former results in some displacement of the latter and vice versa.

Cadmium   Interest in the biological role of cadmium has centered mainly on its toxic properties. It has been known for some time that chronic long-term exposure to cadmium-contaminated air leads to progressive pulmonary and kidney damage. It is now known that prolonged ingestion of relatively large amounts of the element will produce kidney lesions, anemia, necrosis of the testes and the placenta, and stunted growth. Recent studies have also implicated cadmium as a causal factor in human hypertension.

Small amounts of cadmium have been found in the tissues (chiefly the kidney and liver) and fluids of most animal species, but no specific biological function for the element has yet been shown. Studies suggest that the cadmium in both kidney and liver is bound specifically to metallothionein, a protein compound containing approximately 5% cadmium and 2% zinc.

E. J. Underwood states that "an aggregation of cadmium of this size, higher by an order of magnitude than the metal content of any other known metalloprotein, and its specific association with a particular macromolecule, point to a functional role for this element."

The metabolism of cadmium is interrelated with that of other elements—notably zinc, copper, and iron. In fact, it has been said that cadmium is a zinc antimetabolite. This probably because of a competition between cadmium and zinc for protein-binding sites, most likely including those of the zinc metalloenzymes. Studies with rats have pointed to selenium as a protective agent against reproductive abnormalities brought on in both sexes by the ingestion of cadmium.

No cadmium-containing metalloenzymes are yet known, whereas this trace element is thought to interact with the sulfydryl groups of certain enzymes resulting in their inactivation.

Strontium   Interest in the biological role of strontium increased greatly following the discovery that strontium 90 is an abundant and potentially hazardous radioactive by-product of nuclear fission.

Strontium purportedly acts as a growth stimulant in plants, but only one study has suggested it is essential in animal nutrition. In that study, the omission of strontium from a purified diet fed to rats and guinea pigs resulted in a reduced rate of growth, impaired calcification of the bones and teeth, and an increased incidence of dental caries.

This trace element is found in a wide variety of animal tissues in concentrations ranging from 0.01 ppm to 0.10 ppm, but there is no evidence that it accumulates in any particular organ or tissue. However, the strontium content of bone has attracted special attention because the affinity of bone for this element creates a potential for the retention of strontium 90.

Recently, J. L. Omdahl and H. F. DeLuca have suggested that strontium induces rickets by blocking the biosynthesis of 1,25-dihydroxycholecalciferol (1,25-DHCC), the metabolically active form of vitamin D in the intestine.*

---

*Omdahl, J. L., and DeLuca, H. F., *Science* **174** (1971): 949.

The nonessential minerals

Our categorization of minerals (see Chapter 16) included a group of inorganic elements known to be essential to the body, another group whose members display some potential for essentiality, and finally a group of minerals not believed to be essential to the body. Of the latter group, some are of nutritional importance because they possess potentially toxic properties if consumed in sufficiently large quantities or over a relatively long period of time.

All the elements discussed so far in this section are physiologically active. They represent only a small proportion of the total inorganic elements shown to occur regularly in living tissues. Spectrochemical studies have revealed the presence of another 15–20 elements for which no physiological functions have yet been found. The following are the most prominent of these.

Aluminum   Aluminum is universally present in foods and therefore is always found in the animal body in traces. However, there is no evidence for its essentiality. The interest in aluminum lies largely in its possible toxic properties. Aluminum has been shown to be toxic when injected. The extensive use of aluminum cooking utensils, leading to a regular intake of the element, has stimulated research on the effects of feeding large amounts of aluminum. Experiments with rats, dogs, pigs, and humans have shown, however, that even large amounts of ingested aluminum are not harmful. It appears that a low rate of absorption of aluminum is a protective device of the body.

Aluminum can interfere with the absorption of phosphorus. But, not enough aluminum is present in natural foods prepared in a normal way to interfere with the absorption of phosphorus in humans.

However, aluminum can have a detrimental effect in animals fed soft phosphates and colloidal clays as phosphorus supplements; these products contain a significant quantity of aluminum, which may in fact interfere with the absorption of phosphorus.

Lead   Traditionally, interest in the biological role of lead has centered upon the toxic properties which make it an industrial hazard to humans and animals. During recent years, decreased exposure to lead from water pipes, food containers, paints, etc. has been compensated by increased exposure from motor vehicle exhausts, cigarette smoke, and cosmetics. Lead occurs naturally in many plants and enters the body when such material is consumed.

The adult human body contains an average of 100 mg–120 mg of lead, with about 90% found in the bones and teeth. Significant amounts are also present in the liver, kidneys, lungs, spleen, aorta, and hair; much less is present in brain and muscle tissue. If ingested in small, nontoxic amounts, lead is poorly absorbed and is excreted chiefly via the feces. Any lead that is absorbed is carried by the blood to the various tissues of the body, with excesses being emptied into the intestinal tract via the bile. In addition, some lead is lost from the body via hair, sweat, and milk.

Acute lead poisoning is characterized by colic, anemia (probably the result of inhibited heme synthesis), neuropathy, and encephalopathy.

Although the possibility exists that lead in low concentrations performs some useful biological function in the body, no evidence of such a function has been uncovered to date.

Mercury   Mercury has long been known as a toxic element that enters the body through both ingestion and inhalation. The exposure of industrial workers to mercury is now under control, but the entry of mercury into the environment primarily through industrial wastes and the application of organic mercury fumigants and fungicides in industry and agriculture has created new problems. The concentration of mercury has increased in the marine life of rivers and lakes, and in the plant and animal products grown near sources of contamination.

Mercury has been detected in many body tissues, with highest concentrations being found in the kidneys, skin, hair, nails, teeth, liver, and lungs.

Ingested mercury is excreted primarily via the feces and only to a small extent in the urine. After absorption, the concentration of mercury in the kidney rapidly increases, following which the metal is slowly eliminated from the body.

Mercury can influence the absorption and transport of copper, zinc, and cadmium; selenium appears to exert a protective influence against the toxic effects of mercury.

There is no evidence that mercury is biologically essential in any animal species.

Suggested readings

Bazell, R. J., "Lead Poisoning: Combatting the Threat from the Air," *Science* **174**(1971):574.

Frost, D. V. "Arsenic: Science or Superstition," *Food and Nutrition News* **40**(1968):1.

Mitchell, H. H., and Edman, M. "The Fluorine Problem in Livestock Feeding," *Nutrition Abstracts and Reviews* **21**(1951–52):787.

Omdahl, J. L., and DeLuca, H. F. "Strontium Induced Rickets: Metabolic Basis," *Science* **174**(1971):949.

Spivey Fox, M. R., and Fry, B. E. "Cadmium Toxicity Decreased by Dietary Ascorbic Acid Supplements," *Science* **169**(1970):989.

Underwood, E. J. *Trace Elements in Human and Animal Nutrition* (3rd ed.). Academic Press, New York (1971).

Walsh, J. "Mercury in the Environment: Natural and Human Factors," *Science* **171**(1971):788.

Section V
SOME QUANTITATIVE ASPECTS OF NUTRITION

We have now completed the sections of this book that deal qualitatively with the operating needs of the animal body. We have identified the sources of energy and the specific nutrients themselves, and considered their metabolism. This broad picture of the way in which the organism functions provides a general basis for understanding not only why the various nutrients are needed but also what consequences result from deficiencies of them in the diet.

To apply this knowledge to dietetics or to animal feeding it is necessary to supplement it with quantitative considerations. Dietitians, for example, must know how much energy, and how much thiamin and phosphorus and iron to provide for an individual. And because these factors can be, and usually are, supplied through foods that are incompletely digested, they must be able to compute the efficiency of foods as sources of the array of nutrients needed. It is important to understand how the facts and figures in dietetic tables are arrived at, and what accuracy and reliability should be ascribed to them. In short, it is essential for nutritionists to know the comparative nutritive values of foods as well as how to formulate diets that meet the specific needs of various species.

The logical starting point is an introduction to the ways by which quantitative nutritional data are obtained, and a brief consideration of the problem of interpreting such figures in view of the variability inherent in them.

Chapter 20
Animals as tools in
nutrition experimentation

Most of the data describing the gross nutrient makeup of foods and feedstuffs are obtained routinely by chemical analysis. The average or typical composition of commonly used foods may be found tabulated in books and publications in the literature on nutrition. These chemically determined data are an adequate description of some of the nutrients in some foods. But the gross composition of most sources of nutrients must be supplemented with figures indicating the extent of utilization—figures obtainable only from biological analysis, that is, from experimentation with animals. Data for the quantities of nutrients needed by the body, and information concerning the digestibility and the biological usefulness of the energy and of the nutrient components of foodstuffs are necessary before a nutritionist can assemble a diet that meets specific nutritional needs.

In obtaining the required biological information, nutritionists employ various species of animals, including at least seven kinds of so-called laboratory animals, and five kinds of domestic animals. For a limited number of problems, they may also use human subjects.

Experimental groups

Ideally, the kind of animal selected for a given test should be of the same species as and otherwise directly comparable to the animals to which the data are to apply. For example, to determine whether urea can replace half of the feed protein in the ration mixture to be fed to a herd of 100 milking cows, the theoretically ideal procedure would be to choose at random a few (perhaps 10) representative cows of that herd. Those chosen might be divided into two equal groups, one to be fed the regular or control ration, and the other to be fed a modification of it in which urea replaced some of the high-protein feeds in such proportions that half of the nitrogen of the final mixture would be urea nitrogen. After a suitable test feeding period, the milk and/or fat production of the two groups would be compared. If there was no significant difference between the two groups, in production or in health or in other criteria, it would be possible to conclude that urea could be introduced into that herd's ration without adverse results.

Note that we have said the sample of 10 cows from the herd of 100 must be chosen at random. This raises two questions. First, why must the sample be random, and second, how do we choose animals at random?

Necessity for random samples

Animals vary in size, weight, response to feed, and many other attributes. In the scale of values for whatever attribute is under consideration, a few are at the lower end of the scale, most are at the midpoint, and a few are at the upper end. If the sample is to truly represent the majority of the population from which it was drawn and if it is to accurately represent a particular attribute of all of the various individuals in the whole population, it must have the same sort of variability as does the parent group. In other words, the sample must not be biased in favor of the larger individual, or the taller, or those that grow more rapidly. Unless the sample does represent its parent population, there is no legitimate reason to assume that the response of the sample group will be representative of the whole population. In general, and subject to the limitations of size of sample with relation to the original population, the average values of samples drawn at random should be essentially the same as the average values of the larger population.

Choosing random samples

To avoid any tendency to a systematic bias, it is necessary to devise schemes whereby chance alone governs the choice of animals; a representative random sampling cannot be achieved without some randomization plan. To pick animals by just reaching for them as they come, so to speak, usually results in picking them according to the speed or agility of the individual. Many people have an uncontrollable bias toward picking the best looking first, but often the differences between individual animals cannot be detected by observation. Experimental studies have shown that no true randomization of sampling can be achieved unless a scheme that operates entirely on chance is followed.

Statisticians frequently use tables of random numbers; however, for most nutrition studies this is unnecessary. Some workers use numbered cards, which when shuffled are presumably randomly arranged. One of the simplest and still effective methods is to use the page numbers of a book opened without conscious selection of the page.

The latter scheme operates something like this. Open a book, without any conscious attempt to open it at a specific page. Divide the page number by the number of animals to be allotted or chosen for the sample. Calculate the largest whole number in the quotient and record the remainder:

Book page number	156
Animals to be allotted	15
Largest whole number in quotient	10
Remainder	6

In the above example *the remainder* 6 tells us that the sixth animal from one end of the line is to be chosen first. The process is repeated, decreasing the number allotted by 1, since one of the intended sample has now been chosen. For example:

Book page number	98
Animals to be allotted	14
Largest whole number in quotient	7
Remainder	7

The second animal to be chosen will be the seventh in line, counting from the same end as before, but since animal 6 has already been chosen, the second choice will be the eighth animal in line in the population from which the sample is being drawn.

Let us return to our example of drawing 10 animals at random from a herd of 100 milking cows numbered from 1 to 100. For convenience we will have the herd standing in ten rows of ten animals each (as shown in the upper part of Table 20.1).

The sample of 10 animals is to be divided into two groups of 5 animals each, and we shall place the first animal chosen in Lot 1, the second animal in Lot 2, and so on until the 10 choices have been distributed to the two groups.

The tabulation of figures in the lower part of Table 20.1 indicates which animals are chosen and the order in which they are chosen.

The only general assumption that need be made is that the 10 cows tested adequately represent the whole population (herd) of which they are a sample. In practice, a sample seldom reflects all the potential variations of the popu-

Table 20.1
Scheme for choosing a random sample of animals

Population (superscripts represent order of choices for sample)

1	2	3	4	5	6	7	8	9	10
11	12	13	14	15^{10}	16	17^{7}	18	19	20
21^{4}	22	23	24	25	26	27^{9}	28	29	30
31	32	33	34	35	36	37	38^{2}	39	40
41	42	43	44	45	46	47	48	49	50
51	52	53	54	55	56	57	58	59	60^{5}
61	62	63	64	65	66	67	68	69	70
71	72	73^{8}	74	75	76	77^{6}	78	79	80
81	82	83	84	85	86	87	88	89	90
91	92	93	94	95^{3}	96^{1}	97	98	99	100

Book page	Cows remaining	Largest whole number in quotient	Remainder	Cows already chosen up to that number	Number of cow to be taken	Lot to which cow is assigned
296	100	2	96	0	96	1
335	99	3	38	0	38	2
192	98	1	94	1	95	1
312	97	3	21	0	21	2
250	96	2	58	2	60	1
264	95	2	74	3	77	2
111	94	1	17	0	17	1
162	93	1	69	4	73	2
301	92	3	25	2	27	1
288	91	3	15	0	15	2

lation to which the results are to apply. Therefore, investigators describe in detail the breed, hereditary background, size, age, and sex of the cows or pigs or chickens used as experimental animals, as well as their commercial productivity and the type of management used in raising them, in the hope of identifying the populations the animals represent even though they may be scattered over a whole continent. Obviously, there are many uncertainties, for example, how the results of a feeding test in Quebec, Canada, will apply to what seem to be comparable animals in British Columbia, Texas, or Vermont. Table 20.2 lists variations among samples of Yorkshire pigs fed identical rations in four Canadian provinces.

Table 20.2
Variation in attributes between samples of Yorkshire pigs fed identical rations
in four Canadian provinces

Samples from	Initial weight (kg)	Age (days)	Daily gain (kg)	Daily feed (kg)	Dig. energy (therms)	Percentage of Grade A carcasses in group
Alberta	18.2	64	0.66	2.85	8.77	66
Manitoba	18.6	63	0.73	2.87	8.95	47
Quebec	20.9	65	0.64	2.83	8.68	28
Nova Scotia	17.7	59	0.77	3.18	9.77	34
Expected			0.82	3.09		

Source: Bell, J. M., *Can J. Animal Sci.* **38**(1958):73.

Use of pilot animals

The problems described above are minor compared to those encountered where it is impossible or at least impracticable to choose for experimental purposes animals (or subjects) of the same species as that to which the results are to apply. Referring again to the "urea test," that problem could not be studied using pigs or rats, because neither of these species can use urea to any significant extent. The cost of experimental animals and of equipment make the use of large animals impractical in some studies. Also, for ethical reasons, pilot laboratory animals* are employed in many studies of intermediary metabolism or nutrient deficiency, or in tests where procedures that cause temporary discomfort are unavoidable.

Superimposed on the problem of interpreting the actual observations of such experiments is the problem of translating results from one species to another whose anatomy, physiology, and environment may differ widely from those of the test subjects. To many people it is somewhat of a shock to learn how few data concerning human nutrition have been obtained from the observation of biological tests carried out on human subjects. Indeed, our current knowledge of food digestion and its subsequent intermediary metabolism, to say nothing of our present beliefs about the probable nutritional requirements of humans, come to us largely via the laboratory animal and the chemist's test tube.

*Pilot animals are animals of a species different from that to which the results of a test are intended to apply.

It is therefore not only appropriate but almost mandatory that before we undertake quantitative consideration of nutrient requirements we examine, if only briefly, the philosophy of animal experimentation, and some of the features of the planning, conduct, and interpretation of the results of such tests.

Choice of species

Nutritionists make use of at least a dozen different species of animals (including poultry) in their research. The choice of a particular species for a particular study depends on several factors. If the animal is to be used as a pilot, the similarity between its type of digestive system and that of the species to which the results will be applied becomes important, as does the adaptability of the animal to the kind of diet necessarily employed, the physical size of the animals, any unique nutrient requirement, and the amenability of the pilot to the experimental conditions to be imposed. If the study is to be made using the same kind of animals (or human subjects) to which the results are to be applied, the choice of species is of course settled automatically.

The species commonly used in nutrition studies wherein biological tests are involved are listed in Figure 20.1; they are classified according to the anatomy of the digestive system because this feature is of particular importance in determining the nature of the foods that a species normally consumes. For example, herbivorous animals have a more complicated and capacious digestive tract than do omnivora and carnivora; the concentrated rations that are suitable for humans are not bulky enough to allow proper functioning of the multiple "stomach" system of the cow or sheep.

It may be helpful at this point to note a few of the characteristics of animals that help determine the types of studies for which they are especially adapted.

Differences in the anatomy of the digestive system are more significant physically than nutritionally because foods or nutrients in the tract are still technically outside the body. Once digested out from the food of which they were originally a part, the nutrients and energy-yielding molecules enter the body by absorption through the walls of the structures making up the tract. Inside the body the metabolic machinery is essentially the same for all species and actually requires the same operating materials, the amounts being proportional to the size of the body, for maintenance, or being related to the speed-up of metabolism involved, for activity or production.

Among the reasons for using pilot animals in nutrition studies are the inavailability and high cost of the food or nutrients that must be supplied. Vitamins, or enzymes, or amino acids, for example, are sometimes so costly that the use of large animals becomes prohibitive. The solution in the preliminary stages of testing is to employ some species of animal whose reaction

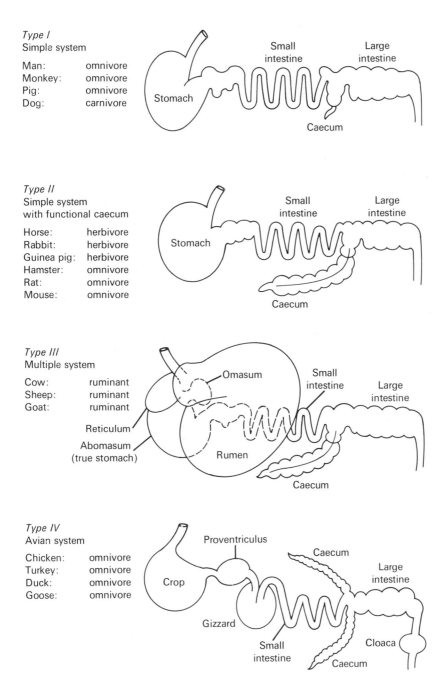

Figure 20.1
Classification of animals according to type of digestive system.

is similar to that of the larger species to which the tests are intended to apply. For example, instead of humans an experimenter may use mice, rats, dogs, monkeys, or pigs. All of these species can readily consume foods and diets normally eaten by humans and digest them to about the same degree. However, the rat appears to be metabolically tolerant of some products that are sometimes toxic to man, whereas the dog often has a strong negative reaction to such materials. Thus, in toxicity studies it is usually necessary to test the food, nutrient, or drug on at least two types of animal, one of which is not a rodent.

The necessary nutrient makeup of the diet or ration can also limit the choice of pilot animal. Humans, monkeys, and guinea pigs must be supplied with vitamin C in the diet. All other major mammalian species synthesize this vitamin. In assaying foods for vitamin C, the pilot animals for humans must therefore be either guinea pigs or monkeys.

The difference between the herbivorous and nonherbivorous animals is another factor determining the choice of pilot animals. Because of the mediation of microorganisms in the rumen or caecum, herbivores do not need a dietary source of certain amino acids that are essential components of the rations of nonherbivores. This peculiarity means of course that among the small animals, only rabbits or guinea pigs can be considered acceptable pilots for studies of the problems of protein metabolism affecting the rations of cattle or sheep. However, even this substitution can lead to problems of interpretation because these small herbivorous species practice copography. Sheep or goats are frequently used in studying the nutritional problems of cattle, providing the most nearly satisfactory employment of pilot animals, except for substitution of small or miniature breeds of dogs or pigs for the larger breeds.

It is difficult for nonprofessionals to grasp the full significance of the use of animals in nutrition studies, and especially the use of laboratory animals as proxies for large animals and humans. No adequate discussion of this problem can be presented in these pages, but we can point out that most of what is known about fundamental nutrition, and much of the information about the metabolism and functions of the nutrients in humans or even in the larger domestic animals, has come to us directly or indirectly from studies on pilot animals rather than from experiments with the larger species themselves. Comparative nutrition has, however, made it clear that the metabolic machinery is essentially the same for all species of mammals. Consequently, the problems arising from the use of proxies are often more quantitative than qualitative, but the necessity of translating the results obtained with laboratory animals still hinders their prompt application to many phases of diet therapy.

Suggested readings

Lane-Petter, W. *Animals for Research. Principles of Breeding and Management.* Academic Press, New York (1963).

Morton, J. *Guts: The Form and Function of the Digestive System.* Edmond Arnold Publishers, London (1967).

National Academy of Sciences–National Research Council. *Defining the Laboratory Animal.* Proceedings of the 4th International Commission on Laboratory Animals, National Academy of Sciences, Washington, D. C. (1971).

Short, D. J., and Woodnott, D. P. *The A.T.A. Manual of Laboratory Animal Practice and Techniques.* Charles C. Thomas, Springfield, Ill. (1963).

Chapter 21
The quantitative description
of animals or animal characteristics

In discussing the use of animals as tools in nutrition research we spoke of comparable individuals, meaning those whose size, age, type, species, sex, physical state, activity, etc. were similar enough to indicate that they would be equally nourished by ingesting appropriate amounts of diets of identical nutrient and energy content. However, each of these factors so obviously affects nutrient needs that feeding standards state requirements separately according to such subgroups.

But between comparable individuals, variability makes it necessary to consider simple averages merely as midpoints of a range of values within which the true figure for each animal lies. For example, the coefficients of digestibility for the dry matter of identical diets for a group of forty senior students at Macdonald College ranged from 82% to 95%, and averaged 91% ± 4%. The variation was due primarily to differences in the inherent efficiency of the digestive machinery of the different individuals. Obviously, the average figure alone gave an imperfect answer to the question of how much energy was available from that diet—it depended on who ate the diet. Evidently we must take a close look at average.

The average as a descriptive term

In dealing with the quantitative aspects of nutrition, we constantly use the terms: an average-sized child, an average rat, average gains, average feed intake, or an average diet. What we sometimes forget is that averages are used in an attempt to describe a population of individuals, some of which will exceed and some of which will fall below the average. Various characteristics—such as weight, height, gain in weight, survival time, or any other characteristic which is describable in numerical terms—are employed in this way.

Implicit in the nutritionist's use of averages is the fact that individuals differ from one another, either in what might be called fixed characteristics or in performance. Not only are there differences between individuals, but there are, obviously, differences between groups of individuals, that is, between averages. Now the question immediately arises: How accurately does an *average* actually describe the group from which it is calculated? It is obvious that the more nearly alike the individuals of a group are, the more accurately will the group average represent each individual. Such groups are of low variation. But if the individuals within a group vary widely, that is, if they differ greatly from the group average, then the average figure may have little use as a description of each individual.

In the everyday use of figures, allowances are made for this sort of variation, and for the inaccuracy of averages, usually by supplementing the figure of average with some further description, such as the range between largest and smallest values. However, in many cases this particular amplification of the average is often indefinite, which makes it of little use in dealing with specific problems. Scientific nutritional studies must include a critical consideration of variation, its causes, its measurements, and its consequences. Biological variability is of sufficient importance to an understanding of the quantitative aspects of nutrition that we will devote the rest of this chapter to its consideration.

Biological variation

There are two fundamental causes of variation among living things: heredity and environment. Strictly speaking, there is also variation due to the interaction between heredity and environment. By this we refer to the fact that good heredity may be limited in its expression by an unfavorable environment, or that mediocre or poor heredity may be considerably helped by a particularly good or suitable environment.

Heredity

In this book we cannot discuss in any detail how heredity background determines differences between individuals within a population; it is enough to say at this point that hereditary variation is a consequence of the mechanism of Mendelism. To develop some understanding of the nature of genetic variation, we will briefly examine the mechanism effecting quantitative inheritance. Any explanation or examples will of necessity be oversimplified, but we hope that they will illustrate how heredity operates to cause variation.

Simple quantitative inheritance   The hereditary factors (genes) of living bodies are located on rod-like structures, called chromosomes, that are an essential part of every cell of an organism. Chromosomes occur in pairs, and the number of chromosome pairs is characteristic of each species. In most of the larger animals there are 20–30 pairs in each cell.

Sexual reproduction consists essentially of:

1. The production by each sex of reproductive cells of that sex.

2. The union of one male with one female reproductive cell.

3. The subsequent division and multiplication of this fertilized cell.

The male reproductive cells are called spermatozoa (sperms) and those of the female, ova (eggs). Each reproductive cell, be it male or female, carries one chromosome of each of the pairs of chromosomes possessed by the individual from which it came; but whichever member of a chromosome pair goes into a particular sperm or ovum is a matter of chance. The union of the male and female reproductive cells restores the original number of chromosomes in the new cell (zygote). After this fertilized cell has started to grow, by cell division and differentiation, it is known as an embryo.

The general mechanism of this reproductive scheme can be illustrated by imagining a male and a female animal each of whose individual body cells carry only two pair of chromosomes. In Figure 21.1 one member of each pair is black and its opposite is white. The pairs of chromosomes are differentiated by length: one pair of chromosomes is long and the other is short. Now let us assume that there is only one gene on each chromosome, and that the gene located on a dark chromosome contributes 100 units to the size of the adult individual, and that the corresponding gene on the light chromosome contributes 50 units to size. This means that the parent female and parent male in our example are each of a 300-unit size because they each have two dark and two light chromosomes.

The female in our example will produce four kinds of reproductive cells or ova. One will contain the dark chromosome of the longer pair and the dark chromosome of the shorter pair. Another will contain a light chromosome of the longer pair and a light chromosome of the shorter pair. The third will contain one light long chromosome and one dark short chromosome. The last will contain a dark long chromosome and a light short chromosome. The male will produce sperm carrying four different kinds of chromosome combinations corresponding to those of the female. When a sperm meets one of

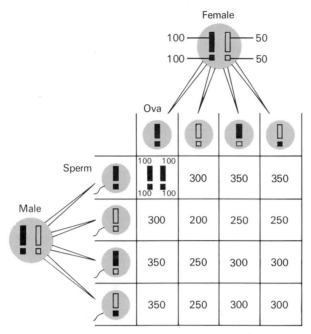

Figure 21.1
Diagram of a simplified quantitative inheritance of size.

the female reproductive cells, the pairs of chromosomes will be restored, but the combinations of dark versus light chromosomes will be matters of chance.

Calculating the combinations possible in the new zygotes or embryos, we find that the potential population of 16 different individuals is made up as follows:

Number of individuals	Dark chromosomes	Light chromosomes	Total size units
1	4	0	400
4	3	1	350
6	2	2	300
4	1	3	250
1	0	4	200

Thus, from a mating of a male and a female of average size (i.e., 300 units each), there is the possibility of progeny ranging in size all the way from 200 to 400 units. This quantitative hereditary mechanism provides for individuals differing from one another over a range of values set by the hereditary minimum and maximum. The example was made simple enough that the numbers can be followed quite easily; it does not represent what happens in practice because it does not include the size classes that are intermediate between those shown. Nevertheless, the distribution of the individuals to groups of different size follows a frequency that is a consequence of the fact that at any given mating, chance alone determines which one of each pair of chromosomes, and hence of each gene pair, will be present in each of the gametes (reproductive cells) produced. The determination of which sperm will fertilize which ovum is also governed by chance.

Probability   This chance determination means that the result of any mating will have to be expressed in terms of probabilities. When an event must occur in one of two ways, and when there are many such events, they tend to be divided equally into two groups. Returning to our example, we will indicate the dark member of the long pair of chromosomes and its gene by A, and the light member of that pair and its gene by a. Similarly, we will call the dark short chromosomes and their genes B, and the light short chromosomes and their genes b.

It is evident from Figure 21.1 that any given reproductive cell (gamete) must contain either gene A or gene a, and the probability that it will be the A is

$$p = \tfrac{1}{2}$$

The probability that either A or a will enter a gamete can be expressed by equation

$$\tfrac{1}{2}A + \tfrac{1}{2}a = 1 \tag{1}$$

For example, suppose we have a female that carries the gene pair Aa. Half the ova she produces will be A and the other half a. Assume also a male Aa. He produces equal numbers of A and of a sperms. If the male and female mate, the probable genotypes of the first filial generation F_1 are:

Female
$(\tfrac{1}{2}A + \tfrac{1}{2}a)$

	A	a
A	AA	Aa
a	aA	aa

Male
$(\tfrac{1}{2}A + \tfrac{1}{2}a)$

The frequency distribution of the four possible genotypes is as follows:

$$AA = \tfrac{1}{4} = 1$$
$$Aa = \tfrac{2}{4} = 2$$
$$aa = \tfrac{1}{4} = \underline{1}$$
$$\text{Total} \qquad 4$$

In equation form this is calculated

$$(\tfrac{1}{2}A + \tfrac{1}{2}a)^2 = \tfrac{1}{4}AA + \tfrac{1}{2}Aa + \tfrac{1}{4}aa \tag{2}$$

Now because each gene pair behaves independently, it follows that with two gene pairs we have a probable genotype distribution in the F_1 generation:

$$(\tfrac{1}{2}A + \tfrac{1}{2}a)^2 \times (\tfrac{1}{2}B + \tfrac{1}{2}b)^2 \tag{3}$$

or if A genes and B genes produce equal effects, we can write

$$(\tfrac{1}{2}A + \tfrac{1}{2}a)^{2 \times 2} \tag{3a}$$

Remembering that

$$(\tfrac{1}{2}A + \tfrac{1}{2}a)^2 = (\tfrac{1}{4}AA + \tfrac{1}{2}Aa + \tfrac{1}{4}aa)$$

we can write

$$(\tfrac{1}{2}A + \tfrac{1}{2}a)^{2 \times 2} = (\tfrac{1}{4}AA + \tfrac{1}{2}aa + \tfrac{1}{4}aa)^2$$

Multiplication gives the following distribution of the genotypes.

AAAA	1/16	1
AAAa	2/16 + 2/16	4
AAaa	1/16 + 4/16 + 1/16	6
Aaaa	2/16 + 2/16	4
aaaa	1/16	1
	Total	16

Generalizing, we arrive at the rule that the genotype distribution of a population is given by the binomial

$$(\tfrac{1}{2}A + \tfrac{1}{2}a)^{2n} \tag{5}$$

where n is the number of pairs of genes involved in determining the characteristic.

Thus, the frequency distribution, in individuals of a population, of a character determined by ten pairs of genes may be calculated as

$$(\tfrac{1}{2} + \tfrac{1}{2})^{20} \tag{6}$$

As an example let us assume a random breeding population of equally frequent, nondominant, additive genes in which each A gene of a pair adds 5 inches to the stature of an adult, and each a gene adds 2.5 inches. A and a are used here to mean dark and light genes, respectively. (To be more explicit, but it would also be more cumbersome, we could write out the ten gene pairs as $Aa, Bb, Cc, Dd, Ee, Ff, Gg, Hh, Ii, Jj$.) Ten gene pairs create the possibility of 21 different gene combinations or genotypes. One genotype or zygote will have all A genes, and the genotype at the other end of the series will have all a genes. Between these we shall have groups whose members have 19 A and 1 a genes; 18 of one and 2 of the other; 17 of one and 3 of the other; etc. The frequency distribution of the approximately one million individuals making up the total population of genotypes possible with ten gene pairs is shown in tabular form in Table 21.1.

Table 21.1
Frequency distribution of heights of genotypes

Genotype 2.5 a	Genotype 5.0 A	Height in inches	Frequency of individuals with n = 10 pairs	Distribution of individual heights
20	0	50	1	
19	1		20	
18	2	55	190	
17	3		1,140	
16	4	60	4,845	$1/6$
15	5		15,504	
14	6	65	38,760	
13	7		77,520	
12	8	70	125,970	
11	9		167,960	
10	10	75	184,756—mean	$2/3$
9	11		167,960	
8	12	80	125,970	
7	13		77,520	
6	14	85	38,760	
5	15		15,540	
4	16	90	4,845	$1/6$
3	17		1,140	
2	18	95	190	
1	19		20	
0	20	100	1	
Total			1,048,576	

The normal frequency curve   We can depict this distribution of individuals by plotting a graph on which the horizontal axis represents the height groups, which will, of course, range from 50 inches to 100 inches, and on which the vertical axis represents the number of individuals in each of the height groups. By connecting the points representing the numbers of individuals in each height group we obtain a curve whose shape approaches the normal frequency distribution (Figure 21.2).

Both the data for the expansion of the binomial to the 20th power, and the graph that represents this expansion indicate that there is the probability that the largest number of individuals in this population will be 75 inches tall. This is the height determined by a genotype consisting of $10A + 10a$ genes (the average type). Potentially there will be one individual that is only 50

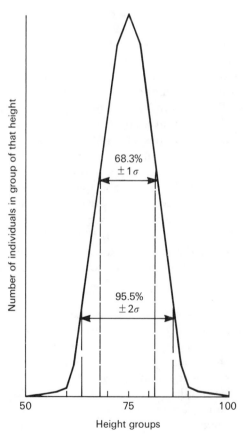

Figure 21.2
Frequency distribution of heights of genotypes.

inches tall; and there will also be one attaining a height of 100 inches. This distribution presumes that there are no other causes of variation and that these genetic possibilities are allowed full expression.

Standard deviation (SD)   If we take the trouble to measure and count the individuals in this population of 1,048,576 we shall find that about 2/3 (67%) of them will be in the height group ranging from 69.4 inches to 80.6 inches. This interval of 5.6 inches above and below the average height of 75 inches marks the limits plus or minus one *standard deviation.** We shall also find that 1/6 of the individuals are taller than the upper limit of the standard deviation and 1/6 are shorter than the lower limit. The number of individuals above and below the mean fall off symmetrically to the final extreme values of 50 inches and 100 inches.

The meaning of standard deviation   Remembering that ⅔ of the total population is between the heights of 69.4 inches and 80.6 inches, and that the other ⅓ of the population is above and below these limits, it follows that if we should pick at random any individual in the population, we would expect that in two cases out of three he would be within the range marked plus or minus one standard deviation; and in one case out of three we would have either an individual that is taller or an individual that is shorter than the limits of one standard deviation. Thus, an average of a group plus or minus one standard deviation (average ± SD) will describe the height, or the weight, or whatever other characteristic we are measuring, with the probability that only once in three times will an individual in the population we have used as an example is 75 inches ± 5.6 inches. This is just another way of saying that the height of two individuals out of three will be between 69.4 inches and 80.6 inches.

Most of the criteria by which we describe groups, such as height, weight, ability to digest food, vitamin levels in blood, ability to run or work, are inherited in such a way that the individuals in a population are distributed around their mean in a symmetrical fashion known as the normal frequency curve.

Random samples   Fortunately we can, by use of relatively simple formulae, determine the standard deviation applicable to the means of small groups whose members are randomly chosen from larger populations. For example, if we know the weights of all the students in one senior college class, we can calculate their average weight and from this, together with the individual weights, calculate the standard deviation. And we can be reasonably sure that our standard deviation figures will be typical of senior students in any university (though the average weights might vary with race and nutritional status).

---

*See p. 299 for example of how to compute standard deviation.

Environment

Superimposed on the genetic causes of variation between individuals are all of the environmental conditions that modify the full expression of the basic genetic factors. The environment, of course, includes a large number of influences, some of which affect individuals imperceptibly. But because these influences include nutritional factors, they are of importance to us.

In combination with hereditary factors, these unidentified causes usually account for the variability between individuals or between groups of individuals in an essentially identical local environment. The sum of the causes of variation contributes to the size of the standard deviation, thereby contributing to the allowance that must be made above and below the average of the group to cover factors that cannot be controlled but which, nevertheless, tend to make individuals less alike than otherwise would be expected.

Experimental groups   In experimental nutrition studies investigators frequently divide a population of animals by random selection into groups. By such division they hope to get groups that are comparable—that is, in which the environmental causes and hereditary factors will operate equally so that between groups there will be about the same amount of variation due to influences which we cannot control. The nutritionists then impose on one or more of the groups some special treatment, such as a particular kind of diet, and try to decide whether or not the experimental treatment has caused one group to become sufficiently different from another group that the observable differences are a true reflection of the imposed condition.

Merely describing each group by the average of its characteristics is not sufficient to give us an accurate idea of whether an experimental treatment has really made any difference. If the difference resulting from a test treatment is not very great, there are almost sure to be some individuals in one group whose performance overlaps that of members of an adjacent group. And, so, even though the averages are different, there may be some individuals that could belong to any group of a population on the basis of their own performance.

Calculation and use of standard deviation   At this point it may be pertinent to recall that the field of nutrition embraces a segment of the discipline of mathematics—more specifically, statistics. We cannot in this book hope to teach statistics. However, it may be possible to illustrate with an absurdly simple example how the standard deviation is calculated, and how it helps investigators to judge whether the averages of two groups being compared differ more than they would had there been no difference in environment.

If a group of 100 college students on a track run for a fixed time, they will arrive at different points along the track because of differences in running ability. To describe how far these students can run in say 2 minutes, the average distance is the most useful single descriptive term. However, the average distance may be a figure that does not represent the distance run by any one student in the group. An average is in fact the midvalue of a band or range over which the observations vary.

If we subtract the actual distance each student has run from the average distance covered by all of them, and (1) square these differences, (2) sum the products, (3) find the average of the products, and (4) extract the square root of this average, we shall find that 67 of the students covered a distance equal to the average plus or minus the square root of the average of the squared deviations. The square root of the average of the squared deviations of the separate values from a mean is the *standard deviation*. Symbols for standard deviation are σ, s, or SD. The Greek letter (σ) is usually reserved for use with infinite populations; the other two symbols are often employed interchangeably with the smaller groups typical of nutrition studies.

To express the above discussion symbolically, we write

$$SD = \pm \sqrt{\frac{S(x - \bar{x})^2}{n - 1}}$$

where

$x =$ an observation, a variate

$\bar{x} =$ the mean of the variates

$n =$ number of variates

The symbol S indicates summation of the values in parentheses; sometimes Σ is used instead. The quantity $(x - \bar{x})$ is a difference, or the deviation of one value x from the mean $\bar{x}$. Sometimes $S(x - \bar{x})^2$ is written $S(d^2)$. See also Table 21.2.

The larger the standard deviation in relation to the mean, the greater the spread between individuals. To return to our example of 100 college students on a track, the nearer alike the performance of the different students, the smaller will be their standard deviation. This is clearly shown if the figures are based on a mean of 100, which gives the standard deviation in percentage, a figure called the coefficient of variation (CV).

$$CV(\%) = \pm \frac{SD \times 100}{\bar{x}}$$

In any case, we can expect that $1/6$ of the students (16 or 17) will be slower than the average minus one standard deviation, and $1/6$ will be faster than the average plus one standard deviation. The same average figures would be

Table 21.2
Two methods of calculating standard deviation from simple arrays of variates

Using formula I	Rewriting formula I	Using rewritten formula

Using formula I

$$SD = \pm\sqrt{\frac{S(x-\bar{x})^2}{n-1}}$$

x	$(x-\bar{x})^2$
5	4
6	1
7	0
8	1
9	4
	10

$S = 35$
$n = 5$
$\bar{x} = 7$

$$SD = \pm\sqrt{\frac{10}{4}} = \pm 1.581$$

Rewriting formula I

$$S(x-\bar{x})^2 = Sx^2 - 2Sx\cdot\bar{x} + S(\bar{x})^2$$

But the sum of an array of numerically equal means is normally expressed as $n\bar{x}$; and since

$\bar{x} = \dfrac{Sx}{n}$ and $(\bar{x})^2 = \dfrac{Sx}{n}\cdot\dfrac{Sx}{n}$ we write:

$$S(x-\bar{x})^2 = Sx^2 - 2Sx\cdot\bar{x} + n(\bar{x})^2$$

$$= Sx^2 - 2Sx\cdot\frac{Sx}{n} + n\cdot\frac{(Sx)}{n}\cdot\frac{(Sx)}{n}$$

$$= Sx^2 - 2Sx\cdot\frac{Sx}{n} + Sx\cdot\frac{Sx}{n}$$

$$= Sx^2 - Sx\cdot\frac{Sx}{n}$$

$$= Sx^2 - \frac{(Sx)^2}{n}$$

and

$$SD = \sqrt{\frac{Sx^2 - \dfrac{(Sx)^2}{n}}{n-1}}$$

Using rewritten formula

$$SD = \pm\sqrt{\frac{Sx^2 - \dfrac{(Sx)^2}{n}}{n-1}}$$

x	x^2
5	25
6	36
7	49
8	64
9	81
$S = 35$	255

$n = 5$
$(Sx)^2 = 1225$

$$SD = \pm\sqrt{\frac{255 - (1225 \div 5)}{n-1}} = \pm\sqrt{\frac{10}{4}}$$

$$= \pm 1.581$$

expected by running 10 students at a time until 10 groups had been run, provided that the 10 students in each group were a random sample of the 100. Furthermore, each group of 10 would show the same average and the same standard deviation as the whole population if they were a random sample of that population. *This is the basis of all nutrition studies in which sample groups are employed to represent a larger population.*

The precision with which the simple average describes how far the students ran in 2 minutes depends on how closely all students approached the average distance. The relative uniformity of performance is also indicated by the standard deviation. If each individual's performance closely approximates the average—that is, if the standard deviation is small—the average itself will quite accurately describe the results. Since plus or minus one standard deviation divides the group so that two individuals are within its limits for every one that is outside, the chances of finding any individual *within* plus or minus one standard deviation are two out of three, and the probability that any particular one of the 100 students did not run a distance within the limits of plus or minus one standard deviation from the mean is 33% (written $P = .33$).

Let us assume that by experiment we find that in 2 minutes college students can run 500 yards on the average, and that the standard deviation of individuals from 500 yards is ± 50 yards. From this we can generalize that of college students comparable to those of our test groups, 66.6% can run 450–550 yards in 2 minutes, 16.3% can run less than 450 yards in this time, and 16.3% can run more than 550 yards in this time. Hence we can predict that two college students out of three picked at random can run between 450 and 550 yards in 2 minutes. Our chance of being wrong is one in three, or $P = .33$.

Statistical significance   The accuracy of a prediction can be increased by using a range equal to plus or minus *two* standard deviations. Reference to Figure 21.2 will show that 95% of the population lies between plus or minus two standard deviations. If we describe the results of our experiment with the 100 college students as 500 yards ± 2 SD, or 500 yards ± 100 yards, we gamble that all but 5 of the students can run between 400 and 600 yards in two minutes; and the chances of being wrong are 5 in 100 times. Our prediction is based on odds of 19 to 1 against being wrong. Statistically we might write our answer as

$$500 \pm 100 \text{ yd at } P.05$$

It has become customary in interpreting biological data to consider odds of 19 to 1 as amounting to practical certainty and, as we shall see shortly, nutritionists use the "$P.05$ point" as the basis of judging whether imposed experimental treatments have really made any difference in the performance of the subjects observed. But first we must refine our statistics a bit further.

Standard error   The same reasoning regarding variability applies to *popu-lations of averages*. The standard deviation of an average is merely the stan-dard deviation of an individual in the group divided by the square root of the number making up the average. The standard deviation of an average is usually called *standard error;* it is abbreviated SE or SD_x (standard deviation of the mean). Its calculation from the standard deviation, s, is

$$SE = \pm \frac{s}{\sqrt{n}} \text{ or } \pm \sqrt{\frac{s^2}{n}}$$

Using our example wherein the SD (or s) was found to be ± 50 yards, we calculate the standard error as

$$SE = \frac{50}{\sqrt{100}} = \pm 5 \text{ yd}$$

The standard error becomes the basis for estimating whether or not the average results of two groups are really different, or whether the same mea-surable difference as that observed might occur from chance variation alone. Let us divide our 100 students by random selection into two groups of 50 each, and have one group wear track shoes in the race and the other group wear rubber boots. We might find that the group wearing track shoes aver-aged 600 yards in 2 minutes, with a coefficient of variation of 10% (i.e., $s = \pm 60$ yards). In the other group (the one wearing rubber boots), we might find that the students were able to average only 400 yards in the same length of time, and with the same variation of 10% (i.e., $s = \pm 40$ yards).

Significance of differences   The difference between these two averages is 200 yards. Now we must judge whether all of this difference is due to the type of shoe worn. Is all of this difference due to the imposed experimental condi-tion, or is some of it due to individual ability within the groups? We may proceed to ascertain this by setting up the hypothesis that there is no real difference. We then test whether or not the observed difference exceeds that which might have occurred by chance. The formula for the standard error was given above as

$$SE = \pm \frac{s}{\sqrt{n}} \text{ or } \pm \sqrt{\frac{s^2}{n}}$$

We have assumed in our comparison that the standard deviation in each of the two groups of 50 students was 10% of their respective mean (average) running distances. We calculate

$$\text{Group I: SE} = \pm \frac{600 \times 10\%}{\sqrt{50}} = \pm \sqrt{\frac{60^2}{50}} = \pm 8.48 \text{ yd}$$

$$\text{Group II: SE} = \pm \frac{400 \times 10\%}{\sqrt{50}} = \pm \sqrt{\frac{40^2}{50}} = \pm 5.65 \text{ yd}$$

The *standard error of the mean difference* (SE_{md}) between two groups is calculated as the square root of the sum of the standard errors of the two means in question, i.e., $\text{SE}_{md} = \pm \sqrt{(\text{SE}_1)^2 + (\text{SE}_2)^2}$. In our example we find

$$\text{SE}_{md} = \pm \sqrt{8.48^2 + 5.65^2} = \pm 10.2 \text{ yd}$$

and we conclude that in two tests out of three, conditions other than the kinds of shoe worn would make an average difference of ± 10.2 yards in the distance two groups of 50 students each could run in 2 minutes. We prefer, however, to base our conclusion on odds of 19 to 1. Accordingly, we multiply the standard error of the mean difference of ± 10.5 by 2, and find that in only one case out of twenty can we expect as much as $\pm 10.2 \times 2 = \pm 20.4$ yards of difference to occur as a result of factors other than the type of shoe worn.

Least significant difference (LSD)   Now, because the boots had the effect of decreasing the running distance, we might answer the question about the real effect of shoe type on the performance of students in a foot race by saying, "Rubber boots can be expected to reduce the distance covered by *at least* $200 - 20.4 = 179.6$ yards." We draw this conclusion at the risk of being wrong once in twenty cases (i.e., $P = .05$). We have used twice the standard error of the mean difference between two groups as the *necessary difference* between the means to cover variation not due to the imposed experimental condition being studied. It is the allowance we make above and below the difference observed between the averages of two groups being compared, to cover possible differences that might occur but that are not associated with the experimental treatment. It is, in effect, a measure of the combined genetic factors and unmeasured environmental influences that cause our subjects to differ among themselves irrespective of the imposed conditions of the trial. The logic and the meaning of the term *least significant difference* (LSD) now become clear. Unless an observed difference between two group means is greater than the LSD, we are not prepared to claim that any effect of experimental treatment has been proven. A difference as great as the LSD might occur from chance once in twenty times! To facilitate their use, and to more easily see the relations between these "standard deviations," we can restate the formulae by which they are computed.

Standard deviation of a variate from its mean:

$$SD = \pm \sqrt{\frac{S(x - \bar{x})^2}{n - 1}}$$

Standard error of a mean from the average of a series of means:

$$SE = \pm \frac{SD}{\sqrt{n}} \text{ or } \pm \frac{s}{\sqrt{n}} \text{ or } \pm \sqrt{\frac{s^2}{n}}$$

Standard error of a difference between two means:

$$SE_{md} = \pm \sqrt{(SE_1)^2 + (SE_2)^2}$$

Least significant difference between two means to cover inherent variation:

$$LSD = SE_{md} \times 2\star = SD \times \sqrt{2} \times 2\star$$

Application of LSD to a nutrition test   Now let us consider an example related to nutrition. In a vitamin A assay designed to determine whether the potency of two vitamin A carriers is the same, the weight gain (in grams) of rats is to be the criterion of vitamin A potency. The rats, 10 per treatment group, are fed for an appropriate length of time and, from a comparison of their initial and final weights, their gains are computed. The results are tabulated in Table 21.3.

The data indicate that the performances of several of the rats in both groups overlap such that these individuals might belong to either of the two treatment groups. The averages of the two treatments are not alike, however, and the problem is to decide whether the difference between the two averages is due to a real difference in vitamin potency, or whether it is due to chance variation. To make this decision, it is necessary to calculate the variation between the rats that received the same vitamin carrier—that is, the variation within each treatment group (SD). This calculation is shown in the lower part of Table 21.3.

---

*This is called the *t* value, and it changes slightly according to the number of variates observed. See textbooks on statistics.

Table 21.3
Comparison of weight gains (*in grams*) **of two treatment groups of rats fed different carriers of vitamin A**

	Group I	Group II
Variates (x)	30	40
	34	42
	38	42
	38	44
	40	44
	40	46
	40	48
	42	48
	44	48
	44	48
Total	390	450
Average ($\bar{x}$)	39.0	45.0
$S(x - \bar{x})^2$	170	82
$SD = \pm \sqrt{\dfrac{S(x - \bar{x})^2}{n - 1}}$	±4.6	±3.0

From these data, the LSD can be calculated as follows:

$$SE_I = \pm \frac{4.6}{\sqrt{10}} = 1.46 \qquad SE_{II} = \pm \frac{3.0}{\sqrt{10}} = 0.95$$

$$SE_{md} = \pm \sqrt{(SE_I)^2 + (SE_{II})^2}$$

$$= \pm \sqrt{(1.46)^2 + (0.95)^2} = \pm \sqrt{2.13 + 0.09} = \pm \sqrt{3.03} = \pm 1.74$$

$$LSD = SE_{md} \times 2 = 1.74 \times 2 = 3.5$$

We are now ready to compare the average treatment gains. From calculating the variability of the rats irrespective of the imposed experimental treatment, we have learned that once in twenty similar comparisons we might find as much as 3.5 g difference in the average gains of a group of 10 rats resulting from causes not related to vitamin carrier. In other words, the *least significant difference* in gains between the two treatment groups is 3.5 g. Because this value is less than the difference between the average gains of the two experimental groups (45.0 − 39.0 = 6.0), we can conclude that the performance of rats consuming vitamin carrier II was in fact superior to that of rats consuming vitamin carrier I. The difference in performance was greater than that attributable to chance variation.

Duncan's multiple range test   The LSD only applies to data drawn from a comparison of two treatment groups. In other words, "*t*" values apply only to data from paired mean differences. Because most comparative feeding trials include comparisons among more than two treatment groups, in analyzing the results of such multiple comparisons, it is necessary to establish the statistical significances of a series or range of means.

The limitation of the LSD caused D. B. Duncan to prepare what might be thought of as modified "*t*" values, which take into account both the number of individual observations (variates) and the number of treatments (means) being compared.* These he called "significant studentized ranges" (SSR). The following example illustrates the use of these values.

Let us assume that 35 sheep were used in a comparative feeding trial involving five varieties of alfalfa hay. Coefficients of digestibility for cellulose were found to be as follows:

Variety of alfalfa	A	B	C	D	E
Digestion coefficient (%)	45	46	44	42	40

To determine whether any of these mean values are significantly different one from the other, "least significant ranges" (LSR) are calculated as follows. Significant studentized range values (found in tabular form in textbooks on statistics) are multiplied by the appropriate standard error of the test involved.

In our example, the significant studentized range values, at the *P*.05 level of significance, using 30 degrees of freedom, and comparing 2, 3, 4, or 5 means, are as follows:

Number of means (*p*)	2	3	4	5
SSR	2.89	3.04	3.12	3.20

Assuming that the standard error is ±1.13, the LSR values are:

Number of means (*p*)	2	3	4	5
LSR		3.27	3.44	3.54	3.62

To test the significance of the range of means it is convenient to arrange them, left to right, in ascending numerical order. Thus, the digestion coefficients for cellulose would be arranged:

40   42   44   45   46

---

*Duncan, D. B., *Biometrics* **11** (1955): 1.

We begin by noting

$$46 - 40 > 3.62, \text{ the LSR for a range of 5 means}$$
$$46 - 42 > 3.54, \text{ the LSR for a range of 4 means}$$
$$46 - 44 < 3.44, \text{ the LSR for a range of 3 means}$$
$$46 - 45 < 3.27, \text{ the LSR for a range of 2 means}$$
$$45 - 40 > 3.54, \text{ the LSR for a range of 4 means}$$
$$45 - 42 < 3.44, \text{ the LSR for a range of 3 means}$$
$$45 - 44 < 3.27, \text{ the LSR for a range of 2 means}$$
$$44 - 40 > 3.44, \text{ the LSR for a range of 3 means}$$
$$44 - 42 < 3.27, \text{ the LSR for a range of 2 means}$$
$$42 - 40 < 3.27, \text{ the LSR for a range of 2 means}$$

Using a scheme of underlining in which the means underlined by the same line are not significantly different, we mark and compare the mean digestion coefficients as follows:

Variety	E	D	C	A	B
Digestion coefficient	40	42	44	45	46

Another scheme of designating significance among a range of means is to use superscript letters. In our example, this would be done as follows:

Variety	A	B	C	D	E
Digestion coefficient	45^{ab}	46^{a}	44^{ab}	42^{bc}	40^{c}

Thus, the digestibility of the cellulose in variety A did not differ from that of varieties B, C, and D, but it was significantly higher than that of variety E. The value for variety B was significantly greater than those for varieties D and E. There was no difference between varieties D and E. To recapitulate, these relationships are shown by the use of common underlines or superscript letters for values that do not differ significantly.

Biological variation and the normal animal

The illustrative examples used in this chapter, and the necessarily abbreviated explanation and discussion of them, do little to elucidate the extent to which individuals are in fact products of variation. On first contact with the subject matter of genetics and with the statistics that apply to it, students are all too often so intrigued and perhaps nonplused with the mathematics that they fail to recognize the biological implications of variation in the behavior and performance of animals.

Most scientists accept the view that in any given species or large population there are a few individuals that possess attributes of form, behavior, or functional capacity far enough out of line from the average to be considered deviates. Conversely, they assume that the characteristics of the vast majority are within the "normal" range. Indeed, biologists accept values for a given attribute lying within plus or minus two standard deviations from the mean as being within this normal range.

Biochemical variation

However, a *normal individual*—normal in each of several measurable attributes—may be so rare as to be nonexistent in any finite group. For example, if 0.95 describes the percentage of the population that is normal for one attribute, only 0.902 ($.95^2$) of the population would be normal for two attributes; and 0.60 ($.95^{10}$) and 0.0059 ($.95^{100}$), respectively, would be normal for 10 and 100 uncorrelated attributes. This means that in fact we are all deviates, that there is no individual who is normal in all respects.

It is interesting and instructive to note the extent of the variations we encounter in the living animal. Many of the variants, singly or in combination, are responsible for the response of individuals to their nutritional environment. For example, the size and shape of the stomach and the intestinal tract, the rate of synthesis and secretion of digestive enzymes, the efficiency of excretory mechanisms all determine how much an organism can digest.

R. J. Williams has assembled data on the magnitude of the variations in the size, shape, location, and functioning of organs of the body. The few examples given in Table 21.4 serve to illustrate the extent of the differences between individuals that undoubtedly affect their response to diets.

Table 21.4
Magnitude of variations between individuals in weight and functioning of various organs of the body

Weights of organ or gland	Fold variation	Endocrine activity	Fold variation
Gastrointestinal mass	6×	Insulin	10×
Heart	2×	Steroid excretion	10×
Liver	5×	Prolactin	4×
Kidneys	5×		
Thyroid	25×		
Parathyroid	22×		

SOURCE: Williams, R. J., *Biochemical Individuality*, John Wiley & Sons, Inc., New York (1956).

The fact that no two individuals are alike, however, does not mean that average performances of groups with respect to one or more functions are not predictable from observational data; or that such performance is not indicative of the effects of one or more conditions under consideration. Variation merely limits the accuracy with which simple unqualified averages describe biological events. Statistics is a method of reducing a mass of data resulting from the interaction of many variable factors to values that are interpretable in terms of cause and effect. As such, it becomes an indispensable part of the discipline of nutrition.

Suggested readings

Dunn, O. J., and Clark, V. A. *Applied Statistics: Analysis of Variance and Regression.* John Wiley & Sons, New York (1974).

Kleiber, M. *The Fire of Life.* John Wiley & Sons, New York (1961).

Snedecor, G. M., and Cochran, W. G. *Statistical Methods* (6th ed.). Iowa State University Press, Ames, Iowa (1967).

Chapter 22
Comparative feeding trials

Most information about nutrient content of food is obtainable by chemical analysis, but chemistry cannot by itself be used to measure the extent to which the nutrients consumed in diets are available to the body. The digestibility of nutrients, their usefullness in intermediary metabolism, the tolerance of the body for various food components, and the quantity of each nutrient that must be made available to the individual are all necessarily determined through a type of biological test referred to as a comparative feeding trial.

As with any other undertaking, there are many ways of organizing, conducting, and interpreting a comparative feeding test. The principles underlying an efficient trial are, however, essentially the same. First it is necessary to consider the objectives: What is the trial expected to do? What questions are supposed to be answered by it? Next an investigator must decide what criteria to use in assessing the effects of treatment. Sometimes the observations or measurements to be recorded are not themselves criteria but are necessary for computing them. For example, a common criterion in feeding tests is *feed efficiency* measured as the gain-to-feed ratio. The two values, weight gain and feed intake, may or may not be criteria in a particular trial, but both must be recorded to compute the feed efficiency.

The criteria must correlate highly with the imposed experimental conditions, but it may not matter whether they are related as cause and effect or whether they are related through some other factor. For example, high intakes of fluorine tend to reduce milk production by dairy cows, but the effect is achieved indirectly through a disturbance in energy metabolism that causes a decrease in appetite. The direct cause of the decline in milk production is not excess fluorine but an inadequate intake of feed. A reduction in milk production will nevertheless correlate statistically with the amount of fluorine ingested, and can therefore serve as one criterion of fluorine intake.

In addition to clarifying the objectives and deciding upon the criteria, an investigator must determine what procedures to follow in carrying out a feeding trial. Because of the variability in response between individuals treated alike, it is necessary to observe more than one subject on the same treatment program and to average their performances. Certain arrangements of the comparative groups of animals enable investigators to obtain more information than they could obtain with less efficient designs. The design of trial is actually a statistical consideration which is significant because it determines the validity of the data produced, the elegance of the analysis that is possible, and the precision of the interpretation that can be placed on the results obtained.

In this chapter we shall elucidate the broad relations between the *objectives* of a feeding test and the *criteria* by which the results can be recorded and on which their interpretation must be based. We shall also examine the main features of the basic plan of comparative feeding trials, known as the *factorial design*.

Precise statement of objective

The objectives of feeding tests are legion, limited only by the curiosity of the nutritionist. This curiosity may have been stimulated as a result of his own thinking, or provoked by the thinking of others. One definition of research says that, "though stealing one man's ideas is plagiarism, acting on those stolen from several is research."

Defining the objectives of a specific nutrition test is not always a simple matter. However, the objective of a particular trial is the key to the organization of that research. The *purpose* of the test is the guidepost for the procedures selected, and is the central idea in the interpretation of results. Researchers take a journey into the unknown, and on their exploratory trip they are likely to uncover so many things of interest, and perhaps of significance, that when they are ready to record their experiences they find they have missed the very thing they set out to discover. They are then in the position of the schoolchild who, in an examination, wrote many interesting things about a topic but failed to answer the specific question itself. A clear, concise statement of the objectives of a research project is the insurance against such a situation.

The objectives must be free of ambiguity. Ambiguous questions addressed to Nature bring only ambiguous answers. The ability to make a clear statement of the objectives of a test enables an investigator to delimit its scope to a manageable unit. The necessity for carefully delimiting the scope of comparative tests, in the interests of insuring unequivocal answers to the questions implicit in the objectives, leads to the danger that the results may not be applicable to circumstances and conditions other than those of the trial itself. The environmental conditions of housing, of animal management, and indeed, of the choice of test animals are sometimes so unique that generalizations from the test results may be unwarranted.

There is a basic problem with research in which the actual feeding trials must use subjects that are not random samples of the population to which the results are to be finally applied. Can the results of nutrition studies conducted with patients of mental hospitals, with inmates of penal institutions, or with members of the armed forces be applied to the general human population whose environment and activity are not comparable to those of the experimental subjects? Can the response of rats, dogs, or pigs justifiably be translated into recommendations for human use? The answers are different in different cases, but the problem must be considered in organizing any research project.

Factorial designs

A partial resolution of the problem can be effected by experimental designs that permit several comparisons to be combined in one test and, while preserving the separate measurement of each, at the same time allow measurement of interactions between them. Such arrangements are called factorial designs, perhaps because they permit us to factor out and measure separately each direct comparison in the test, and in addition to determine whether or not and to what extent the several comparisons differentially influence each other.

As a simple example, let us suppose we wish to devise an experiment to determine the effect on the daily gain in weight of pigs of (1) the introduction of wheat bran into the finishing ration, (2) the sex of the pigs, and (3) the season of the year during which they are fed. If we use 40 pigs we might arrange them into two main treatment lots and four secondary lots, as indicated in Table 22.1. The figures in this table represent the hypothetical average daily gains (in kilograms) made by the pigs during the test feeding period.

In this design we have four pairs of lots among which the only difference is the addition of bran to the control ration. The data in Table 22.2 show that the pigs whose rations contained bran gained an average of 0.105 kilograms less per day than the pigs on bran-free rations.

Table 22.1
Plan of a 2 × 2 × 2 factorial design for a feeding trial using 5 pigs per sublot
(*average weight gain shown in kilograms per day*)

| | Ration | | | | |
| | Control–no bran | | Bran added | | Seasonal average |
Season	Males	Females	Males	Females	
Spring farrowed	0.77	0.73	0.68	0.64	0.70
Fall farrowed	0.82	0.80	0.70	0.68	0.75
No-bran vs bran	0.78		0.68		General
Male vs female	0.74 (male)		0.70 (female)		average 0.725

Table 22.2
Comparison of daily gain in weight of eight sublot of pigs on two different rations
(*in kilograms per day*)

| Season of farrowing and sex | Comparable lots | | Differences in daily gains |
	No bran	Bran fed	
Spring-farrowed males	0.77	0.68	0.09
Spring-farrowed females	0.73	0.64	0.09
Fall-farrowed males	0.82	0.70	0.12
Fall-farrowed females	0.80	0.68	0.12
		Average	0.105

The data also enable us to calculate that males gain an average of 0.04 kilograms more per day than females, whether or not bran is fed, and that fall-farrowed pigs tend to gain about 0.03 kilograms more per day than spring-born litters, independent of the change in ration. We can therefore conclude that the addition of bran reduced the weight gains of market pigs and we can generalize that this applies to both sexes of both spring- and fall-fed pigs even though females gained less than males on either ration.

By this design we have been able to compare the effects of both fall and spring farrowing on the weight of two lots of 20 pigs each, to measure the effects of the ration change, and also to compare the response of 20 males with 20 females where sex was the only difference. We have "factored out" separately the effects of bran, season, and sex. In addition, we have obtained evidence that each sex reacts similarly to the addition of bran and to season.

A somewhat more elaborate example may be drawn from a research project conducted in our laboratories in 1955 and 1956. We were interested in learning how variations in fat content affect the ingestion and utilization of a diet. Accordingly we fed 42 sublots of various animals diets of similar formulation, except for a content of 20% by weight of one or another fat from animal or plant sources and analyzed the detectable differences in (1) the amounts of the diets voluntarily eaten, (2) gains in live weight, and/or (3) the ability of the experimental animals to digest the rations.

The information was wanted in connection with child feeding, but children were not available for the tests. We therefore employed, in three separate series, 2-week-old baby pigs, 4-week-old puppies, and 2-day-old guinea pigs. Thus we used animals at ages when their chief natural source of energy was the fat of their mothers' milk. We knew that orphans of these species could be raised on cow's milk. We also had three species whose natural food habits, from the standpoint of diet, are quite unlike after weaning. One, the dog, is remarkably similar to man. If all three species reacted similarly, we felt reasonably safe in generalizing to predict similar results with children. The design plan, simplified for use here as to the range of fats tested, is given in Table 22.3.

The design of the test shown in Table 22.3 makes possible valid comparisons between:

> 3 species of animals
>
> 2 levels of fat
>
> 7 kinds of fat

and any interactions between all combinations of them. In addition, there is the possibility of subgrouping the fats to examine separately those of long-, medium-, and short-chain fatty acid makeup. Of necessity, the animals were started on test at differing calendar dates, but because all were individually penned, the "confounding" effects of feeding period dates were negligible.

Suitable designs of all trials do not follow exactly the model patterns described here as examples. Detailed consideration of experimental designs of feeding tests is more appropriately subject matter for a course in statistics; the two plans mentioned above are intended only to illustrate the relation between the general design and the objective of a trial. The full advantages of experimental allotment plans are realized only if a statistical examination of the data they make possible can also be undertaken. The two examples show the general scheme by which several specific but independent comparisons can be made within a single trial, and a measure obtained as well of the interrelations between them if such interactions prove to pertain. Suitable statistical analysis would allow an assessment of the probable significance of any effects of the treatments imposed.

Table 22.3
Plan of a 3 × 2 × 7 factorial design for a feeding trial

Sources of fat \ Species \ Fat (%)	70 pigs, 5 per lot		70 guinea pigs, 5 per lot		70 puppies, 5 per lot	
	0	20	0	20	0	20
Butter (cow)						
Lard (pig)						
Corn oil						
Soybean oil						
Rapeseed oil						
Linseed oil						
Sunflower seed oil						

Criteria

Once the objective of a test has been defined, a decision about the criteria that might be useful is the next logical step. Such a decision must depend on a knowledge of physiology, chemistry, enzymology, bacteriology—in short, on a knowledge of nutrition. The following example will illustrate this use of nutritional knowledge.

Suppose we are to set up a biological test to determine whether grain starch can be utilized as a source of energy by 3-week-old pigs. We begin by asking ourselves what criteria might be used to measure the utilization of starch as energy. Our thinking might proceed somewhat as follows.

We know that starch is a pure, noncellulosic carbohydrate. We also know that the principal carbohydrate in the natural diet of the 3-week-old pig is milk sugar, lactose. A pig is a monogastric animal. To furnish energy to a monogastric animal, a noncellulosic carbohydrate must be digested to a simple sugar (galactose, glucose, or fructose). We know that, per unit of weight, starch and lactose contain essentially the same gross energy. We also know that neither lactose nor its component monosaccharides, glucose and galactose, are found in the feces of healthy young mammals. This means that milk sugar is completely digested and absorbed. The products of digestion eventually appear as glucose in the blood stream. Soon after ingestion, carbohydrates that are digested and absorbed cause temporarily a measurable and

Box 22.1   E. B. Hart and comparative feeding trials

Edwin Bret Hart (1874–1953) was born in Ohio, the youngest of a family of fourteen children. Following undergraduate studies in chemistry at the University of Michigan, he went in 1897 to the New York State Experiment Station at Geneva, and from there to study in Germany under the famous biochemist Albrecht Kossel. He then returned to Geneva for four years, where he first carried out research on milk and other dairy products.

In 1906, Hart went to the University of Wisconsin as head of the Department of Agricultural Chemistry, a position he held for thirty-eight years. During that period some forty-six students received Ph.D.'s under Hart, though he himself never completed that degree. He was awarded an honorary D.Sc. from the University of Wisconsin in 1949.

No individual has contributed more to research on the role of minerals and vitamins in nutrition than Professor Hart. Over the years he worked with phosphorus, iodine, iron and copper, manganese, zinc, cobalt, boron, and fluorine. Although he worked in the vitamin field most of his life, he did not discover any specific vitamin. However, he collaborated with E. V. McCollum in differentiating fat-soluble A from water-soluble B, and with Steenbock in his early research on vitamins A and D.

Like his predecessor at Wisconsin, Dr. Stephen Babcock, and along with such junior colleagues as McCollum and Steenbock, E. B. Hart became disenchanted with chemical analysis as a sole means of predicting the nutritive value of rations for farm animals. They emphasized the theory that there might be nutritionally important substances in rations that chemical analyses might fail to reveal. This theory was almost heretical at the time.

A few years before Hart arrived at the University of Wisconsin, Babcock had experimented with growing heifers on restricted rations. The results of these experiments were not conclusive, and when Hart arrived in 1906, Babcock suggested to him that a more comprehensive experimental plan should be inaugurated. The results of the subsequent studies of Hart and his associates were published in the famous University Bulletin 17, *Physiological Effect on Growth and Reproduction of Rations Balanced from Restricted Sources*. This has become a classical report in that it laid the foundation for modern applied nutrition research, and was the first break with traditional research based strictly on chemical analyses. Edwin Bret Hart could be considered the father of comparative feeding trials in nutrition experimentation.

For further information, see *J. Nutr.* **51**(1953):3.

characteristic rise in the level of blood glucose. Eventually any carbohydrate consumed in excess of the needs for maintenance and activity is converted to fatty acids and glyceride and deposited as neutral fat in adipose tissue. If the amount of carbohydrate absorbed is less than that needed for metabolic purposes, and if it is lower than optimum in amount with respect to the quantities of amino acids absorbed from the diet, an increased proportion of amino acids will be diverted to supply the deficiency of energy from carbohydrate. This will result in an increase in urinary nitrogen over that normally obtained from that same protein when consumed in a properly balanced, energy-adequate ration.

From this nutritional knowledge we can now make some deductions about suitable criteria for use in the test. At the outset we can assume that because lactose is the natural food carbohydrate of the 3-week-old pig, this sugar can be taken as the standard or the *control* against which our cereal starch may be tested. Here, of course, we are at once implying a comparative feeding test.

If, on feeding equal amounts of starch in one case and lactose in another, we find more starch in the feces than we find lactose, we could conclude that starch does not yield as much energy to the body as does lactose, since to yield its potential energy it must be digested and absorbed. If these products, starch and lactose, are the only carbohydrates fed, we can obtain information about the extent of *digestibility* by comparing the total carbohydrate of the feces with the quantity consumed.

We have another possible criterion in the behavior of *blood glucose* following the ingestion and absorption of carbohydrate. If in comparable feeding trials equal amounts of lactose in the one case and of starch in the other are ingested, there should be an equal rise in blood glucose if both are equally well utilized to this stage. We can assume that once in the form of blood glucose they will yield energy (or fat) to the body, if there are no other limiting factors operating such as a vitamin deficiency or disturbed enzyme function.

There is still another possible criterion that we might employ: the physiological change expected following the ingestion of a liberal amount of lactose—that is, the synthesis and *deposition of body triglyceride*. In other words, we can think of this as a storage of carbon. Stored carbon can be detected and measured by recording total carbon intake and total carbon output—that is, by a *carbon balance test*. The only source of carbon will be the food ingested. The amount of carbon is easily determined by chemical analysis of the diet. Carbon will be discharged from the body mainly through urinary and fecal excretion, plus the CO_2 in respiration. The sum of the carbon output (through urine, feces, and as CO_2) subtracted from that ingested in food will be the carbon balance. In our comparative test, if starch is utilized as fully as lactose, we should find carbon balances of equal magnitude.

We can go still further by combining the carbon balance with a *nitrogen balance* to make our comparison more precise. A positive nitrogen balance indicates nitrogen retention and protein synthesis. From the positive nitrogen balance, we can calculate the amount of protein synthesized (assuming protein to be 16% nitrogen). We can also assume that protein is 52% carbon, and compute the carbon stored as protein. Finally, by deducting from the total carbon stored (i.e., the positive carbon balance) the carbon accounted for as protein, we arrive at the carbon that must have been stored as body fat. Assuming fat to be 76.5% carbon, the *weight of fat stored* is easily estimated.

Some approximate values obtained from a *carbon-nitrogen balance* test with a steer will help visualize how to use these latter criteria (see Table 22.4).

Table 22.4
Typical carbon–nitrogen balance data for a steer (*in grams*)

	Nitrogen balance		Carbon balance	
Product	Intake	Output	Intake	Output
Food	390		5668	
Feces		106		1457
Urine		263		283
Gases				3248
Gain to body		21		680
Total	390	390	5668	5668

Protein gain: $21/0.16 = 131$ g
Carbon gain in protein: $131 \times 0.52 = 68$ g
Carbon gain in fat: $680 - 68 = 612$ g
Fat gain: $612/0.765 = 800$ g

To return to our problem of determining whether 3-week-old pigs can utilize grain starch as a source of energy, if from our feeding trial we find less fat formed by the starch-containing ration than by the lactose diet, we can conclude that starch does not yield as much useful energy as lactose to the baby pig.

And so we see how both the design of comparative feeding trials and the criteria that can be employed in measuring the response of the experimental subjects to the imposed condition are directly dependent on the objective or objectives of the test. The objectives chosen for a given study are in no small degree an indication of the ingenuity and nutritional competence of the researcher.

Suggested readings

Cochrane, W. G., and Cox, G. M. *Experimental Designs* (2nd ed.). John Wiley & Sons, New York (1958).

Crampton, E. W. "Design for Comparative Feeding Trials." In *Techniques and Procedures in Animal Production Research*. American Society of Animal Production Monograph (1959):122.

Chapter 23
Coefficients of apparent digestibility

Nutritionists conduct comparative feeding trials to obtain data pertaining either to a food or to the needs of an animal. Regardless of what other criteria are also employed, most studies of the nutritive properties of foods include an examination of their digestibility and/or of the biological nitrogen balance and/or carbon balance as fundamental criteria. In this chapter we shall consider some of the problems of determining the apparent digestibility of a food, and of interpreting such data.

In considering the nutrients necessarily supplied to the body through the food eaten, we pointed out that the Weende proximate analysis is the most commonly used chemical scheme for describing the quantities of protein, fat, and carbohydrate foods contain. No such proximate scheme is available for analyzing the mineral and vitamin content of foods, and we therefore depend on specific analyses for each entity.

The nutrient composition of most of the foods and feeds used around the world has been determined by the above methods. However, it would be wrong to assume that these figures give an accurate picture of the nutritive values of foods, because the nutrients found in foods by chemical methods are not completely available to the body when such foods are eaten. There is no extensive information about the availability of most of the minerals and vitamins, but insofar as carbohydrate, fat, and protein are concerned, it is known that the greatest factor in their incomplete utilization is imperfect digestion. It is reasonable to suppose that the major reason for imperfect digestion is failure in the intestinal tract of complete breakdown of the walls of the food cells. Until these cells are disrupted, their contents (i.e., the nutrients themselves) are protected from attack by digestive enzymes. The cell wall in plant material is cellulose, whereas that of animal or marine foods is usually a resistant type of protein.

It may also be reasonable to assume that the proportion of the minerals and vitamins in food that is "available" (not including purified or synthetic sources) parallels that of the available carbohydrates, fats, and proteins, on the grounds that once a food cell is "opened" its contents will be digested and absorbed. Nutritionists do not normally refer to digestible calcium, or thiamin, or cobalt; but they do express human dietary and animal feeding standards on the basis of digestible or metabolizable energy, and digestible or usable protein. They also attempt to compound diets and rations to yield specified quantities of "useful" energy and protein. Dietitians commonly employ specific factors for calculating from proximate composition data the usable calories from carbohydrate, fat, and protein, and agriculturalists use a comparable scheme to accomplish the same objective.

In both of these schemes, digestibility is the key factor, as is shown in Table 23.1.

Table 23.1
Calculation of useful energy in the organic matter of human and animal diets

	Human diets	
Fraction	Amount × kcal/g × digestibility	Useful metabolizable energy
Carbohydrate	60 × 4.10 × .97	238 kcal
Fat	20 × 9.39 × .95	178 kcal
Protein	20 × (5.65 − 1.25) × .92	81 kcal
	100 g Total/100 g	497 kcal

	Animal diets	
Fraction	Amount × digestibility	Total digestible nutrients (TDN)
N-free extract	70 × .80	56 lb
Crude fiber	10 × .50	5 lb
Fat	5 × .80 × 2.25	9 lb
Protein	15 × .75	11 lb
	100 lb TDN/100 lb	81 lb

The influence of digestibility on the final usefulness of foods to the body is shown in Table 23.2, which shows the extent and the variability in the proportions of carbohydrate, fat, and protein lost through incomplete digestion of different types of foods. Depending on the specific foodstuff, we may

Table 23.2
The partition of food energy

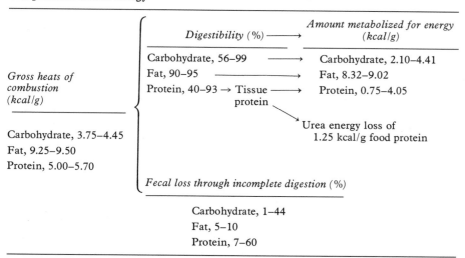

Gross heats of combustion (kcal/g)		Digestibility (%) ⟶	Amount metabolized for energy (kcal/g)
		Carbohydrate, 56–99 ⟶	Carbohydrate, 2.10–4.41
		Fat, 90–95 ⟶	Fat, 8.32–9.02
		Protein, 40–93 → Tissue protein ⟶	Protein, 0.75–4.05
Carbohydrate, 3.75–4.45			Urea energy loss of 1.25 kcal/g food protein
Fat, 9.25–9.50			
Protein, 5.00–5.70			
		Fecal loss through incomplete digestion (%)	
		Carbohydrate, 1–44	
		Fat, 5–10	
		Protein, 7–60	

find in the feces up to 10% of the calories from its fat, 44% from its carbohydrate, and 60% from its protein. Occasionally, high digestion losses are welcomed, as in certain dietary regimens intended to restrict the intake of metabolizable calories. Most often, the losses resulting from incomplete digestion have an economic importance. In either case, the nutritionist must understand them in order to use foods correctly.

Some problems of determining and interpreting coefficients of digestibility

Coefficients of digestibility are not determined for nutrients or for food components that are found in the feces as normal excretory products following previous absorption. In practice, this means that digestibility is determined only for

> Dry matter
> Protein
> Fat
> Carbohydrate
> > Crude fiber
> > Nitrogen-free extract
> > Cellulose
> > Hemicellulose
> Total energy

In principle, determination of the digestible portions of a nutrient is exceedingly simple. If 100 units of one of the above food components are ingested and subsequently 25 units are recovered in the feces, the 75 units unaccounted for are considered to have been digested. The coefficient of digestibility is merely the quantity ingested that is subsequently not recovered, expressed as a percentage of the intake. In practice, however, the procedure poses problems.

Quantitative identification of feces   The first technical problem is one of determining quantitatively the fecal output belonging to a given measured intake of the diet or nutrient. Various devices and procedures have been proposed to permit identification of the fecal material resulting from a given intake. In one of the simplest, the experimental animals are fed markers just prior to, and again immediately following, a test meal or series of test meals. Such markers color the fecal output so that the feces produced by the diet eaten previous to, and immediately following, the test period are distinguishable from the fecal output of the test meal(s). Commonly used markers are iron oxide, bone black, carbon, and chrome green. The marker procedure works quite satisfactorily for animals with simple digestive systems, in which there is very little mixing of fecal material from adjacent meals.

Markers do not work satisfactorily in ruminants, where the food consumed at different times is not kept in serial order during its passage through the digestive tract. For such species it is necessary to resort to a sampling scheme, and to make certain assumptions. The basic assumption made in all studies of digestion in which markers are not used is that if a constant daily intake of a diet can be arranged over a sufficiently long period, the daily output of feces will also remain constant, and that the feces collected between fixed time intervals will contain the output from an intake over an equal time period. (See Figure 23.1.) This assumption is valid only if the collection period lasts several days so that the day-to-day fluctuations balance out.

Index method   The determination of digestibility can sometimes be greatly simplified by the use of index substances. Index substances are materials that can be readily consumed by an animal but that are entirely inert during their stay in the digestive tract and are completely excreted by the animal uniformly mixed with the fecal material. The most commonly used index substance is chromic oxide in the form of chrome green, Cr_2O_3.

If the whole diet is mixed together for feeding it is usually possible to add a known quantity of chrome green, and thus arrange for an intake of the index material as a fixed proportion of the diet. Otherwise, chrome green is fed by capsule, either once a day or with each feeding. In using the index method, investigators determine the digestibility of the diet (or of a nutrient in the

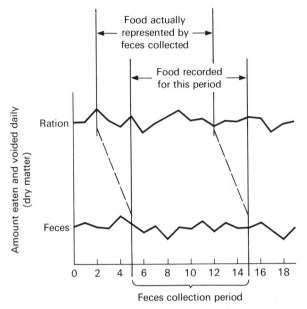

Assumption: Feces between days 5–15 represents equally
well the amount and kind of food eaten
between days 2–12 or 5–15.

Figure 23.1
Time relations of food intake and feces output.

diet) from the ratio of the concentration of the index material in the feed to its
concentration in the corresponding fecal output. Table 23.3 gives data from a
digestion trial in which the digestibility of protein was to be determined, and
shows the computations used.

Although the chief technical problems in determining digestibility are
related to the recording of food intake and subsequent fecal output, sometimes the difficulties are a consequence of a lack of cooperation by the animals rather than of the accuracy of the technician.

Refused feed   Experimental animals frequently refuse to consume completely all of the food offered. The problem then is how to deal with the
refused feed. If such refused food is a true sample of the food that was
consumed, as might be the case with a ration that cannot be sorted, it is
possible to make satisfactory adjustments merely by subtracting the weight of
the refused food from the total amount offered to the animal. If, however, the
refused food is inedible material that the animals will consistently refuse, it
is expedient to include it as part of the feces rather than subtract it from the
food offered.

Table 23.3
Calculations of coefficient of digestibility of protein

	Relevant data	
Feed eaten	100 g	from quantitative feed record
Nitrogen in feed	2.5%	from chemical analysis of feed sample
Chromic oxide in feed,	1.0%	from chemical analysis of feed
or	10 mg/g	
Feces voided	20.0 g	from quantitative feces collection
Nitrogen in feces	2.0%	from chemical analysis of feces sample
Chromic oxide in feces,	5.0%	from chemical analysis of feces
or	50 mg/g	

Calculations, using quantitative collections

$$\text{Intake} = 100 \times 2.5\% = 2.5 \text{ g N in feed}$$
$$\text{Feces} = 20 \times 2\% = 0.4 \text{ g N in feces}$$

$$\text{Digestibility} = \frac{100(2.5-0.4)}{2.5} = 84\%$$

Calculation, using index method

$$\text{Digestibility} = 100\,\frac{(a-b)}{a} \quad \text{where } a \text{ and } b \text{ are the ratio of the nutrient to the index substance in feed and in feces, respectively}$$

$$= 100\,\frac{\dfrac{1\text{ g} \times 2.5\%}{10\text{ mg}} - \dfrac{1\text{ g} \times 2\%}{50\text{ mg}}}{\dfrac{1\text{ g} \times 2.5\%}{10\text{ mg}}}$$

$$= 100\,\frac{\dfrac{.025}{10} - \dfrac{.02}{50}}{\dfrac{.025}{10}}$$

$$= 100\,\frac{.0025-.0004}{.0025}$$

$$= 84\% \text{ of protein is digestible}$$

Assume a trial in which 100 g of feed are offered, of which 5 g are uneaten, and from which 10 g of feces are recovered. If we deduct the waste feed from the intake, we calculate a digestibility of 100 [(95 − 10)/95] = 89%; but if, instead, we add the refused feed to the feces we find a digestibility of

[(100 − 15)/100] = 85%. Obviously, refused feed cannot be ignored. The question of how to deal with it must frequently be settled by the experimenter for each individual case.

Indirect digestibility   So far we have discussed the digestibility of foods or mixtures that constitue the entire ration of an animal. Relatively few individual foods can alone constitute an entire diet and consequently it is impossible to determine the digestibility of a majority of foods by the direct procedure of feeding the food and measuring the fecal residues. For most foods it is necessary to determine their digestibility indirectly. In theory the procedure is as follows.

To determine the digestibility of some dietary component by indirect procedures, two or more digestion trials are necessary. In one, a basal diet without the foodstuff in question is fed and the digestibility of its nutrients determined.

Subsequently, the same basal diet but with the addition of the food to be tested is fed and the fecal output measured.

Then on the assumption that the nutrient content of the original basal diet shows the same percentage digestibility as it did in the first test, the amount of the nutrient in the feces presumably belonging to the basal portion of the ration in the second digestion trial is estimated.

The remaining fecal nutrient is presumed to come from the food being tested.

Two examples will suffice. First, in a domestic animal ration:

Test I: Animals fed alfalfa alone—40% of dry matter eaten recovered in feces.

Test II: Animals fed 10 lb of alfalfa plus 10 lb of meal—5 lb dry weight of feces produced.

From the 10 lb of alfalfa fed in Test II there would be 10 × 40% = 4 lb of dry feces, and therefore 1 lb of feces resultant from the 10 lb of meal.

Digestibility of meal = 100 (10 − 1)/10 = 90%.

Or in a human diet:

Test I: From 600 g (dry weight) of a standard diet fed—30 g dry weight of feces produced.

Test II: From 600 g of standard diet plus 100 g of molasses—32 g dry weight of feces.

If 30 g of feces came from standard diet, then 2 g came from the molasses.

The digestibility of the 100 g of molasses is then 100[(100 − 2)/100] = 98%.

Figure 23.2 illustrates the facts and assumptions used in digestibility calculations.

In actual trials to determine the digestibility of a supplement (that is, of a single food making up a part of the mixed ration) it is necessary to proceed somewhat differently. In the first trial some convenient normal diet is fed, if the trial is to be carried out with humans or animals that do not consume roughage; herbivores might receive a forage that would be suitable as the entire ration. This diet is ration A. In the second trial, ration A is again fed but to it is added a specified quantity of the single food or feed for which we wish to determine the digestibility. The single feed, the supplement, is designated S, and the combination of A plus S, the total ration, is designated by T. The corresponding small letters indicate the proportions of A and S in

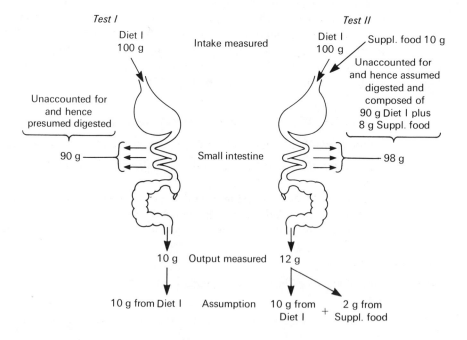

Figure 23.2
Schematic representation of the facts and assumptions involved in the calculation of the digestibility of food. [From *Applied Animal Nutrition* (2nd ed.), by E. W. Crampton and L. E. Harris. San Francisco: W. H. Freeman and Company, 1969.]

ration T. After determining the coefficient of digestibility of ration A from Trial I and that of ration T from Trial II, we compute the digestibility of supplement S as the weighted mean of the digestibilities of A and S.

If the digestibilities of A and T are 85% and 90%, respectively, and if mixture T is composed of 50 parts of a and 50 parts of s, we calculate the digestibility of the supplement under consideration as indicated in Table 23.4 (which corresponds to the method outlined in Table 23.3), using A and T to mean the coefficients of digestibility of rations A and T, and S the digestibility of feed S.

Table 23.4
Calculation of digestibility of a single food of a mixed ration

Basic equation

Where $a = 50$ and $s = 50$, and therefore $a = 100 - s$,

$$(A \times a) + (S \times s) = T(a + s)$$
$$(S \times s) = T(a + s) - (A \times a)$$
$$(S \times s) = T(100) - A(100 - s)$$

whence

$$S = \frac{100T - A(100 - s)}{s}$$

$$= \frac{100T - 100A + As}{s}$$

$$= \frac{100(T - A)}{s} + \frac{As}{s}$$

$$= \frac{100(T - A)}{s} + A$$

Inserting values of A = 85, T = 90, s = 50

$$\text{Digestibility of supplement} = \frac{100(90 - 85)}{50} + 85$$

$$= \frac{500}{50} + 85$$

$$= 95\%$$

The result is the same as would have been calculated by the method mentioned earlier:

Test I, ration A:

$$Intake, A = 100$$
$$Output, A = 15$$
$$Digestibility\ of\ A = (100 - 15)/100 = 85\%$$

Test II, T = mixture of ration A 50 parts plus single feed S 50 parts:

$$Intake, T = 100$$
$$Output, T = 10$$
$$Digestibility\ of\ T = (100 - 10)/100 = 90\%$$

$$Intake\ from\ A = 50$$
$$Feces\ from\ A = 50 \times 15\% = 7.5$$
$$Feces\ from\ S = 10 - 7.5 = 2.5$$
$$Intake\ from\ S = 50$$
$$Digestibility\ of\ S = (50 - 2.5)/50 = 95\%$$

To show clearly that we are actually calculating the digestibility of the supplement by the method of weighted means, we can tabulate our figures as follows.

Ration or food	Digestibility (%)	Relative weight
A	85	50%
S	—	50%
T	90	100%

therefore

$$S \times 50 = (90 \times 100) - (85 \times 50)$$
$$S = (9000 - 4250)/50 = 4750/50 = 95$$
$$S = 95\%$$

The indirect method described in Table 23.3 was used in computing all the coefficients of digestibility applied in deriving the current physiological fuel values of foods.

There are three values that affect our estimate of the digestibility of the single food in the preceding example: the digestibilities of the two diets actually fed, and the proportion of the test feed in the ration containing it.

Variability of coefficients of digestibility

Researchers must also take the variability of coefficients of digestibility into consideration. Data from our laboratory show standard deviations for coefficients of digestibility of the dry matter of diets to be about

Human   ±1.00

Rat   ±0.85

Swine   ±0.50

The effect of variation on the reliability of coefficients of digestibility can best be shown by an example. We do not expect to base conclusions concerning digestibility on the observation of a single subject. Therefore, in our example, we shall use a group of nine subjects whose performance is to be averaged in arriving at a valid coefficient of digestibility for our test food; and we shall demand a 95% probability of having a true value (i.e., $P.05$).

Let us return to our equation for the digestibility of S (see Table 23.4). Perhaps the meaning of the equation will be more evident if it is written:

$$S = A + \frac{100(T - A)}{s}$$

which says that the digestibility of the supplement S is equal to the digestibility of diet A plus whatever difference there is between the digestibilities of diets T and A. If there is no difference in digestibility between T and A, the digestibility of the supplement is the same as that of A!

It follows, therefore, that we must be certain whether there is a real difference between T and A—that is, between the coefficient of digestibility of the original ration A and that found when the test food is mixed with it to form ration T. This we do by taking into account that the digestibilities of each of these diets is subject to a variability measured by a standard deviation of ±1.0 (for humans).

Using nine subjects per test, we can calculate the least significant difference between the average coefficients for T and A (see Chapter 21):

$$\text{LSD} = \sqrt{\left(\frac{1}{\sqrt{9}}\right)^2 + \left(\frac{1}{\sqrt{9}}\right)^2} \times 2$$

$$= \frac{1}{\sqrt{9}} \times \sqrt{2} \times 2$$

$$= .33 \times 1.414 \times 2$$

$$= \pm .94 \text{ percentage units}$$

Box 23.1   William Beaumont and "friend"

William Beaumont (1785–1853) was born in the town of Lebanon, Connecticut. The son of a farmer, he left home at the age of twenty-one to seek fame and fortune. He left equipped with a horse and sleigh, a barrel of cider, and $100. Traveling northward, he arrived at the little village of Champlain, New York, in the spring of 1807. He taught school in Champlain for about three years, and devoted his leisure time to the study of medical works from the library of the local doctor.

From Champlain, Beaumont went to St. Albans, Vermont, where he entered the office of the St. Albans doctor and began a regular course of medical reading. This continued for two years, until the war of 1812 broke out. He applied and was appointed assistant surgeon to the 6th Infantry, joining this regiment at Plattsburgh, New York, in September 1812.

At the close of the war in 1815, Beaumont resigned from the service; in 1816 he settled in Plattsburgh and remained there four years in successful practice. In 1820 he joined the army again and was sent, as post surgeon, to Fort Mackinac located on an island at the junction of Lakes Michigan and Huron. The fort was occupied by U.S. troops, whose assignment was to keep the Indians "in check" and generally to police the frontier. The fort had become a rendezvous for Indians and voyageurs in the employment of the American Fur Company.

On the morning of June 6, 1822, a young French Canadian, Alexis St. Martin, was standing in the store of the American Fur Company when a shotgun was accidentally discharged with the muzzle about three feet from him. William Beaumont was summoned immediately and he described the wound later as follows:

> The wound was received just under the left breast, and supposed, at the time, to have been mortal. A large portion of the side was blown off, the ribs fractured and openings made into the cavities of the chest and abdomen, through which protruded portions of the lungs and stomach, much lacerated and burnt, exhibiting altogether an appalling and hopeless case. The diaphragm was lacerated and a perforation made directly into the cavity of the stomach, through which food was escaping at the time I was called to his relief.

St. Martin did recover, and after one year the wound had healed with the exception of the fistula in the stomach; six months later a fold of gastric mucous membrane had developed which acted as a valve that rendered external dressings unnecessary. During this period St. Martin was declared a "common pauper" by the American civic authorities who recommended his return to Lower Canada, more than 1500 miles away. Beaumont, feeling that this trip would be critical for St. Martin, took him into his home and kept him for about two years.

In 1825 Beaumont began his physiological experiments on St. Martin, made possible because of the external access to the stomach. When Beaumont was moved back to Burlington and Plattsburgh, he brought St. Martin with him. St. Martin eventually returned to Canada, without Beaumont's consent, where he remained for four years, working as a voyageur; there he married and had two children.

In 1829 Beaumont succeeded in tracking down St. Martin, and the American Fur Company hired the Canadian and transported him to Fort Crawford on the upper Mississippi. The side and wound into the stomach were in the same condition as in 1825 and hence Beaumont continued experiments until 1831 when St. Martin's wife became homesick and convinced her husband to return to Canada. In 1832 Beaumont again engaged St. Martin and convinced him to submit to another series of experiments in Plattsburgh and Washington, D.C. The last recorded experiment was in November 1833.

St. Martin returned to Canada, became a farmer, and died in 1880 at the age of 83. His family resisted all requests by members of the medical profession for an autopsy.

As a record of his experiments on Alexis St. Martin, William Beaumont published a book in 1833 entitled *Experiments and Observations on the Gastric Juice and the Physiology of Digestion.* His work made the following contributions to our knowledge of digestion in the simple stomach:

1. Described the gastric juice.
2. Confirmed that the acid of the gastric juice is HCl.
3. Recognized the fact that the essential elements of the gastric juice and the mucus are separate secretions.
4. Established that mental disturbances directly affect secretion of the gastric juice and digestion.
5. Presented accurate and complete comparison of the digestion in the stomach with digestion external to the body.
6. Refuted many erroneous opinions relating to gastric digestion.
7. Reported the first significant study of the motions of the stomach.
8. Determined the digestibility of different dietary components in the stomach.

For further information, see *J. Nutr.* **44**(1951):3. Beaumont's book has been reprinted by Dover Publications, New York (1959).

It will be interesting now to see just what this means. If we write the last radical of our equation by replacing the quantity $(T - A)$ with the necessary difference between these two coefficients, we may calculate the LSD between the digestibility of the mixture T and that of diet A to be LSD $= 100(\pm.94)/s$. A few values are of interest:

Proportions of test food in diet (%)	LSD between coefficients for A and T, where $n = 9$ and SD $= \pm 1$
5	± 18.8 percentage units
10	9.4
20	4.7
30	3.13
40	2.35
50	1.88

Now let us assume that the digestibility of diet A $= 90\%$, of diet T $= 89\%$, and $s = 20$. We compute the probable digestibility of S to be:

$$S = 90 + \left[\frac{100(89 - 90)}{20} \pm \frac{100(0.94)}{20} \right]$$

$$= 90 + \left[\frac{100(-1)}{20} \pm 4.7 \right]$$

$$= 90 + (-5 \pm 4.7)$$

This may be written:

$$S = (90 - 0.3) \text{ to } (90 - 9.7)$$

$$= 89.7 \text{ to } 80.3\%$$

or, as usually reported:

$$S = 85 \pm 4.7\%$$

Of course, changing the proportion of the supplementary food S whose digestibility we wish to determine alters its influence (i.e., the arithmetic weight) on the digestibility of the diet of which it is a part. However, the variability of the response of the test animals is not changed. Where the proportion of the supplement in the mixed diet fed (i.e., in T) is small, the *uncertainty* of the computed average digestibility of S will be relatively great, since the arithmetic weight of the digestibility of the supplement will be small, while at the same time the variability will remain unaffected by the value of s.

The figures in our examples illustrate the difficulty in interpreting the coefficients of digestibility of many of our human foods. This problem is especially serious with foods that constitute but a small proportion of the diet eaten. In interpreting published values, if the test food is not likely to make up more than about 10% of the ration, we must allow about 10 percentage units above and below the reported digestibility merely to cover variation between animals that is not related to the nature of the foods.

Once a coefficient of digestibility has been determined for a food, the circumstances under which it was determined (the digestibility of the original test ration and of the mixture fed, which we have called T), are forgotten. It now stands alone as though it were a constant. Unfortunately, this is not the case. The problem is not that average values are not essentially correct as averages, but rather that we can be so much in error when we start to deal with specific foods expected to furnish some specified quantity of metabolizable energy.

Chapter 24
Energy value of foods

In Section II we described in detail the metabolic pathways involved in the metabolism of carbohydrates, fats, and proteins and discussed how these metabolic conversions effect the orderly transfer of energy to ATP—the ultimate source of energy for all activities essential to life. To summarize, energy is a primary requirement of living organisms, and a major function of most foods is to serve as a source of energy for bodily processes. The optimal amount of many nutrients in the diet is related to the energy content of the diet. In fact, there is considerable evidence to suggest that the nutrient requirements of many animals can best be related to kilocalories of available energy rather than to units of weight of diet.* Thus, information on the usable energy in foodstuffs is important not only as a measure of the overall value of the food but in formulating diets that provide the optimal ratios of nutrients to energy. In general, nutrient-to-energy ratios depend upon the purpose for which the diets are intended.

---

*Crampton, E. W., *J. Nutr.* **82** (1964):353.

The importance of coefficients of apparent digestibility for various nutrients as a criterion of the usefulness of foods was discussed in the previous chapter. In applied nutrition a quantitative statement of the "available or usable" energy of a food is often more useful than a knowledge of the digestibility of the major nutrients contained in the food. Available energy comes from the biological oxidation of carbohydrates, fats, and proteins. Because absorbed carbohydrates and fats are completely oxidized, the available or useful energy from these nutrients is identical to their digestible energy. Oxidation of protein, however, leaves a nitrogenous residue that is excreted via the urine. To compute the available energy in protein, it is necessary to correct its digestible energy for the energy lost in the urine. In general, the available energy of a food is its gross energy minus the energy in fecal and urinary residues. Several measures that take account of these losses in the feces and urine have been used to determine the useful energy in specific foods and feeds. Examples of such measures are digestible energy, metabolizable energy, total digestible nutrients, and physiological fuel values. An understanding of the origin, nature, and limitations of the various measures used to express the energy value of a food is helpful in making the fullest use of the energy values published for the various foodstuffs.

Gross caloric values of foods

The energy of foods is contained in the four proximate principles, crude protein, ether extract, crude fiber, and nitrogen-free extract. Because the last two are carbohydrates and the gross energy of one is not distinguishable from the gross energy of the other, we shall deal only with their total, as carbohydrate (by difference).

The gross energy of a food—in other words, of the three fractions, carbohydrate, fat, and protein—can be determined by combustion in a bomb calorimeter. The heat released during complete combustion to water, carbon dioxide, and other gases is called the *heat of combustion*. Heats of combustion of pure substances (i.e., of identical chemical molecules) are constants. However, the proximate fractions of the Weende food analysis are mixtures. Even if ether extract were composed entirely of triglycerides, there could be appreciable differences between the energy values of this fraction in different foods because of differences in the fatty acid composition of the triglycerides characteristic of each foodstuff. In general, heats of combustion vary directly with the carbon and hydrogen content and inversely with the oxygen content. We will not describe how various methods of chemical determination affect the energy values of specific foods nor will we present extensive data for different specific foods. However, we will provide examples to illustrate how composition affects the heat of combustion of nutrients and of foods.

Heats of combustion of fat   Nutritionists have known about the variation in the heats of combustion of the ether extract of different foods for three-quarters of a century. A few examples from data obtained by W. O. Atwater in the 1890s illustrate the differences that have been observed among fats from different sources (see Table 24.1).

Box 24.1   The calorie and the joule

The calorie has been used as a unit of energy for at least two centuries, having been used by Lavoisier in measurements of the heat production of guinea pigs. It is actually a unit of heat, since according to its definition, one calorie is the amount of heat required to raise one gram of water one degree centigrade at atmospheric pressure. This is also the specific heat of water, which varies slightly with temperature. The 15° calorie is defined as the amount of heat required to increase the temperature of water from 14.5°C to 15.5°C, the specific heat of water at 15°C at constant pressure being defined as unity. The electrical energy required to increase the temperature of water from 14.5°C to 15.5°C has been determined, and averages out to 4.1855 joules per 15° calorie.

The joule is defined as "the work done when the point of application of a force of one newton (1 N) is displaced a distance of one metre (1 m) in the direction of the force." Thus, the joule can be used to measure heat, mechanical, and electrical energy, and can replace such measures as the calorie, erg, British thermal unit, electrovolt, foot pound-force, and therm.

Years ago the Conférence Générale des Poids et Mesures worked out a Système Internationale d'Unités (SI), which it formally approved in 1960. A refinement of the metric system, the new system has dropped many units (including the calorie) of the older system. The joule is the unit for measuring all forms of energy in the SI, whereas the calorie is a valid unit only in the metric system. The SI has already been approved for use in about thirty countries, which has created pressure to replace the calorie with the joule as a unit of energy.

This pressure has resulted in controversy among nutritional scientists about the pros and cons of discarding the calorie and adopting the joule. Proponents of the change emphasize that the joule is a completely coherent unit for measuring energy in all the branches of science upon which nutritional science ultimately depends, and that efforts by nutritionists to retain the calorie as the unit of energy will isolate nutritional science from the other sciences, in particular from physics and chemistry. Those opposed to the change claim that the negative effect of the upheaval caused by revising the basic nutritional literature will outweigh the gain of the refinements possible from using the joule as a measurement of energy. Some opponents, such as Dr. Thomas Moore of Cam-

It is evident from these examples that the gross energy of nontriglyceride material in ether extract is lower than the gross energy of triglycerides themselves. However, the energy value of triglycerides also varies according to the structure of the fatty acids they contain. The heat of combustion of the triglycerides in butter is lower than that of the triglycerides in lard. This

bridge University, suggest that the calorie be retained as a unit of food energy rather than of heat, but in deference to international standardization, that the calorie be redefined as that amount of any food which can, if used exclusively by an animal as a source of energy, produce 4.180 joules.

It is not our intention to take a specific position on the controversy taking place at the time of writing, but we do wish to alert the reader to the fact that many countries have adopted the SI, and that conversion to the joule may be inevitable with time. Although the calorie has been retained throughout this text, the values given can be converted to the joule by using the conversion factor 4.1855 kilojoules = kilocalorie. In nutritional work, kilocalories are often rounded off to the nearest 50, which would be approximately to the nearest 200 kilojoules. Representative converted values are shown below.

Kilocalories	Kilojoules (exact)	Kilojoules (rounded to nearest 200)
500	2,093	2,000
1,000	4,186	4,200
1,500	6,278	6,200
2,000	8,371	8,400
2,500	10,463	10,400
3,000	12,556	12,600
3,500	14,649	14,600
4,000	16,740	16,800

Comparisons of physiological fuel values are as follows:

	Kilocalories	Kilojoules
Protein	4	17
Fat	9	38
Carbohydrate	4	17

Table 24.1
Heats of combustion of food fats

	Kilocalories per gram	
Food	Ether extract	Triglyceride
Beef	9.24	9.50
Mutton	9.32	9.51
Pork	9.13	9.50
Lard		9.59
Butter		9.27
Olive oil		9.47
Corn oil		9.28
Wheat	9.07	
Oats	8.93	
Barley	9.07	

difference is explained by the fact that butter contains appreciable quantities of short-chain fatty acids. The heat of combustion for butyric acid, for example, is 6.0 kcal per gram whereas the heat of combustion of palmitic acid is 9.4 kcal per gram. Atwater proposed the following average heats of combustion for the ether extract from various classes of foods.

Class of food	Heat of combustion of its ether extract
Meats, fish, eggs	9.50 kcal/gram
Dairy products	9.25 kcal/gram
Cereals, vegetables, fruits	9.30 kcal/gram
Average	9.35 kcal/gram

The average of these figures, 9.35 kcal per gram ether extract, does not agree with the figure of 9.40 kcal per gram frequently quoted as the gross energy value of fat in human diets. This discrepancy stems from the fact that Atwater never proposed that average heats of combustion be applied to individual foods. Rather, he arrived at the value of 9.40 kcal per gram as the weighted average for fat in a mixed diet—weighted according to the typical quantities of foods containing the different types of fat represented. Clearly we cannot accurately compute the physiological fuel value of fats of different types of foods on the basis of a single general heat of combustion for the ether extract in food.

Heats of combustion of carbohydrate   The carbohydrate fractions of foods differ widely in the proportions of starch, sugar, cellulose, and hemicellulose they contain. The heats of combustion of seven carbohydrates as given in Atwater's data are assembled in Table 24.2.

Table 24.2
Heats of combustion of food carbohydrates

Material	Kilocalories per gram
Starch	4.20
Glycogen	4.19
Dextrose	3.75
Cane sugar	3.96
Milk sugar	3.86
Cellulose	4.20
Hemicellulose	3.72–4.38

Having determined that foodstuffs contain variable proportions of these carbohydrate components, and using such information as he had concerning this variability, plus his own reasoning, Atwater proposed and used the following values:

Class of food	Heat of combustion of its carbohydrate
All animal and fish products	3.90 kcal/gram
Cereals, legumes, vegetables, and starch	4.20 kcal/gram
Sugars	3.95 kcal/gram
Fruits	4.00 kcal/gram
Average	4.01 kcal/gram

Heats of combustion of protein   Atwater distinguished between true proteins (proteids) and nonprotein nitrogenous compounds (nonproteins) in foods, and his heats of combustion for crude protein are weighted averages of the caloric values of these two types of nitrogenous compounds in the food.

The gross energy of protein varies with the nitrogen content or, in other words, the amino acid composition of the protein. The heat of combustion for glycine, for example, is 3.1 kcal per gram compared to 5.9 kcal per gram for tyrosine. Table 24.3 illustrates how the nitrogen content of the protein and the proportions of protein nitrogen and nonprotein nitrogen affect the caloric value of crude protein. Because there is a limited amount of data on

Table 24.3
Atwater's method of calculating the heats of combustion of food protein

Food	Nitrogenous fraction	Proportion in food protein (a)	Protein per gram nitrogen (b)	Grams protein equivalent in food (c) = (a × b)	Kilocalories per gram of protein equiv. (d)	Kilocalories in protein equivalent (e) = (c × d)	Heat of combustion (kcal/g) of crude protein (f) = (e ÷ c)
I	True protein	0.96	5.7	5.47	5.90	32.27	
	Nonprotein N	0.04	4.7	0.19	3.45	0.65	
	Crude protein	1.00		5.66		32.92	5.80
II	True protein	0.60	6.25	3.75	5.80	21.75	
	Nonprotein N	0.40	4.7	1.88	3.45	6.49	
	Crude protein	1.00		5.63		28.24	5.02

the proportion of protein nitrogen to nonprotein nitrogen in the crude protein of specific foods, it is customary to treat all nitrogen in food as protein nitrogen and to weight heats of combustion for the protein in foods of plant origin in a somewhat arbitrary way. For this purpose the heats of combustion of the principal protein of the food and that of asparagine, representing the nonprotein nitrogen (NPN) compounds, have been used (see Table 24.4).

Atwater's proposal for computing the caloric values of the protein of foods was based on figures such as those shown in Tables 24.4 and 24.5.

Table 24.4
Heats of combustion for protein of foods

Material	Kilocalories per gram
Beef muscle	5.65
Veal	5.65
Mutton	5.60
Gelatin	5.25
Egg albumin	5.71
Egg yolk	5.84
Milk casein	5.63–5.86
Gliadin	5.92
Glutelin	5.88
Legumin	5.79
Plant fibrin	5.89
Asparagine as NPN of plant products	3.45

Table 24.5
Heats of combustion for protein in different classes of foods

Food	Kilocalories per gram
Meats, dairy products	5.65
Eggs	5.75
Cereals, 4% NPN	5.80
Legumes, 4% NPN	5.70
Vegetables, 40% NPN	5.00
Fruits, 30% NPN	5.20
Average	5.52

Calculation of gross caloric value from proximate analysis   In view of the variations in heats of combustion, it is necessary to ask if the gross caloric value of a food can be computed with acceptable accuracy by applying appropriate heats of combustion to data obtained by proximate analysis. If it cannot, calculated available energy values, such as physiological fuel values and total digestible nutrients (TDN), are of little value in predicting the useful energy of foods and feeds. Data indicate that when appropriate heats of combustion are used, the computed gross caloric values of common foodstuffs in

---

Box 24.2   Wilbur O. Atwater and physiological fuel values

Wilbur O. Atwater (1844–1907) has been called the founder of the science of nutrition in the United States. Born in New York state, Atwater moved to Vermont with his family as a young boy. He entered the University of Vermont, but transferred to Wesleyan University, Middletown, Connecticut, where he received his baccalaureate degree. His Ph.D. degree in chemistry, received in 1869, was from the Sheffield Scientific School of Yale University. From Yale, Atwater went to Germany, studying agricultural and physiological chemistry in Berlin and Leipzig. Following brief appointments at what are now the Universities of Tennessee and Maine, Atwater returned to Wesleyan University in 1873 as Professor of Chemistry, a position he held until his death.

Influenced by his experience in Germany, W. O. Atwater was largely responsible for establishing the first agricultural experiment station in the U.S. This was set up at Wesleyan in 1875. Following the lead of Connecticut, certain other states established experiment stations in the following years. Atwater helped campaign for federal support for these stations, and eventually such support was provided through the Hatch Act of 1887. A new station was set up at the Agricultural School (now the University of Connecticut) at Storrs, with Atwater as director. During this period, however, he maintained his headquarters at Wesleyan, some thirty-five miles away. Atwater became director of the USDA Office of Experiment Stations for three years, and hence held three positions concurrently during this time.

With the support of federal funds for investigations into human nutrition, a cooperative project was initiated to obtain data on the composition and nutritive value of American foods, similar to the information then available in European tables. As a result, Atwater and C. D. Woods in 1896, and Atwater and A. P. Bryant in 1899 published data on American foods, which included maximum, minimum, and average values for "refuse," water, protein, fat, total carbohydrates, ash, and "fuel values" calculated by Rubner's factors.

Beginning in 1890, Atwater along with such associates as Woods, Bryant, and H. B. Gibson was involved in a number of dietary surveys in different regions of

the human diet agree well with those determined directly by bomb calorimeter methods. Discrepancies as great as 5% may occur in a few instances, but on the average the agreement is usually within 2%. Selection of the appropriate heat of combustion is the critical step in obtaining accurate gross caloric figures, and it should be evident that general figures for carbohydrates, fats, or proteins cannot be applied to the composition of individual foods. Similarly the average caloric value for TDN in a variety of feedstuffs appears to be about 4.4 kcal per gram of TDN. Values for the TDN of individual feeds vary

the U.S. Atwater also established dietary standards resembling those already formulated in Europe. He had the perception to state that dietary standards are estimates only and that although "tables of composition of food materials and dietary standards are rational and useful, the housewife who attempts to bring the daily meals of herself and her family into exact mathematical accord with any given standard will not be making the best use of what the science of nutrition has to offer."

W. O. Atwater's basic contributions to the science of nutrition originated in his metabolic studies. In 1887 he visited C. Voit's laboratory where he learned about Rubner's experiments with a respiration calorimeter. In 1897 Atwater, along with E. B. Rosa, a physicist at Wesleyan, completed the construction of a calorimeter for the direct determination of the amount of heat given off by the human body, as well as for the conduct of digestion trials and nitrogen–carbon–balance studies to measure the gain or loss of protein and fat. Before he died, Atwater carried out about 500 experiments in the calorimeter, most of them in collaboration with F. G. Benedict.

Using the results of many digestion trials and of bomb calorimeter determinations, Atwater arrived at factors for calculating the "fuel values" of individual foods, food groups, and mixed diets. Having determined the factors for various individual foods, he summarized 185 dietary studies made in the U.S. to arrive at the food and nutrient composition of the "average American diet." He then applied his factors for individual foods to the makeup of this diet and arrived at the general factors: protein, 4 kcal/g; fat. 8.9 kcal/g (later rounded to 9); and carbohydrates, 4 kcal/g. These values were lower than those of Rubner because they accounted for losses in digestion. Eventually a table of fuel values for specific foods was published, based on calculations using the individual factors.

Atwater's painstaking work and keen analytical mind combined to provide a vast amount of important basic nutrition information. His place in the history of nutrition is well established.

For further information, see *J. Nutr.* **78**(1962):3.

depending on their proximate composition so that an average value would have to be used with discretion in predicting the available energy in a specific feed.

Physiological fuel values

The portion of gross energy from each gram of carbohydrate, fat, or protein in a human diet that is ultimately available for use in the nourishment of the body is commonly referred to as the *physiological fuel value*. By definition, physiological fuel values are digestible energy values adjusted in the case of protein to account for energy loss in the urine. Actually physiological fuel values represent metabolizable energy, because the energy loss in urine is from incomplete metabolism rather than from incomplete digestion.

Carbohydrates, fats, and proteins have characteristic heats of combustion, and in a typical North American diet their digestibility has often been assumed to be constant. In addition, a fixed value of 1.25 kcal per gram of dietary protein has been accepted as the energy loss in the urine. The figures that are often used to compute physiological food values for carbohydrate, fat, and protein are given in Table 24.6.

Table 24.6
Computation of the Atwater physiological fuel values from often-cited figures

Source	Heat of combustion (a) (kcal/g)	Apparent digestibility (b) (%)	Urinary energy loss (c) (kcal/g protein)	Atwater physiological fuel values $(a - c) \times b$ (kcal/g)	"Rounded" (kcal/g)
Carbohydrate	4.15	97	0	4.03	4
Fat	9.40	95	0	8.93	9
Protein	5.65	92	1.25	4.05	4

The figures 4, 9, and 4 in the far right column of Table 24.6 are known as the Atwater physiological fuel values. To use them in estimating the useful calories in a diet, it is theoretically necessary merely to have the proximate analysis of the diet. An example of such a calculation is shown in Table 24.7.

From the figures in Tables 24.6 and 24.7 it would seem that there is an easy solution to the problem of computing the useful caloric value of diets; and by ostensibly good logic the scheme also gives us the equivalent data for the separate foods making up such diets. Unfortunately, estimation of the metabolizable energy of foods is not so simple. The difficulty begins with the

Table 24.7
Calculations of useful energy in 100 grams of a diet

Proximate principle	Amount in 100 g		Fuel value (kcal/g)	Useful (or metabolizable) kilocalories in 100 g of diet	
	As eaten (%)	In dry matter (%)		As eaten (kcal)	In dry matter (kcal)
Water	15.0	0			
Carbohydrate	42.5	50	4	170	200
Fat	25.8	30	9	232	270
Protein	14.4	17	4	58	68
		Total useful kcal in 100 g diet		460	538

unwarranted acceptance of the Atwater figures 4–9–4 as constants. This *a priori* acceptance assumes not only that the digestibility coefficients involved are constants but also that they are applicable to individual foodstuffs. Furthermore deduction of a constant 1.25 kcal per gram from the heat of combustion of protein rests on the assumption that the amount of nitrogen in the urine over a period of time is equal to the amount of nitrogen digested over a comparable time (i.e., that the subject is in nitrogen equilibrium).

Kilocalorie–to–nitrogen ratios in urine have been computed in many metabolic studies, and the figures vary widely, ranging from about 5:1 to as high as 12:1. Atwater obtained an average of 7.9 kcal per gram of urinary nitrogen in his studies, or 1.26 kcal per gram of absorbed protein, but proposed and used 1.25 kcal per gram as the basis of adjusting the digested energy from protein to its metabolizable or useful value. In 100 feeding trials tabulated by A. L. Merrill and B. K. Watt,[*] the average and standard deviation of the ratio was 8.12 ± 1.00 kcal per gram of urinary nitrogen or 1.30 kcal per gram of absorbed protein.

The method for computing the physiological fuel values of food protein is illustrated in Table 24.8. These calculations show that digestibility as well as heat of combustion enter into the physiological fuel value of food protein. Statistical analysis by partial regression indicates that digestibility is the more important factor, accounting for nearly half of the variability in physiological fuel values.

[*]Merrill, A. L., and Watt, B. K., *Agriculture Research Service*, USDA Agriculture Handbook No. 74 (1955).

Table 24.8
Computation of physiological fuel values of protein

Source of protein	Grams food protein (a)	Gross kilocalories per gram protein (b)	Percentage digestibility (c)	Grams digested protein (d) = (a × c)	Digested kilo-calories (e) = (b × c)	Kilocalories lost per gram digested protein (f)	Kilocalories lost per gram diet protein (g) = (f × c)	Physiologic fuel value of protein (h) = (e − g)*
Meat	1	5.65	97	0.97	5.48	1.25	1.21	4.27
Cereal	1	5.80	85	0.85	4.95	1.25	1.06	3.87

*For actual computation note that $h = (b \times c) - (f \times c) = c(b - f)$. Thus, $(5.65 \times .97) - (1.25 \times .97) = .97(5.65 - 1.25) = 4.27$.

Metabolizable energy

As mentioned in the preceding section, physiological fuel values estimate that portion of gross energy which is available for metabolic processes, taking into account not only energy lost in digestion but also protein energy lost in the urine. Thus physiological fuel values are analogous to metabolizable energy values. Physiological fuel values, however, are not used in calculating the available energy of a particular feedstuff or of a diet for species other than the human. The system used for estimating useful energy in the rations of farm animals varies with the species. *Metabolizable energy* (ME) is the system used with avian species. The appropriate ME values for a variety of feeds have been determined for poultry by the standard digestibility procedures. Because birds void urinary and fecal wastes together, the values obtained are direct estimates of metabolizable energy. Poultry scientists at the University of Connecticut[*] have published a fairly complete list of ME values for the ingredients commonly used in poultry rations.

In the conventional system used to describe the energy value of feeds, metabolizable energy is defined as gross energy minus losses of energy in the feces, urine, and gaseous products of digestion.

$$ME = \text{Gross energy} - (\text{Fecal energy} + \text{Urinary energy}$$
$$+ \text{Energy in gaseous products of digestion})$$

For birds and mammals with simple stomachs, the gaseous products of digestion need not be considered. The gaseous products of digestion include the combustible gases, such as methane, ethane, acetone, and carbon monoxide, produced in the digestive tract as a result of fermentation of the ration. Methane makes up the largest portion of the combustible gases, and although methane is produced in nonruminants, loss of energy in methane gas reaches appreciable proportions only in ruminants.

Digestible energy

Digestible energy (DE) is defined simply as gross energy minus fecal energy. Because fecal energy includes the heat of combustion of metabolic products of the body, such as digestive fluids and sloughed intestinal mucosa, as well as that of undigested food, digestible energy measurements made simply by subtracting fecal losses from gross energy are frequently termed "apparent digestible energy values." Fecal energy represents a considerable percentage of gross energy, particularly in animals fed roughages. Even in pigs fed

---

[*]Matterson, L. D., Potter, L. M., Stutz, M. W., and Singsen, E. P., Research Report No. 7, Agricultural Experiment Station, University of Connecticut, Storrs, Conn. (July 1965).

well-balanced rations, fecal losses account for 15%–20% of the gross energy. As a general rule fecal energy losses increase as digestibility of the diet decreases.

Digestible energy values are commonly used in determining the energy requirements of growing and finishing pigs and in describing the energy content of feeds for swine. However digestible energy values determined by direct measurement have been described for only a limited number of swine feeds.* Most of the digestible energy values of feeds for swine reported in feed composition tables have been calculated from data on the total digestible nutrient content of these feeds for swine.

Digestible energy values are subject to the same variables that affect the digestibility of a ration or feedstuff. As digestibility decreases digestible energy decreases, particularly in ruminants fed roughages. In calculating digestible energy, theoretically all of the energy losses that accompany digestion are taken into account. Actually this is not the case because appreciable amounts of energy are lost as combustible gases during ruminant digestion. For this reason, the utility of DE values in describing available energy values for ruminants is limited.

Total digestible nutrients

Until recently the system most often used to describe the energy value of livestock feeds in North America was based on computation of *total digestible nutrients* (TDN). TDN values are similar to physiological fuel values except that they express available energy in terms of carbohydrate equivalents. In other words, the useful or digestible portion of each proximate principle in a feedstuff or diet is adjusted to the same energy base as carbohydrate. The equation for computing TDN may be written as follows:

TDN = (% Protein × Digestibility) + (% Fiber × Digestibility)
     + (% N-Free ext. × Digestibility) + 2.25(% Fat × Digestibility)

The first three terms are of equal weight whereas digestible fat is assumed to yield 2.25 times as much energy per unit of weight. Thus like physiological fuel values, TDN takes account of the fact that fat yields more than twice as much utilizable energy as nonfibrous carbohydrate. In addition, the values for digestible protein are added directly to the values for digestible carbohydrate and digestible fat multiplied by 2.25 on the basis that the metabolizable energy of protein is the same as that of carbohydrate. The basis used to calculate TDN combines the use of digestible nutrient figures for animal feedstuffs and the Atwater system of arriving at physiological fuel values for

---

*Diggs, B. G., Becker, D. E., Jensen, A. H., and Norton, H. W., *J. Animal Sci.* **24**(1965):555.

foods in human diets. Thus the term "total digestible nutrients," which implies that only losses of digestion are taken into account, is a slight misnomer because the value for protein takes account of urinary losses as well as digestive losses and the value for fat (ether extract) is adjusted according to the Atwater system for computing physiological fuel values in which fat has a value of 9 kcal per gram compared to 4 kcal per gram for carbohydrate.

Both physiological fuel values and TDN figures are based on the percentage of digestibility of the proximate principles of the Weende food analysis. Physiological fuel values (4–9–4) are "constants" to the extent that the digestibilities of the carbohydrate, fat, and protein in all human foods are 97%, 95%, and 92%, respectively, whereas TDN values are calculated for individual feeds according to the determined specific digestibility of their energy-yielding Weende fractions.

TDN, like digestible energy, does not account for important losses such as those in combustible gases in herbivorous animals. These losses, which are relatively large for roughages, become especially important if poor-quality roughages are substituted for concentrate. In fact, TDN values for roughages consistently overestimate the utilizable energy of these feeds for ruminants. As a consequence, agricultural scientists are using the TDN system less and less.

Digestible energy values have been determined for only a limited number of feeds. Many of the digestible energy values given in feed composition tables have been calculated from TDN values by use of the factor 4.4 kcal per gram. Experimental evidence obtained by Crampton et al.[*] with swine and by Swift[†] with sheep and cattle indicate that the digestible energy of most feedstuffs was approximately 4.4 kcal per gram or about 2000 kcal per pound of TDN. As might be expected, there was some variation in the value 4.4 depending on species of animal and type of ration used in the determination, although the variation was generally small. Nevertheless, a general factor such as 4.4 must be used with discretion in computing the energy value of specific feedstuffs.

Net energy

Net energy (NE) is defined as metabolizable energy minus heat increment where heat increment[‡] is the cost in energy associated with the assimilation of food. The energy cost of assimilating food manifests itself as heat lost from

---

[*]Crampton, E. W., Lloyd, L. E., and MacKay, V. G., *J. Animal Sci.* **16**(1957):541.

[†]Swift, R. W., *J. Animal Sci.* **16**(1957):753.

[‡]Harris, L. E., Publication 1411, National Academy of Science, U.S. National Research Council, Washington, D.C. (1966).

the body and can be measured directly by using a respiratory calorimeter. Although the concept of net energy was introduced early in this century, application of this system was limited because direct determination of net energy values is slow and expensive. However, a few years ago a relatively simple slaughter technique was developed at the University of California at Davis for determining the net energy requirements for growing and finishing cattle and the net energy value of feeds for this class of livestock.* The system includes separate estimates for energy depending on whether it was used for maintenance (NE_m) or for body weight gain (NE_g).

In this system NE_m measures the heat produced by fasting animals. Estimates of NE_m for beef cattle range from 72 kcal to 82 kcal per unit of metabolic size ($W_{kg}^{.75}$), the mean value being 77 kcal. The equation expressing the energy of maintenance is

$$NE_m = 77 \text{ kcal}/W_{kg}^{.75}.$$

Because it allows for basal metabolism plus the heat produced as a result of activity, the net energy of maintenance is slightly higher than the value of 70 $kcal/W_{kg}^{.75}$ generally accepted as a good estimate of basal metabolism. Determination of the NE_m of a ration or a specific feed simply depends on an estimation of the amount of energy required to maintain energy equilibrium—in other words, the quantity of feed required to produce 77 $kcal/W_{kg}^{.75}$.

Net energy for the production of weight gain is determined by calculating the amount of energy stored in the body as a result of a particular gain in body weight. In both steers and heifers, energy deposited in the body as a result of body weight gain correlates highly with empty weight gain. In addition, energy concentration in the weight gain increases as the rate of gain increases. Part of this increase in energy concentration is related to body weight. Lofgreen and Garrett† found that the relationship between NE_g and weight gain could be expressed by the following equations:

$$NE_g = (52.72\, a + 6.84\, a^2)(W_{kg}^{.75}) \text{ for steers}$$

$$NE_g = (56.03\, a + 12.65\, a^2)(W_{kg}^{.75}) \text{ for heifers}$$

where NE_g is in kilocalories, a is daily weight gain in kilograms, and W_{kg} is body weight in kilograms.

The NE_g of a feed or ration is generally determined by feeding it at two levels and measuring the amount of energy deposited as a result of the increase in feed intake between the two levels. Any two levels of feeding above

---

*Lofgreen, G. P., in K. L. Blaxter (ed.), *Energy Metabolism*, European Association of Animal Producers, Publication No. 11, Academic Press, New York (1965):309; Lofgreen, G. P., and Garrett, W. N., *J. Animal Sci.* **27**(1968):27.

†Lofgreen, G. P., and Garrett, W. N., *J. Animal Sci.* **27**(1968):793.

that required for maintenance can be used to determine the NE_g of a ration but the greater the difference between the two levels the more accurate the estimate of NE_g.

One of the main advantages to estimating NE_m and NE_g separately is that computations based on this system produce a higher ratio of maintenance energy to weight-gain energy for roughages than for concentrates. The system thus overcomes one of the common criticisms of net energy systems, namely that they frequently underestimate the capacity of roughages to supply energy for maintenance in comparison to the capacity of concentrates.

Some nutritionists have criticized the California Net Energy System, challenging the theoretical validity of its measures, particularly the method of determining the energy required for maintenance (NE_m). Nevertheless the system has been widely accepted by the feed industry, which is convinced it works.

Suggested readings

Knox, K. L., and Handley, T. M. "The California Net Energy System: Theory and Application," *Journal of Animal Science* **37**(1973):190.

Kromann, R. P. "Evaluation of Net Energy Systems," *Journal of Animal Science* **37**(1973):200.

Moe, P. W., and Tyrell, H. F. "The Rationale of Various Energy Systems for Ruminants," *Journal of Animal Science* **37**(1973):183.

Chapter 25
Nutritional balances

The determination of nutrient balance is a widely applied method for assessing nutritional status (i.e., evaluating whether the needs of the body for essential nutrients are being met) and for appraising the value of various foods. To determine nutrient balance, intake is compared with the sum of the losses from the body through all channels. If less is lost than is ingested, an individual is in positive balance with respect to the nutrient under consideration. A negative balance reflects greater output than intake. Healthy adults should maintain equilibrium, whereas growing individuals should show a positive balance.

Nutritional balances are commonly ascertained for energy, carbon, and nitrogen.

The nutrient balance method is also useful in determining the utilization of such nutrients as calcium and phosphorus, where the fecal excretion includes not only unabsorbed material from the diet but also material that has served its metabolic function. Because of this phenomenon we cannot speak of digestible calcium or phosphorus.

To illustrate the essential steps in determining nutrient balance and in interpreting data on nutritional balance, we shall consider only balances of energy and nitrogen.

The balance of energy in nutrition

As we have already pointed out, proteins, fats, and carbohydrates are all potential sources of energy. Energy is the most significant factor in the "nutritional status" of the body. Proteins, fats, and carbohydrates consumed as foods are, in the metabolic processes which utilize their energy, degraded to CO_2, H_2O, and in the case of protein a nitrogenous residue; or converted temporarily to some form of body tissue (such as body fat, muscle); or synthesized into some product (such as milk, eggs, or wool). Substances in the last category are of no further use to the body, but adipose, glandular, and muscle tissues are eventually further degraded and their potential energy used in metabolism. Thus, protein in the diet eventually yields its energy to the body, even though its molecules first serve as a part of some tissue or as an enzyme.

Significance of the energy balance By quantitatively comparing energy intake with energy output in all forms, we can measure the nutritional status of the body. If intake and output are equal, energy is in equilibrium. This is the normal condition in adults. If outgo is less than intake, energy must have been stored as body tissue of some kind—a positive balance. If the storage is solely in protein tissue, a determined nitrogen balance would be positive whereas the carbon balance might be at equilibrium. However, neither the nitrogen balance nor the carbon balance can be interpreted in any simple way to indicate directly the total quantity of food energy that must be consumed by the body to establish energy equilibrium under specific conditions of age, body size, productive capacity, reproductive status, and physical activity.

However, because it accounts for heat losses from the body as well as for losses resulting from incomplete utilization of dietary energy, the energy balance can become the basis for determining the caloric intake necessary to maintain the particular nutritional status desired. Because requirements for noncaloric nutrients are correlated closely with caloric requirements, the energy balance can in fact be the basis for establishing dietary and feeding standards for humans and animals.

Partition of dietary energy To consider the problems of energy balance, it is necessary to know the several channels through which energy is lost to the body (see Table 25.1).

Although we shall deal with basal metabolism in detail in Chapter 28, we can point out here that whereas that portion of the energy lost to the body as heat which is traceable to basal metabolism is a constant for all homeotherms, all other energy losses vary with the type of food and with the balance of nutrients in the diet eaten. The age of animal (beyond weaning) and/or the species of animal probably affect the extent of these losses chiefly because of differences in the types of food that naturally make up the rations.

Table 25.1
Partition of energy in nutrition

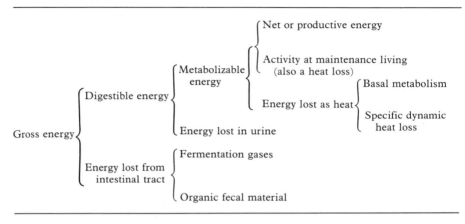

It has been shown, for example, that humans, growing swine, guinea pigs, rats, and sheep, fed essentially identical low-roughage diets, digest them to about the same extent. The herbivorous species digest cellulose more completely, but this is offset by greater fermentative gas losses which, incidentally, arise largely from the cellulose component of the ration. Urinary losses correlate with the intake of protein, and though the ratio of urinary calories to nitrogen is not identical for all species, urinary energy loss is not an important factor of difference between them.

Specific dynamic heat loss is a variable that is dependent on suitability of ration, and hence it is largely independent of age or species. *The sum of the energy lost as heat plus that required for the activity at maintenance living represents the energy required for maintenance in terms of metabolizable energy.*

The amount of net energy from a diet—that is, the quantity that is available for production and/or work—is that left after deduction of the maintenance needs plus the sum of urinary, gaseous, and fecal losses from the gross energy intake.

Measuring heat losses from the body   The technical problem in determining energy balance is that of measuring the heat losses. These measurements are carried out in either of two ways; one is referred to as direct calorimetry, the other as indirect calorimetry. In the former method the subject is placed in a closed, box-like chamber fitted with recording devices that measure the escaping body heat; such an apparatus is called a calorimeter. The indirect method is based on the fact that the source of body heat is the "oxidation" of carbon compounds. Consequently, oxygen consumption correlates almost perfectly with body heat production and can be used as an index of it. The apparatus used to measure oxygen consumption is called a respirometer. With animals whose body temperature is a constant, heat production in the body is a satisfactory measure of heat loss from the body.

Use of C–N balance in indirect calorimetry The carbon–nitrogen balance also can be used to calculate indirectly total heat loss (as shown in Table 25.2). The losses of energy from feces, urine, and gas are determined by standard procedures. The sum of the losses is corrected by adding or subtracting the energy value of the carbon–nitrogen balance, assuming average caloric values for the protein and the fat. This corrected total energy loss is subtracted from the total energy intake to give a figure for the heat loss. The calculation of heat loss, in terms of the partition of energy given in Table 25.1, is shown in Table 25.3. This method is more difficult than that of measuring total heat loss from the record of oxygen consumption.

Direct calorimetry is not commonly employed in nutrition studies with humans or large animals because there are but a few suitable calorimeters in the world today. Indirect calorimetry, by contrast, is relatively simple, and respirometers are common items of equipment in nutrition laboratories.

The order of magnitude of the several channels of energy loss for adults at maintenance energy equilibrium are of some interest, and sample values are shown for humans and for cattle in Table 25.4.

Table 25.2
Typical carbon–nitrogen balance for a steer

	Nitrogen (g)		Carbon (g)	
Item	Intake	Output	Intake	Output
From feed	390		5668	
Feces		105		1457
Urine		265		283
Gases: CO_2, CH_4				3248
Total	390	370	5668	4988
Gain to body		20		680

20 g N ÷ 16% N in protein = 125 g protein gained.
125 g protein × 5.65 kcal per gram = 706 kcal stored as protein.
125 g protein × 52.5% carbon = 65.6 g carbon in the protein gained.
680 g − 65.6 g = 614.4 g carbon gained as fat.
614.4 g carbon ÷ 76.5% carbon in fat = 803 g fat gained.
803 g fat × 9.35 kcal per gram = 7508 kcal stored as fat.

Table 25.3
Calculation of heat loss by a 432-kg steer

Energy intake, 31,291 kcal
- Absorbed, 20,339 kcal
  - Metabolized, 18,149 kcal
    - Stored as protein, 706 kcal ⎫ From C–N balance
    - Stored as fat, 7,508 kcal ⎬ (Table 25.2)
    - Heat loss, 9,935 kcal ⎭
  - Urine loss, 2,190 kcal (7% of gross kcal)
- Intestinal tract loss, 10,952 kcal
  - Gases, 3,129 kcal (methane, 10% of gross kcal)
  - Solids, 7,823 kcal (25% of gross kcal)

Computation

kcal intake	=	31,291
kcal losses, feces	= 7,823	
kcal losses, gas	= 3,129	
kcal losses, urine	= 2,190	
kcal stored	= 8,214	
	21,356	
Heat loss by diff.	= 9,935	

Table 25.4
Approximate energy partition (in kilocalories)
of adults at maintenance energy equilibrium

Source		Man, 65 kg	Percentage loss	Steer, 432 kg	Percentage loss
Intake in ration		2,500		17,290	
Feces		175	7.0	4,325	25.0
Urine		120	4.8	1,200	7.0
Gas (CH₄, CO₂)		——		1,790	10.3
Activity		375	15.0 ⎫	2,625	15.2 ⎫
SDA*	Expressed as heat	160	6.2 ⎬ 88.2	700	4.0 ⎬ 57.7
BM†		1,670	67.0 ⎭	6,650	38.5 ⎭

*SDA = specific dynamic action
†BM = basal metabolism

Measurements of fecal and urinary energy loss are made by a bomb calorimeter, and the methane energy loss can be calculated by one of several formulae from the dry matter, the digested carbohydrates, or the digested crude fiber of the ration. One formula is

$$Y = 1083 \, X^{0.638}$$

where Y is methane energy, and X is digested carbohydrate in kilograms.*

Measurement of heat loss by O_2 consumption   Total heat loss is calculated from the respirometer record of oxygen consumption and its average caloric equivalent of 4.825 kcal per liter. In studies with humans, an ordinary metabolor, used in hospitals for determining the basal metabolic rate, is conveniently employed. It consists of a face mask, which is worn in such a way that all respiration occurs within an enclosed oxygen-rich atmosphere, the exhaled CO_2 being absorbed by soda lime. The quantity of oxygen used is indicated on a scale calibrated with the volume capacity of the canister of the metabolor.

The total heat loss for a particular individual can quite easily be computed from the record of his oxygen consumption. The difference between the total energy lost (i.e., feces, urine, gas, and heat) and the total energy ingested indicates whether the body is gaining or losing energy and thus measures the "overall" nutritional status of the body. The total of the energy losses is also a measure of the quantity of energy that must be returned to the body in food in order to maintain energy equilibrium.

*Axelson, J., *Ann. Royal Agr. College, Sweden* **16**(1949):405.

Heat loss and body size   Total heat loss is not, however, a suitable basis for determining maintenance energy needs, because caloric requirements depend so much on body size. Nevertheless, since heat loss (see Table 25.4) in adult humans at maintenance represents nearly 90%, and in cattle nearly 60%, of the total energy intake, and, further, since the basal metabolism accounts for two-thirds to three-quarters of this, it is evident that the energy lost as heat can serve as an important general index of the maintenance energy needs of animals. To make this index useful it is necessary to find some measurement of body size, some unit of reference to which that requirement is proportional. This problem will be considered in more detail in Chapter 28.

The nitrogen balance

The most common balance used in nutrition studies, and technically the simplest to ascertain, is that for nitrogen. A quantitative statement of the intake and excretion of nitrogen is one measure of the amount of protein utilized. Table 25.5, which gives figures for a steer, illustrates the bookkeeping necessary to compute a nitrogen balance.

Table 25.5
Nitrogen balance for a steer (*in grams*)

Average daily nitrogen	*Income*	*Outgo*
In feed (by analysis)	70	—
In feces (loss in digestion)	—	28
In urine	—	58
Negative balance	16	
Total	86	86

The steer represented in this table lost 16 g of nitrogen daily, which means that the animal was in negative nitrogen balance and was losing the equivalent of 100 g of protein daily. This nitrogen loss does not necessarily indicate the animal was losing weight. For example, it might have had a large enough positive carbon balance that the body was actually gaining weight from simultaneous fat storage. In lactating animals, the record of nitrogen output must include a record of that in the milk secreted. Precise estimates must also account for losses through the skin and hair. If a nitrogen balance is being run alone, urine and feces may be collected and analyzed together, but ordinarily a nitrogen balance is run in conjunction with a digestion test, which of course necessitates separate treatment of urine and feces.

Use of nitrogen balance   Data from a pig feeding trial* will serve to illustrate the use and interpretation of a nitrogen balance.

Four rations, each consisting of 85% of one or another of four cereal grains (No. 3 barley, No. 1 screenings, No. 1 oats, No. 3 oats), plus 15% of a protein supplement were fed to pigs confined in metabolism crates. Feed intake was held constant over a collection period of 10 days. Urine excretion was measured for this period, and 1/200 of the urine output every 12 hours was saved for nitrogen analysis. The feeds were also analyzed for nitrogen. Typical 24-hour data for one of these feeds (No. 3 barley) are given in Table 25.6.

Comparable data and the computed equivalent protein obtained for each of the four feeds examined are:

Feed	N balance	Protein gain
No. 3 Feed barley	+ 21 g	131 g
No. 1 Screenings	+ 19 g	120 g
No. 1 Feed oats	+ 17 g	106 g
No. 3 Feed oats	+ 0.25 g	1.5 g

Relative value of foods as sources of useful protein   One measure of the usefulness of the protein of a food is the percentage of the digestible protein retained in the body. Another way of expressing biological value of protein is the percentage of the total intake retained in the body. In either case, the positive nitrogen balance measures the quantity of nitrogen (and thus, protein) retained in the body.

The relation between these ways of using the nitrogen balance data is clarified in Table 25.7, which uses the figures for No. 3 barley (given in Table 25.6).

The data for the four feeds studied are tabulated for comparison below.

Feed	Digestibility of nitrogen (%)	Nitrogen balance as percentage of nitrogen digested	Nitrogen balance as percentage of nitrogen ingested
No. 3 Feed barley	75	43	32
No. 1 Screenings	78	37	29
No. 1 Feed oats	83	33	28
No. 3 Feed oats	69	3	2

*Crampton, E. W., and Whiting, F., *Sci. Agriculture* **23**(1943):12.

Table 25.6
Nitrogen balance (for a 24-hour period) in pigs consuming a diet composed of No. 3 Canadian Western barley (85%) and a protein supplement (15%)

Pig no.	Intake (feed)			Output (feces)			Output (urine)			Nitrogen balance (g/24 hr)
	Amount eaten (g) (a)	Nitrogen (%) (b)	Nitrogen (g) (a×b)	Excreted (g)	Nitrogen (%)	Nitrogen (g)	Excreted (cc)	Nitrogen (%)	Nitrogen (g)	
1241	1766	3.01	53	555	2.55	14	3711	0.52	19	+20
1256	2148		64	641	2.31	14	5798	0.49	28	+21
1252	2563		77	806	2.48	20	5942	0.59	35	+22
Average			65			16			28	+221

NOTE: All data except percentage of nitrogen, to whole numbers.
SOURCE: Crampton, E. W., and Whiting, F., *Sci. Agriculture* **23**(1943):12.

Table 25.7
Relation between digested and metabolized protein

Intake, 65 g $\begin{cases} \text{Digested, 49 g} \begin{cases} \text{Metabolized, 21 g (i.e., grams nitrogen retained per day)} \\ \text{Urine, 28 g} \end{cases} \\ \text{Feces, 16 g} \end{cases}$

$$\text{Proportion of digestible protein in ration} = \frac{100(65-16)}{65} = 75\%$$

$$\text{Proportion of digested protein retained} = \frac{21 \times 100}{49} = 43\%$$

$$\text{Proportion of ingested protein retained (metabolized protein)} = \frac{21 \times 100}{65} = 32\%$$

The differences in the nitrogen balances generated by these feeds reflect differences in both biological value and digestibility of their protein.

Nitrogen balance as an index of dietary needs   The nitrogen balance also provides one basis for indicating the protein status of the body. Subject to some qualifications to be mentioned later, the requirement of the body for protein is represented by an amount that will maintain nitrogen equilibrium, in the case of adult maintenance, or will permit a positive balance of certain size, in the case of growing animals. A method of utilizing results of nitrogen balance studies for determining the probable amount of dietary protein necessary for maintenance equilibrium has been proposed by Leitch and Duckworth.* It presumes that the dietary protein intake level which results in positive as often as in negative balance is the intake most likely to keep the body in nitrogen equilibrium (see Chapter 29).

The meaning of nitrogen balance   The concept that nitrogen balance can serve as an index of the protein status of the body is based on the storage or loss of nitrogenous materials in the body. There are two types of protein metabolism. Endogenous metabolism consists of irreversible reactions involving proteins and other nitrogenous materials in the body tissues. Exogenous metabolism is the metabolism of nitrogenous constituents present in amounts exceeding the needs of the animal for maintenance, and of those which cannot be utilized by the body for synthesis or productive purposes. Although the concept of exogenous and endogenous proteins is useful in understanding nitrogen metabolism, it is not actually possible to distinguish the two types of protein metabolism because dietary and body nitrogen meet in a common metabolic pool of blood and tissues.

---

*Leitch, I., and Duckworth, J., *Nutr. Abstr. and Revs.* 7(1937):257.

Depletion of body protein stores is reflected by a decrease in the excretion of urinary nitrogen. When an animal is placed on a protein-free diet, urinary nitrogen excretion decreases—rapidly at first and then more slowly. The initial rapid loss of nitrogen represents the catabolism of the labile protein reserves. The decrease in urinary nitrogen loss as protein depletion continues represents a decrease in the rate of turnover of tissue protein. Eventually a minimum excretion level is reached, which is referred to as the obligatory urinary nitrogen loss. In regeneration, the process seems to be reversed, and when the body is in a greatly depleted state, a relatively small amount of dietary protein can result in nitrogen retention. As the body becomes more and more nearly fully repleted with protein, larger daily intakes of protein are necessary to maintain the positive balance.

The relation between nitrogen balance and the nitrogen stores of the body can be demonstrated experimentally. If an animal is placed on a nitrogen-free diet, after having been fed normally, a large negative balance will result. The magnitude of the urinary loss while on the nitrogen-free diet will depend on the previous nitrogen intake under the normal feeding regimen. If the animal is then given a small quantity of protein, the negative balance will be much reduced because of the partial restoration of dietary nitrogen intake. If the animal is again placed on a nitrogen-free diet, a negative nitrogen balance will result, but this time it will be less than in the first case because the nitrogen metabolism will have been reduced. If, following the second nitrogen-free feeding, the same small quantity of protein is again given, the amount of negative balance during this second period of nitrogen feeding will again be less than it was in the first instance. If further periods of nitrogen-free feeding followed by the same low intake of protein are continued, it will be found that ultimately this small protein intake will be sufficient to maintain a positive nitrogen balance. However, this small intake of protein will maintain positive balance only if it is adequate to meet the obligatory nitrogen loss of the animal.

Thus the amount of dietary protein necessary to achieve nitrogen balance is variable and changes as protein stores of the body are increased or decreased. In practice, animals can achieve nitrogen equilibrium with different amounts of protein in the diet. This explains many of the apparent discrepancies in the amount of protein required by an individual. Nutritionists now consider that an animal which is maintained in nitrogen equilibrium on less protein intake than another comparable animal is actually operating with less than full protein reserves in the body. As long as health is normal, this is perfectly satisfactory; but should some condition of stress arise which places demands on these reserves (such as a wasting disease or a disease involving fever), the animal with the smaller body reserve of protein is likely to succumb to the stress more quickly than one having a greater reserve.

This relation between nitrogen balance and body stores of protein affects the comparison of the biological values of proteins from different sources. If test animals have the same relative protein stores, the problem is not serious, but if the same animal is used for comparing different foods in succession, the amount of nitrogen in its feed may have altered its protein stores, causing successive tests to differ in the magnitude of the nitrogen balance.

Relation between caloric intake and nitrogen balance   Caloric intake is another important factor that influences body stores of protein. At constant levels of protein intake, nitrogen balance decreases regularly as the caloric intake decreases. The interpretation has been that a restriction in calories increases the catabolism of exogenous reserves of both body and dietary nitrogen. Presumably, the purpose of this catabolism is to obtain energy from metabolized amino acids. Animals with adequate body protein reserves can resist the depleting effects of caloric restriction over long periods of time, whereas those with inadequate stores deteriorate rapidly. In the absence of abundant labile protein stores in the body, animals drift from a high to a low positive balance and eventually into negative nitrogen balance. Thus, the nitrogen integrity of the body cannot be maintained unless the caloric intake is adequate.

Maintenance of body tissues   The balance between protein and calories is a particularly important one in the maintenance of normal body tissues. Diets that are relatively high in calories but low in quality and quantity of protein cause depletion of the dispensable protein reserves of the animal. Depletion of the protein stores of the body, either through lack of calories or through lack of protein, or both, results in changes in tissue proteins and enzyme systems, which can markedly alter the physiology of the animal.

As an example, plasma albumin is depleted more rapidly than plasma globulins. The activity of the succinic-oxidase system of the citric acid cycle is thereby reduced whereas that of the cytochrome-oxidase system is not.

Nitrogen balance an overall measurement   Thus, there can be a differential depletion and repletion of many types of protein systems, depending on the physiological state of the animal and the nature of the diet. The nitrogen-balance method does not describe these shifts among the various protein components of the body, but instead measures the overall status of nitrogen retention in the animal. It is possible for an animal to be in positive nitrogen balance, and yet be depleting some of its labile stores of protein.

It would be impractical to go further into the problem of nitrogen balance or protein metabolism here. Enough has been said to suggest that the problem is not a simple one, and also that the interpretation of nitrogen-balance figures is by no means a matter of addition or subtraction alone.

Suggested readings

Food and Agriculture Organization/World Health Organization. *Energy and Protein Requirements*. WHO Technical Report Series No. 522, World Health Organization, Geneva, or FAO Nutrition Meeting Report Series No. 52, Food and Agriculture Organization of the United Nations, Rome (1973).

Forbes, G. B. "Another Source of Error in the Metabolic Balance Method," *Nutrition Reviews* **31**(1973):297.

Hegsted, D. M. "Balance Studies," *Journal of Nutrition* **106**(1976):307.

Malm, O. J. *Calcium Requirements and Adaptation in Adult Men*. Oslo University Press, Oslo (1958).

Wallace, W. M. "Nitrogen Content of the Body and Its Relation to Retention and Loss of Nitrogen," *Federation Proceedings* **18**(1959):1125.

Section VI
THE NUTRIENT NEEDS
OF ANIMALS

It is not particularly difficult to determine experimentally an individual's approximate daily requirement for most of the nutrients that nutritionists must consider in assembling an adequate diet. Feeding diets in which the quantity of a particular nutrient is varied systematically over some suitable range will disclose the level at which the health, growth, or some performance criterion appears to be normal or most desirable. This is in fact the basis for arriving at the figures that constitute the dietary or animal feeding standards. A much more difficult problem is how to describe or translate the experimentally determined data to make them applicable to other individuals whose heredity, size, age, sex, climatic environment, physical activity, and/or production performance may differ from those of the observed experimental subjects.

The several factors that affect nutrient needs are not of equal effect or significance with each nutrient, and there are well-known differences between species. Consequently, the figures found in feeding standards for different species are often quite different. Within each species there are groupings that permit a more specific statement of the nutrient needs of the individuals according to the common characteristic (such as sex or activity) defined by the classification. We shall not attempt to evaluate the relative effects on nutrient requirements of the many factors known to cause variations. However, there are three biological factors that are of particular importance because they occur universally. Before dealing specifically with nutrient requirements, we shall therefore consider (1) growth, (2) reproduction, and (3) lactation as biological functions affecting nutrient needs.

In addition to these primary factors, we have some evidence that nutrient needs may be influenced by other conditions, such as the provision of adequate levels to allow for optimum (1) immunity and protection against specific diseases, (2) longevity, and (3) mental development.

Box VI.1 Immunity and nutrient needs

There is a long history of inquiry into the relationship between nutrition and immunology. Much of the recent research into the role of nutrition in the immune response undoubtedly stems from a desire to improve human resistance to infectious disease. However, animal scientists have also been concerned with the relationship between nutrition and resistance to infection.

Immunology deals with the specific responses of a host to the entry of foreign materials called *antigens* or *immunogens*. There are two main types of response: *humoral immunity,* which is transferred by the serum, is responsible for the production of antibodies; *cell-mediated immunity,* which is transferred not by the serum but by sensitized cells, is primarily responsible for certain delayed immune responses and for resistance to transplants and tumors. The duality of the immune system is well illustrated in the chicken where removal of the bursa of Fabricus from the chick embryo seriously impairs antibody production, whereas removal of the thymus results in a defect in cell-mediated immunity. It is important to distinguish between these two defense mechanisms when considering the effect of nutrition on acquired immunity.

Specific nutrients have been found to play an important role in antibody production. Deficiencies of protein, pyridoxine, pantothenic acid, and folacin produce the most consistent deleterious effects on antibody production, perhaps because of the biochemical functions of these nutrients in the synthesis of DNA and protein. Studies of other nutrients have produced less consistent results. A deficiency of vitamin A, for example, has been shown to have a deleterious effect on antibody formation in chickens and swine, although the effects of the deficiency varied with the particular antigen employed. Large amounts of vitamins A and E have been found to stimulate antibody response, whereas a deficiency of vitamin E had no uniform effect on antibody production. The function of minerals in the synthesis of antibodies has been sadly neglected.

Cell-mediated immunity is usually depressed in animals by general under-nutrition as well as by specific nutritional deficiencies. Protein–calorie malnutrition (PCM) increases a child's susceptibility to infection. Although cell-mediated immunity is depressed in children suffering from PCM, the levels of antibodies circulating in their serum is not always low, and in some cases these levels are even elevated. The clinical significance of these findings is that malnourished children may be more prone to fungal and gram-negative infections. Investigators have reported that deficiencies of specific nutrients also impair cell-mediated immunity. Deficiencies of pyridoxine, vitamin C, and folacin have been found to inhibit delayed hypersensitivity to a variety of stimuli and to impair allograft rejection.

The actual effect of nutritional status on the defense mechanisms of the host is still unclear in spite of a great deal of interest and research into the relationship in recent years. This lack of precise knowledge applies particularly to humans, in whom nutrient deficiencies are more complex than in experimental animals, often creating multiple problems. Of particular concern with humans, however, is the vicious cycle that may be set in motion when malnutrition predisposes to infection, which in turn intensifies the severity of malnutrition.

The role of nutrition in the immunological response may be broader than simply affecting resistance to infection. Nutritional deficiencies and imbalances may also contribute to aging and tumorogenesis.

Chapter 26
Growth as a biological function affecting nutrient requirements

Max Rubner called growth and its regulation "the supreme riddle of life." Growth is a complex and intriguing phenomenon, which is a source of some difficulties to the nutritionist; to interpret intelligently many of the data collected in nutrition research, it is necessary to understand the nature of growth.

How should growth be measured? In previous chapters we have pointed out that an increase in body weight, although usually related to growth, is by no means an accurate or critical measure of it. In review, an animal not gaining in weight may actually be enlarging its skeleton while losing fat or water. Therefore, tests that reveal nutritional balance and composition of the body, from which investigators can determine the actual increase in the various tissues of the body, are more accurate measures of growth. Weight plus another measurement, such as height, is often better than weight alone.

In spite of its recognized limitations, live weight change is used as the important criterion of the effects of an imposed experimental condition in a large proportion of nutrition studies. Live weight changes are more valid reflections of growth in young than in more mature animals. It is well, therefore, to note some of the characteristics of growth.

Characteristics of growth

Growth results from the anabolic, rather than catabolic, processes of the body. In general, nutrient requirements are measured in terms of nutritive material stored in tissues during the growing period, and in skin and its appendages which continue to grow throughout life. However, in addition to storing vital nutrients, the body deposits nutrients consumed in excess of current needs, as in fattening and in storage of protoplasmic and mineralized tissues. This storage of excess nutrients is also the result of anabolic processes and is measured by the amounts retained in the tissues above basal or minimal needs.

Growth is a much more complex process than merely an increase in size. As an animal grows, two fundamental things happen:

1. Weight increases until a mature size is reached: this is defined as growth.

2. The shape or conformation of the body changes: this is called development.

In 1911 Schloss defined growth as a "correlated increase in the mass of the body, in definite intervals of time, in a way characteristic of the species." This implies that, subject to individual variability, there is a characteristic rate of growth for each species and a characteristic adult size and conformation. Whereas growth in some tissues continues throughout life, growth in body size and change in shape depends largely on skeletal growth. The latter reaches a maximum in early life, the exact magnitude of which depends upon species, the immediate hereditary background of the individual, and the environmental conditions during the growing period.

Maximal size and development are fixed by heredity. However, nutrition is one of the important environmental factors that determines whether this maximum will be reached; an optimal level of nutrition is one that enables an organism to take full advantage of its heredity. However, maximal growth fixed by heredity cannot be *exceeded* through nutrition.

Cellular growth

Growth takes place by an increase in the number of cells (*hyperplasia*) and an increase in the size of cells (*hypertrophy*). In early embryonic life, both processes occur in all cells; but in adults, there are three types of cells differentiated:

1. *Permanent cells* (e.g., nerve cells) cease to divide early in prenatal life and their numbers are therefore fixed early in life.

2. *Stable cells* (e.g., those of most organs) continue to divide for a variable but major part of the growth period, but their numbers are fixed in the adult.

3. *Labile cells* (e.g., those of the epithelial and epidermal tissues) continue to divide throughout life, but the process in the adult is limited to the replacement of worn-out cells.

All three types of cells undergo hypertrophy during growth. Some of them may also increase in size even after growth ceases, as a consequence of special physiological demands. For example, the muscular development induced through exercise is produced by hypertrophy, and an enlargement of kidney cells results from a continuing burden on this organ.

Differential growth of tissues and organs

Let us examine a little more closely this phenomenon of growth and differentiation. Even from casual observation, it is evident that the body does not grow as a unit. The differential growth of various parts of the body is indicated by the following figures, which represent the number of times the tissue increases in size from birth to maturity.

Muscles	48	Heart	12
Skeleton	26	Brain	4
Lungs	20	Eye	2
Liver	14		

In general, prenatal growth is characterized by a marked and early proliferation of nervous tissue; at birth the head is relatively large, the legs long, and the body small. The rate of postnatal growth is greatest in the cephalothoracic region so that in the mature animal the head is small, the legs relatively short, and the body large. Thus, in farm animals the head, legs, and feet develop early and attain their final size while other parts are still actively growing. The body, particularly the hindquarters and loin region, develops very late.

With this background, we can now proceed to resolve the problem of analyzing the time relation of growth as measured by weight change.

The growth curve

If changes in live weight are plotted against time and the points joined, a curve results which is often referred to as the normal growth curve. The curve is sigmoid in shape for both animals and plants *if it covers the full growth period* from conception to maturity.

In its simplest form, growth may be thought of as a first-order chemical reaction—basically, the result of cell division (multiplication). One cell divides to make two; these mature, and in turn divide to make four, and so on. In the absence of any inhibiting force, and if the rate of cell maturation and division is constant, the total number of cells present at any one time will determine the total increase in weight over a given period. It is believed that cell division repeats itself at a constant rate, and that somatic cells are potentially immortal. If such is the case, this situation would lead to an increased slope of the normal curve.

Eventually the situation becomes complicated by factors or forces that inhibit the growth processes. What these forces are is not known specifically. In chemical reactions an accumulation of end products can inhibit the reaction. In animal growth it has been suggested that cellular competition for food or nutrients, or perhaps the limitation of nutrient transport, may be involved. In any case, it appears that during the self-inhibitory stage of growth, weight still to be attained in order to reach the final or adult size regulates the rate of weight increase.

The trend of weight change with increasing age can be illustrated by assuming an initial weight of 100 units which accumulates at an increasing rate of 25% for each equal period of time (or age) to puberty, and then at a decreasing rate of similar magnitude until a final or mature weight of 1,000 units is attained. The calculations and the plot of these data appear in Table 26.1 and Figure 26.1.

Table 26.1
Accumulated weights with increasing age
with rate constant at 25% per unit of time

Time	Initial wt., w_1	Wt. to be made	K (%)	Increment	Attained wt., w_2
t_0	100		25	25	125
t_1	125		25	31	156
t_2	156		25	39	195
t_3	195		25	49	244
t_4	244		25	61	305
t_5		695	−25	174	479
t_6		521	−25	130	609
t_7		391	−25	98	707
t_8		293	−25	73	780
t_9		202	−25	55	835
t_{10}		165	−25	41	876
t_{11}		124	−25	31	907
t_{12}		93	−25	23	930
t_{18}		70	−25	18	948
t_{14}		52	−25	13	961
t_{15}		39	−25	10	971
t_{16}		29	−25	7	978
t_{17}		22	−25	6	984
t_{18}		16	−25	4	988

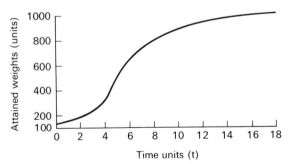

Figure 26.1
Accumulated weights with increasing age, with rate of
change constant at 25% per unit of time.

Box 26.1   Nutrition, brain development, and behavior

In 1973 a position paper of the Food and Nutrition Board of the National Academy of Sciences (National Research Council, Washington, D.C.) on "The Relationship of Nutrition to Brain Development and Behavior" was introduced as follows:

> The physical, chemical and physiological development of the brain and consequent behavior in all species of higher animals evolve from the continuous interaction of genetic and numerous environmental factors. Among the latter are nutritional, disease, psychological, learning and cultural variables. Of these, nutrition is concerned directly with providing energy and nutrients needed for cellular structures and various metabolic systems. Indirectly, food may serve as a stimulus for behavior as well as providing a basis for social interaction.
>
> In most instances, the specific effects of sub-optimal nutrition on brain development in man are inseparable from those of other environmental factors. Adequate nutrition generally is part of a good environment; malnutrition occurs primarily within poor environments in which many other forces may also limit the individual's development. In any event, malnutrition is detrimental in both good and poor environments but not necessarily equivalently so.
>
> In some instances—such as when nutrients are imperfectly utilized owing to inborn errors of metabolism, or when nutrients are lacking, as in specific nutrient deficiencies—malnutrition, *per se*, clearly alters the central nervous system by acutely or chronically limiting its metabolic, structural, and functional capabilities and performance. In other circumstances, malnutrition, reflected in chronic limitation of amounts of food consumed, may result in general stunting of growth accompanied by reduced brain size, decreased brain cell number, and immature or incomplete biochemical organization of the brain.

The maturation of the brain and central nervous system progresses in an orderly sequence in which the synthesis of DNA (a reflection of cell division) stops prior to the cessation of net protein synthesis. The rate of cellular growth varies within specific areas of the brain and between brains of different species.

Brain development has been divided into three phrases of growth dependent upon DNA synthesis: (1) hyperplasia, a stage representing a proliferation of cells, and where there is an increase in the weight of the brain and in its protein and DNA content; (2) hyperplasia plus concomitant hypertrophy, a stage where the increase in DNA content falls behind the increase in brain protein content and weight; (3) hypertrophy, a stage where there is no additional increase in DNA content, but where net protein synthesis and brain weight continue to increase at the same rate; the consequence of these events is an enlargement of existing cells.

The different stages of brain development vary among species. In humans, the greatest "growth spurt" takes place during the last trimester of fetal life and continues for at least 18 months postnatally, with the maximal rate of growth of the brain occurring prior to birth. Thus, the importance of maternal and infant nutrition as major environmental factors influencing brain development becomes obvious.

A widely accepted theory is that malnutrition inflicted during hyperplastic growth results in a brain with a permanent defect in cell number, with biochemical recovery being relatively difficult upon the provision of adequate nutrition. However, malnutrition imposed during the hypertrophic phase results in a reduction of cell size—a situation that can be more easily rectified by correcting the nutritional problem.

The effect of nutritional deficiencies on behavior and learning capacities has been studied in both animals and humans, but as yet the results are not conclusive. Because other environmental factors can be controlled more easily with experimental animals, more definitive results are found in the literature on the influence of malnutrition upon subsequent behavior and learning abilities in species such as rats, monkeys, etc. Human malnutrition is frequently accompanied by a variety of inferior environmental circumstances—high incidence of disease, cultural deprivation, overcrowded living conditions, parental indifference, etc.

However, in spite of the many serious methodological shortcomings of the studies that have been reported, there appears to be good indication that *early* and *severe* malnutrition is an important factor in subsequent behavior and intellectual development, above and beyond the effects of social, familial, and other such influences. The effect of *mild* to *moderate* malnutrition on later behavior and intellectual development is less clear. Studies that have attempted to assess the relative contribution of moderate malnutrition and other environmental factors to subsequent intellectual performance have often suggested that malnutrition of this order also can play a role quite apart from factors related to social status. The Food and Nutrition Board has emphasized that this is a tentative conclusion, and that more systematic research is required for its confirmation.

For further information, see *Dairy Council Digest* **44,** No. 6 (1973).

Age equivalence in growth

It is interesting, and nutritionally significant, that if the attained weights of animals of different species are plotted against percentage of mature weight on an age equivalent basis, the curves coincide, with the exception of the human, whose long juvenile period is unique (Figure 26.2).

In general, nutritional needs of animals are similar at equivalent physiological ages. This is roughly indicated by the equivalence of the percentage of their mature weight at a given chronological age.

The growth curve can be divided into two major segments. The first segment is one of increasing slope, and, except in humans, extends from conception to a time when about one-third of the mature weight has been attained. The first segment of the human growth curve extends to a point where two-thirds of mature weight has been attained. The age at which other organisms reach this point is variable with species. The second segment is one of decreasing slope, extending from the end of the first segment to the conclusion of the growing period (i.e., to maturity). Within each of these two major segments, growth may be cyclic with differing growth rates. The junction of the segments is called the *point of inflection.*

The point of inflection is of interest for several reasons: (1) It is the age or time of most rapid growth, and in animals it is probably the time of most economical gains in weight in terms of feed cost. (2) It is the point at which the rate of acceleration of growth is zero, and also the point of age equivalence between species with respect to growth. This is significant because at an equivalent physiological age, animals of different species pass through the same physiological stages of development. (3) With children, and possibly also with animals, the curve of specific mortality (i.e., the ratio of number dying to the number living of the same age), passes through a minimum at approximately the same age the growth curve passes through the point of inflection. (4) Finally, the point of inflection coincides with puberty in most species. For example, in humans it occurs at a time when a little more than 60% of mature weight has been attained, or at an age of 12–15 years. With rats the point of inflection occurs at about 30% of mature weight, or at an age of 2½ months. With cattle it occurs at about 30% of mature weight, or at an age of 10 months. Of note is the fact that in the human, for some reason, puberty is delayed until about two-thirds of the mature weight has been attained. This is in contrast to most other species, in which puberty occurs at about one-third of mature weight.

When attained weights of animals are plotted against time (age), the smoothed growth curve appears to indicate a regularly changing rate of gain.

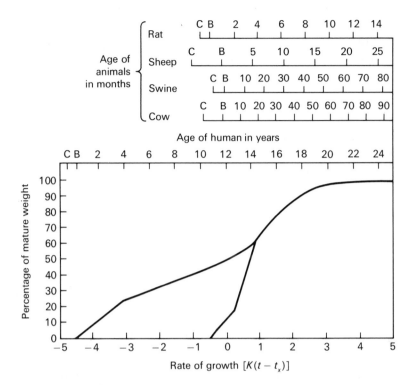

Figure 26.2
Weight and growth equivalents of farm animals, laboratory animals, and humans.

If, however, the rate of gain is plotted against time, it will be seen that growth is really a series of cycles or periods differing in rate but within which rate k is constant. These cycles of constant rate of gain are often surprisingly long. In rats these rates are:

	Rate of gain of body weight (%)
Conception to birth	53
Birth to 10 days	11
10 days to 25 days	4.7
25 days to 65 days (puberty)	3.1 (this period used for growth tests)

The existence of these differing cycles is of importance in nutrition studies because of the usual practice of comparing gains over some period of time. If the animals being compared are in different stages of growth, differences in gains credited to experimental conditions may in reality be due to differing physiological ages.

Calculation of rate of growth

Rate of growth may be calculated in several ways. The most common is to merely compute the change in weight over some period of time:

$$\text{Average absolute growth rate} = \frac{w_2 - w_1}{t_2 - t_1}$$

where w and t represent weight and time.

Technically, this value (gain per unit of time) is only hypothetical. Although it is useful in making some comparisons, it does not acceptably describe the facts of the progress of growth if $t_2 - t_1$ is of any considerable duration, because it gives no accurate idea of the change in weight at any specific age. For example, a Yorkshire pig may weigh 200 pounds at an age of 300 days from conception. According to the above method of calculation, this pig gained an average of 0.66 pound per day; but there may have been no one day when it gained exactly 0.66 pound. In fact, shortly following conception the gain was only a small fraction of a pound per day; at 150 days the gain reached 0.5 pound per day; and at 300 days the animal was gaining about 1.8 pounds per day.

Rate of growth is sometimes calculated relative to initial weight as:

$$\text{Average relative growth rate} = \frac{w_2 - w_1}{w_1}$$

If the gain thus computed is multiplied by 100, gain becomes a percentage of initial weight. This measurement of rate of growth is nearly identical to the true value if the gain $(w_2 - w_1)$ during the interval $(t_2 - t_1)$ is small compared to the weight of the animal (w_1). However, if the gain is relatively large, this formula gives an erroneously high figure, since the initial weight (w_1), the denominator, will be too small to represent the true basis for expressing the rate of weight change.

Some improvement in accuracy may be effected by relating the gain to the midweight during the time period.

$$\text{Average relative growth rate} = \frac{w_2 - w_1}{\frac{1}{2}(w_2 + w_1)}$$

These relationships are evident in the examples given in Table 26.2.

Table 26.2
Two methods of calculating rates of gain
according to values of initial and final weights

				Method I
				Rate of gain $100\,(w_2-w_1)$
w_2	w_1	w_2-w_1	w_1	w_1
100	90	Small	Small	11%
200	90	Large	Small	122%
200	190	Small	Large	5%

				Method II
				Rate of gain $100\,(w_2 - w_1)$
w_2	w_1	w_2-w_1	$\frac{1}{2}(w_2 + w_1)$	$\frac{1}{2}\,(w_2 + w_1)$
100	90	Small	Small	10.5%
200	90	Large	Large	75.9%
200	190	Small	Large	5.1%

The above expressions of rate of growth are unsatisfactory physiologically because they assume growth rate to be a linear function of time. True growth rate is correctly measured by using "instantaneous" gain and time figures. Thus, in the formula $(w_2 - w_1)/(t_2 - t_1)$ we replace $w_2 - w_1$ by dw, and $t_2 - t_1$ by dt. Then dw/dt corresponds to $(w_2 - w_1)/(t_2 - t_1)$ when $t_2 - t_1$ approaches zero, and so represents instantaneous weight gain. To obtain true relative growth rate, this ratio is divided by the weight (w) at the time of the gain. Therefore

$$\text{Instantaneous relative (true) growth rate, } k, = \frac{dw/dt}{w}$$

It is not physically possible to measure the instantaneous rate of growth, because of the finite time intervals required for making the measurement. To solve this equation for k requires the use of abstract mathematics, details of which may be found in an appropriate text.

Growth curves as standards

Much research has been undertaken to determine normal growth curves; in fact, such curves have been published for nearly every species of animal. Normal growth curves are used primarily as standards against which to gauge the adequacy of dietary allowances. Indeed, they provide the entire basis of most feeding or dietary standards for growing individuals. Unfortunately, not all published growth curves agree, and hence feeding standards do not necessarily agree.

Many growth curves represent trends of weight at different ages. It has been shown, however, that a more accurate picture of normal growth can be obtained if the gains are plotted against weight attained. This is so because gains still to be made depend more on size attained than on age. For example, normal, healthy pigs of the same age differ widely in gains per day, whereas pigs of similar initial weights are likely to gain similarly. This means that normal growth is not merely a function of age. Rate of growth for an individual is partly hereditary, and so individuals of one age may be widely different in size, and the variability increases as age increases. The data of Figure 26.3 illustrate the variability of gains in pigs with advancing age or weight. What is true for growing pigs is true also for other species. This is evident in the data for boys and girls shown in Table 26.3.

The use of weight as the basis of expressing nutrient needs in all dietary and feeding standards is based more on a recognition of the direct relationship between rate of gain and weight attained than on that between rate of gain and age.

Limitations of weight as an index of nutritional status

The use of weight alone as a measure of nutritional status is, however, subject to several objections:

1. Normal growth is ill-defined.

2. The "allowable" variation from normal has not been established.

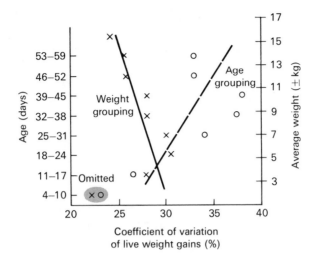

Figure 26.3
Change in variability of weight gains in pigs with
advancing age or weight.

Table 26.3
Weight in kilograms for age of early- and late-maturing individuals

Age (yr)	Boys		Girls	
	Early	Late	Early	Late
8	29	21	27	22
10	36	26	35	27
12	48	30	49	32
18	71	56	56	52

3. Weight is a nonspecific and nonsensitive index of health. It cannot be assumed that because individuals who are underweight may be undernourished, those who are not underweight are well nourished.

4. Satisfactory growth may continue for some time after poor nutrition is in effect.

5. The finding that growing rats receiving a diet restricted as to calories will have a greatly lengthened life span suggests that maximal gains are not necessarily optimal gains for general well-being.

The rate of increase in height is practically constant up to puberty, and thus the curve for attained height to this age is linear, whereas that for weight is concave. Following puberty, both curves take similar paths. Linear measurements, such as height, are influenced more by heredity than by nutrition and other environmental conditions (i.e., they are not complicated as much by body fat deposits). However, different parts of the body normally mature at different ages, and thus the use of height standards alone is also unacceptable.

Growth and the nutrient requirements of the body

Growth, in the sense used here, is a consequence of a normal increase to maturity in the mass of those body parts that might be thought of as "nonexpendable." The only tissue not in this category is adipose tissue, which is primarily a deposition of surplus energy and which is largely expendable without damage to the economy or functioning of the body.

Growth therefore involves synthesis and deposition of minerals and protein, which must be supplied by the food eaten in quantities in excess of the needs for merely operating the machinery (as in the maintenance of idle adults). In addition, the energy needs of the growing body increase for one or more of three reasons. First, the ultimate building stones of the tissues do not come to the body already cut and shaped, needing only to be placed in position as in the prefabricated house. Rather, for the most part, the precursors must be digested out of the food, the bits put together into appropriate molecules, and these then assembled into tissues. All of these processes require energy, protein (amino acids), vitamins, and minerals, irrespective of the fact that the tissue formed may actually be composed of some of these same "units."

This is just another way of saying that in order to grow the young animal needs more of all parts of the diet than would be necessary for maintenance only; and that with the increase in amounts of protein and minerals needed for deposit in the tissue itself, there is an obligatory increase in the "operating necessities" involved in growth metabolism.

Second, growing animals synthesize and store in varying amounts tissue that is lipid in nature. The "depot storage" is normally relatively small, but some fat is always formed as reserve energy to carry the animal between feedings. This synthesis also requires energy. The efficiency of food for body fat formation is only about 56% in terms of weight of materials.

Finally, as a young animal grows, his activity normally increases, often very markedly. This in turn demands extra energy because it requires a speedup of metabolism and an increase in operating needs. The Food and

Nutrition Board, author of the U.S. Recommended Dietary Allowances,* states: "The dominant factor leading to variability in energy needs is the proportion of time an individual devotes to moderate and heavy work tasks in contrast to light or sedentary activities." It is known that there are wide variations in the physical activity of children and adolescents. For this reason energy allowances must be individually adjusted to guarantee adequate energy for all physiological processes, including growth.

The situation is less marked in farm animals that are sold for food while still in the growing stage (hogs, poultry, and baby beef) because such stock are normally confined in pens to restrict their activity and hence divert more of their intake to tissue growth and fat deposition.

Because some of the factors governing the energy needs of growing animals do not contribute to growth *per se,* growing animals may not need a large increase in the concentration of protein and minerals as much as they need an increase in total daily allowance of food. We shall deal with this deduction in more detail when we consider requirements quantitatively in Chapters 28 and 29.

*NAS–NRC (U.S.), *Recommended Dietary Allowances* (8th ed.), National Academy of Sciences–National Research Council, Washington, D.C. (1974).

Suggested readings

Lodge, G. A., and Lamming, G. E. *Growth and Development of Mammals.* Butterworth & Co., London (1967).

Needham, A. E. *The Growth Process in Animals.* Sir Isaac Pitman & Son, London (1964).

Chapter 27
Nutritional aspects of reproduction and lactation

Reproduction and lactation represent two biological functions that require a synthesis from dietary nutrients of materials ultimately lost to the female; they necessitate therefore an augmentation of her diet. The minimal quantities of such "extra" nutrients are equal to those of the products synthesized plus whatever additional amounts are needed to cover the "cost of synthesis." Because pregnant and lactating females produce new tissue daily for growth of the fetus or for synthesis of milk, their day-by-day diet must supply additional nutrients to meet their augmented demands.

Quantitatively, nutrient needs correlate with the stage of development of the fetus or with the stage of lactation. Reproduction and lactation are parts of a repeating female sexual cycle. With the intervention of pregnancy, the recycling period is extended. Lactation occurs as a consequence of reproduction, and the same mechanisms regulate both functions.

Reproduction and lactation are physiological processes, the development of which is brought about in specified sequence by the action and interaction of a series of hormones arising in four glands or organs of the adult female mammal's body: the pituitary, the ovary, the uterus, and the mammae. In addition, at least two temporary "endocrines," the corpus luteum and the placenta, take part in reproduction; and during the lactation phase the thyroid, parathyroid, and adrenals also play specific, though indirect, roles. Details of the processes involved may be found in many textbooks on reproductive physiology.

The nutrient demands of reproduction and lactation

Demands of pregnancy   The nutritional burden of reproduction in mammals is borne by the female and is related to the events occurring in the uterus subsequent to fertilization and continuing at an increasing rate up to the time of parturition; and the effect of these events on maternal behavior and metabolism. Pregnancy is characterized by a series of marked physiological adaptations that enable the female body to accommodate the rapid growth of the products of conception. The total nutrient requirements of pregnancy, however, cover much more than the nutrients contained in the fetus or fetuses.

One of the obvious changes that occurs as a consequence of pregnancy is an increase in the weight of the gravid female. It is common knowledge that some of this increased weight is due to fluid and some to an increase in body tissues. The type and weight of the different tissues formed vary not only with stage of pregnancy but with the kind and amount of diet ingested by the gravid female. The components of the average weight gained in normal pregnancy by women at different stages of pregnancy are shown in Table 27.1.

The data in Table 27.1 indicate that 5,200 of the grams gained during pregnancy are not accounted for by the products of conception and the expansion of tissues directly associated with the reproductive process. Most

Table 27.1
Average weight gained (*in grams*) by women at various stages of normal pregnancy

Component	Weight gain at			
	10 weeks	*20 weeks*	*30 weeks*	*40 weeks*
1. Total body weight gain	650	4,000	8,500	12,500
2. Weight gain accounted for by reproductive process	320	2,100	5,000	7,300
Fetus	5	300	1,500	3,300
Placenta	20	170	430	650
Liquor amnii	30	250	600	800
Increase in: Uterus	135	585	810	900
Mammae	34	180	360	405
Blood	100	600	1,300	1,250
3. Weight gain not accounted for by reproductive process (1. − 2.)	330	1,900	3,500	5,200

SOURCE: Adapted from NAS–NRC (U.S.), *Maternal Nutrition and the Course of Pregnancy*, National Academy of Sciences–National Research Council, Washington, D.C. (1970).

nutritionists postulate that this "unaccounted-for" weight represents stores of fat that are laid down as an energy reserve, presumably in anticipation of lactation.

An accumulation of fatty tissues is one of the objectives of proper feeding during pregnancy in domestic animals. Unless body fat stores are built up considerably during pregnancy, the female will lose weight after beginning to lactate for the simple reason that she will be unable to consume sufficient energy and nutrients to maintain the peak of milk production that comes early in the lactation cycle. Pregnant farm animals increase their consumption of feed during the latter part of pregnancy.

Fat deposition occurs at a maximal rate about midpregnancy, and the fat is deposited principally at central, rather than peripheral, sites of the body. There is normally a decrease in physical activity after the middle of pregnancy, which obviously releases some of the dietary energy for fat storage. The net result, in the human, is an actual extra average daily caloric requirement of about 200 to 300 kcal during the last half of pregnancy. This amount is relatively small, and may not be recognized by the pregnant female herself as an increase in her daily consumption.

However, this additional allowance is particularly important for the active young woman during her first pregnancy, especially if she is still growing.

ACCUMULATION OF NUTRIENTS IN THE PRODUCTS OF CONCEPTION   H. H. Mitchell et al.* have reported what amounts of various nutrients accumulate in the fetus and placenta of sows during gestation. Other investigators have used these data to prepare curves showing relative rates and extent of the increases in body weight and nutrients as percentages of their total at parturition (Figure 27.1). These data are representative of the trends in all species.

When computing an animal's requirements for nutrients during pregnancy, it is necessary to exercise care in transposing data from one species to another. Some of the obvious reproductive differences between species are: (1) prolificacy—some species (e.g., rat and pig) are multiparous, whereas others (e.g., dairy cow and human) are primarily uniparous; (2) length of gestation; and (3) the birth weight of the offspring in relation to the weight of the mother. The rat, for example, synthesizes 10 times as much protein per unit of time per unit of body weight as the human.

Nevertheless attempts have been made to arrive at generalized expressions (or equations) that relate weight of offspring to maternal body size and length of gestation. In general, the larger the species the smaller the offspring relative to maternal size; the weight of the offspring increases as a fractional power of the weight of the adult of the species.

---

*Mitchell, H. H., Carroll, W. E., Hamilton, T. S., and Hunt, G. E., *Illinois Agricultural Experiment Station Bulletin No. 375* (1931).

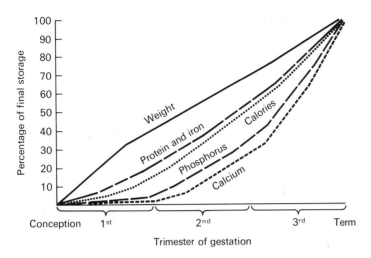

Figure 27.1
Trends of energy and nutrient accumulation in placenta and fetus during pregnancy.

Similar generalizations apply to the duration of pregnancy in relation to the size of the offspring. For example, the longer the gestation period, the smaller the offspring relative to the time required to complete fetal growth.

DIETARY CHANGES NECESSARY DURING PREGNANCY   From the trends of nutrient deposition (Figure 27.1), it is clear that most of the needs for extra food as a result of pregnancy occur during the last third of the gestation period. Even here the necessary change in food intake may be minor because, concurrent with advancing pregnancy, there is often a progressive reduction in the physical activity of the female so that there is a change in the use of at least some of the nutrients rather than an increase in the overall quantity required. In dairy cows, advancing pregnancy usually coincides with a decrease in milk production such that there may even be a reduced requirement for feed prior to parturition. Because of these complicating circumstances it is not possible to generalize between species as to the effect of pregnancy on the needed daily ration intake. Feeding standards for different species take these factors into account to some extent in the description of feeding groups. Some of the pertinent data will be presented in Chapter 30. Here, we shall comment primarily on the requirements for energy and for protein during gestation.

ENERGY REQUIREMENTS IN PREGNANCY   The demands of the pregnant female for energy to meet her increased metabolism plus the deposition of nutrients in the fetus, placenta, and in her mammae is a continuous variable starting at zero and increasing at an accelerating rate until at term it amounts to an increase of about 20% over maintenance. Because individual circumstances affecting energy requirements are so variable, it is more satisfactory to adjust actual food allowances in accordance with expected or desired increases in body weight during gestation.

For example, for an average 55-kilogram woman a weight gain during pregnancy of about 10 kg is considered normal, and the extra daily caloric requirement to cover the increased basal metabolism at the increased weight resulting from the pregnancy *per se* can be estimated as follows.

> Nonpregnant
> Basal metabolism, $70(55^{.75})$ 1,400 kcal
>
> At end of pregnancy
> Basal metabolism, $1.20 \times 70(65^{.75})$ 1,920 kcal
>
> Extra daily energy needed during latter
> part of gestation for pregnancy *per se*   520 kcal

In practice this would represent the maximum.

Table 27.2 gives some idea of the desirable gains during pregnancy for three species of adult females of normal body weight, and is a rough guide to corresponding extra daily energy allowances.

Table 27.2
Normal increases in body weight during pregnancy and
estimated corresponding daily requirements for extra energy during last trimester

Species	Normal adult weight (kg)	Expected gain during pregnancy (%)	(kg)	Length of gestation (days)	Extra energy per day in last third of pregnancy* (kcal)
Dairy cow	545	16	87	282	10,000
Sow	205	10	21	113	5,000
Woman	55	20	11	280	500

*These amounts will be lowered by whatever reduction there may be in energy requirement as a result of reduced physical activity or decreased milk production.

DESIRABLE WEIGHT GAIN DURING PREGNANCY   The key to desired weight gain in pregnant females is proper modification of the diet to guarantee this change. The current practice is to recommend an increase in body weight of 11 kg–12 kg in humans. Many studies clearly demonstrate that dietary practice aimed specifically at restricting gains to appreciably less than this figure of 11 kg–12 kg is correlated with low birth weight and increased neonatal mortality. However, excessive weight gains during gestation are also to be avoided in the interest of complication-free parturition. An interesting example of the effect of the level of nutrition on growth of the fetus is found in the experience of workers in Utah who provided supplementary feeding during pregnancy of desert range beef cattle. Raising the nutrition level caused enough of an increase in size of the fetus at term to greatly increase difficulties at parturition among the mothers, who were themselves undersized from an habitual low plane of nutrition.

PROTEIN REQUIREMENTS IN PREGNANCY   Pregnancy necessitates not only an augmentation in energy intake but also an increase in the daily intake of protein. There is no well-defined mechanism for storing protein, equivalent to the process of storing energy in deposited fat. However, there is some evidence that maternal tissues store protein early in pregnancy and then mobilize this protein later when fetal demands are greatest. Nutritionists recommend that the diet of the pregnant female contain an adequate allowance of protein of high biological value at all times.

The problem of protein nutrition during pregnancy is often overemphasized. It is true that there is a marked increase in protein content of the uterus and its contents as pregnancy progresses. In addition, a considerable amount of protein can be stored in the extrauterine tissues of the body. (There is fairly good evidence that species such as the rat, mouse, and perhaps the pig retain more nitrogen in their bodies during pregnancy than they deposit in the fetuses.) Furthermore, insufficient dietary protein during pregnancy markedly impairs the reproductive performance of the rat; severe protein deficiency in pregnant rats results in fetal resorption, a high percentage of stillborns, and low birth weight of the offspring. By contrast, however, feeding a low-protein diet to female pigs during gestation was not found to affect the number of offspring or their postpartum growth, although the average weight of the offspring at birth was low and lactation was impaired. In fact, even the feeding of a protein-free diet did not seriously impair the reproductive performance of the pig.

Nutritional scientists have estimated that about 925 g of protein are deposited in the fetus and adnexal tissues of the human female during pregnancy. The bulk of this deposition occurs during the last half of pregnancy when 5.5 g to 6.0 g of protein are deposited daily. These data raise questions about the adequacy of the protein in the diets of many pregnant women, even in affluent countries.*

Evidence suggests that the efficiency of protein utilization in pregnant women is considerably lower than in adults utilizing protein solely for

---

*NAS–NRC (U.S.), *Maternal Nutrition and the Course of Pregnancy*, National Academy of Sciences–National Research Council, Washington, D.C. (1970).

maintenance. In addition, there is evidence that considerably more than 925 g of protein are stored during pregnancy. Consequently, the recommended daily allowance for protein during pregnancy increased from 65 g per day in the 7th edition of the *Recommended Dietary Allowances* to 76 g per day in the 8th edition.* However, epidemiological studies reporting impaired reproductive performance in association with low-protein intakes are usually confounded by the fact that energy intake also was inadequate in those diets. Protein intake of people on self-selected diets usually accounts for 12%–14% of the total calories ingested.

DESIRABLE CHANGES IN DIET VARY   Recommendations such as those reported in the preceding sections on energy and protein requirements must be used carefully because they are predicated on two assumptions, both of which are variables: (1) the activity of the pregnant female is such that her daily energy intake does in fact require augmentation to the full "pregnancy" allowance, and   (2) consumption of protein prior to pregnancy was no more than that *needed* for maintenance.

We have already pointed out that reduced physical activity (or a decline in production of milk) concurrent with pregnancy may be such that no extra energy intake is needed to ensure the desired weight gain.

Studies on humans in North America show that most adults eat an appreciable excess of protein in the "regular" diet, and that no increase over this is necessary to meet the demands of pregnancy. Nutritionists agree that there is little virtue in ingesting more nutrients than are adequate to meet the needs of the condition. The real problem is to define "adequate."

The nutrient needs of pregnant farm animals are analogous to those of humans. It is necessary to increase total feed by some 20% and protein concentration by about two percentage units during the last third of gestation to ensure normal body gain and to maintain the protein status of the mother.

It is possible to assess the adequacy of the energy and protein content of the diet of a pregnant female by evaluating the outcome of the pregnancy in terms of the weight of the newborn relative to that of the mother. Several studies have shown a strong positive relationship between the weight gained by a woman during pregnancy and the birth weight of the infant. A special Committee on Maternal Nutrition in the United States† recommended that women gain an average of 11 kg during pregnancy; this committee strongly discouraged the prevalent practice of restricting weight gain during pregnancy to 5.5 kg.

---

*NAS–NRC (U.S.), *Recommended Dietary Allowances* (8th ed.), National Academy of Sciences–National Research Council, Washington, D.C. (1974).

†NAS–NRC (U.S.), *Maternal Nutrition and the Course of Pregnancy*, National Academy of Sciences–National Research Council, Washington, D.C. (1970).

Workers in a number of countries have shown that insufficient protein and energy in the maternal diet can have especially damaging effects on the baby.* It is important to note that there is a considerable increase in the number of brain cells in the human fetus during the third trimester of pregnancy. Indeed, the rate of brain growth reaches a maximum just prior to parturition. The reduction in the number of cells in the brain that occurs during fetal growth as a consequence of maternal malnutrition is not corrected by remedial feeding after birth. It can cause permanent brain damage that frequently leads to mental retardation in the child.

This problem, which is of paramount importance to humans, is difficult to study experimentally because the same situation does not prevail in all species. In the rat and dog, for example, brain growth takes place primarily following parturition. The guinea pig, on the other hand, shows most of its brain development prior to parturition. Therefore, the consequences of undernutrition differ strikingly from species to species.

In farm animals, an increase in the diet toward the end of pregnancy helps the animal prepare for successful lactation.

REQUIREMENTS FOR OTHER NUTRIENTS IN PREGNANCY   Requirements for energy and protein during pregnancy can be specified with reasonable accuracy. It is much more difficult to describe quantitatively the increased requirements for many of the other nutrients. Balance studies are difficult to carry out for nutrients other than protein.

In addition, there is a lack of precise information on the requirements for maintenance for many nutrients, as well as a lack of information on efficiency of absorption and the degree to which the nutrient can be stored. Finally, it is difficult to determine the amount of storage at the start of pregnancy. The magnitude of the problem can be illustrated by considering requirements for calcium, iron, and vitamin A.

The recommended daily allowance for calcium usually increases by 50%–100% during pregnancy. The actual requirement varies with the species and the nutritional status of the female prior to pregnancy. The high-producing dairy cow, for example, must restore a considerable amount of calcium lost during the previous lactation as well as build up stores for the forthcoming lactation.

The provision of supplemental iron during pregnancy is a problem limited almost exclusively to humans. Iron-deficiency anemia occurs in many pregnant women, and obstetricians universally recommend an iron supplement during pregnancy. This practice is necessitated by the fact that it is virtually impossible for a pregnant woman to meet the increased requirement for iron of about 4 mg per day during the later stages of pregnancy even if she con-

---

*Cravioto, J., and DeLicardie, E. R., *Nutr. Rev.* **29**(1971):107.

sumes a well-balanced diet containing large amounts of meat. The problem of iron deficiency during pregnancy is particularly acute in the developing countries where the intake of meat is low and intestinal parasites are invariably present.

Successful reproduction in a number of species requires considerable stores of vitamin A in the liver. Vitamin A deficiency during pregnancy has been a particularly troublesome problem to cattle raisers. The primary manifestation of the deficiency is the birth of weak calves that readily develop

---

Box 27.1   Breast milk—Is it unique?

"Cow's milk is for calves. Human milk is for babies." "The human is the only species known to utilize milk other than its own to nourish its young."

Statements such as these are common proclamations of the advocates of breast feeding. Although catchy, these statements, until recently, had been largely ignored or rejected by nutritionists and medical practitioners.

The marked decline in breast feeding over the past 40 years has resulted from a lack of any convincing evidence that human milk was definitely superior to a variety of infant formulas, together with the social stigma associated with breast feeding, and the ready availability of easily prepared formulas. Recent evidence that breast milk may be important in protecting the infant against several forms of *E. coli* infection and the finding that the chemical composition of human milk differs appreciably not only from that of cow's milk, but also from that previously reported for human milk, has stimulated renewed interest in breast feeding.

Colostrum and mature human milk contain several immunoglobulins that are active against viruses and bacteria. Immunoglobulins of the IgA, IgG, IgM, and IgD classes have been identified in human milk. The concentration of these antibodies is particularly high in colostrum. IgA, reported at levels of 17 mg/ml in the initial colostrum, decreases to levels of 1 to 2 mg/ml in mature breast milk. Since IgA is not absorbed to any appreciable extent from the gastrointestinal tract, at least following "closure" of the small intestine, the action of the immunoglobulins is thought to be associated primarily with the formation of a local defense in the gastrointestinal tract. In addition to the immunoglobulins, human milk contains other anti-infective agents, such as lysozyme, the bifidus factor, and lactoferrin. The relatively high concentration of lactose and relatively low concentration of phosphate and protein of human milk ensure a low pH in the gut of breast-fed infants, which in turn promotes the growth of lactobacilli and inhibits the growth of coliforms, shigellae, and sal-

scours. The problem appears to arise from the fact that the vitamin A intake of the mother during pregnancy has a limited influence on vitamin A storage in the fetus. However, liberal intakes of vitamin A during pregnancy will result in considerable storage of the vitamin in the mother's liver from where it is easily mobilized and transferred to the colostrum and milk.

It is interesting to reflect on the differential transfer of iron and vitamin A across the placenta and through the mammary gland. The ready mammary transfer of vitamin A is in contrast to the relatively poor transfer of iron to

monellae. Surveys have shown that breast feeding reduces not only the incidence of and mortality due to gastrointestinal tract infections, but deaths due to respiratory infections as well. The replacement of breast feeding by bottle feeding may be particularly hazardous for infants born of parents in lower socioeconomic groups in industrialized countries and for nearly the entire infant population in developing countries.

Evidence that the nutrient analysis of human milk may vary from that reported previously, together with evidence that the individual constituents may differ appreciably from those in cow's milk, has also cast some doubt on the advisability of displacing the breast with the bottle. Reports from the University of Uppsala in Sweden,* for example, suggest that the mean protein content of human milk is around 0.88 mg/100 ml rather than the 1.1 mg/100 ml usually reported in the literature. These studies found that approximately 25% of the nitrogen in human milk is nonprotein in nature. Investigators have also found that the methionine-to-cystine ratio in human milk is much lower than that in cow's milk, which may be particularly important to the immature infant in whom the activity of cystathionase—an enzyme involved in the conversion of methionine to cystine—is low. Reports such as these, together with the finding that the spatial arrangement of fatty acids in the triglycerides of human milk differs from that in cow's milk, have stimulated considerable interest among pediatricians and nutritionists in reevaluating the health benefits of breast feeding.

Whether human milk is unique, however, is open to debate. Certainly it is different from cow's milk, but there are marked differences in the composition of the milk of most species.

*Lönnerdal, B., Forsum, E., and Hambraeus, L., *Nutr. Rep. Internat.* **13**(1976):125.

milk. The situation is reversed with the placenta through which iron crosses relatively freely, whereas vitamin A traverses it with difficulty and is therefore poorly transmitted to the fetus.

Demands of lactation   Lactation imposes a greater stress on the female than does pregnancy, not so much because of the increase in metabolism as because of the direct loss to the body of nutrients that must be replenished by increased dietary intake. The efficiency of energy utilization for milk production is of the order of 61%, compared to an efficiency of 50% for body weight gain. However, whereas the dry weight of a newborn calf and its adnexa is about 7 kg, the dry matter in subsequent lactation, of say 6,000 kg of milk, amounts to about 780 kg; this ratio of slightly more than 1:100 of product formed during gestation and lactation is about the same for humans.

Thus, even with a greater efficiency of energy conversion in lactation, the stress from lactation is strikingly greater than that from reproduction.

CALCULATION OF THEORETICAL NEEDS   The theoretical nutrient needs for lactation in excess of maintenance are relatively easy to estimate. The milk leaves the body and thus its amount can be recorded and its nutrient content analyzed. Cow's milk of 4% fat contains about 750 kcal per kg, and represents about 1,230 kcal of food energy. Thus, to produce 1 kg of 4% milk a cow must consume about 1,200 kcal in excess of her maintenance allowance. A woman who daily produces 850 ml of milk containing 0.75 kcal per ml, and whose energy conversion efficiency is 80%, has an extra daily requirement of about 750 kcal ($850 \times 0.75 \div 0.80$).

PROTEIN REQUIREMENT   The protein requirement can also be computed by the same procedures. One kilogram of milk contains 35 g of protein, which represents 75% of the digestible dietary protein intake required. Hence, 1 kg of milk requires 47 g of usable food protein. Another way of arriving at the protein needed in the milking cow ration is to calculate that for each kilogram of protein in the daily milk yield there will be required 1.33 kcal of digestible protein in the ration above the daily maintenance allowance.

For the human, 100 ml of milk contains 1.2 g of protein. With an assumed efficiency of conversion of 75%, the necessary daily metabolizable protein intake would be 1.6 g of protein per 100 ml of milk.

The actual augmentation of the regular diet to meet the extra needs of lactation is directly dependent on the level of milk production, and can easily be adjusted periodically. In this connection it should be noted that increasing food or specific nutrient intake will not stimulate greater milk production. On the other hand, food restriction will result at first in a loss of body weight, and then in a drop in milk production.

CONCLUSIONS REGARDING NUTRITIONAL DEMANDS OF LACTATION   Lactation imposes a heavy extra nutritional demand on the female. The nutrient makeup of the diet of the lactating mammal is not unlike that of a well-balanced mintenance ration. However, in the human female the quantity required to maintain the nutritional status of the female may represent as much as a 50% increase over the maintenance allowance. In farm animals the milking ration is often double that needed for maintenance alone. The amounts of extra diet needed daily are proportional to the quantity of milk produced. The necessary amounts must be provided regularly if lactation is to be maintained.

Suggested readings

Austin, C. R., and Short, R. V. *Reproduction in Mammals. 3. Hormones in Reproduction.* Cambridge University Press, London (1972).

Blaxter, K. L. "Protein Metabolism and Requirements in Pregnancy and Lactation." In H. N. Munro and J. B. Allison (eds.), *Mammalian Protein Metabolism*, vol. II. Academic Press, New York (1964).

Cole, H. H., and Cupps, P. P. *Reproduction in Domestic Animals* (2nd ed.). Academic Press, New York (1969).

Kon, S. K. *Milk and Milk Products in Human Nutrition.* FAO Nutrition Studies No. 27, Food and Agriculture Organization of the United Nations, Rome (1972).

National Academy of Sciences–National Research Council. *The Relationship of Nutrition to Brain Development and Behavior.* National Academy of Sciences, Washington, D.C. (1973).

Schmidt, G. H. *Biology of Lactation.* W. H. Freeman and Company, San Francisco (1971).

Chapter 28
Energy requirements of the body

Basal metabolism

A large though variable fraction of the rations of all animals is needed for the maintenance of the body. Superimposed on this need are all the additional nutritive requirements—for growth, production of energy, wool, milk or body fat. It is from the maintenance requirement that nutritionists calculate the total nutrient requirements. The best indication of the energy required for maintenance, or at least the starting point in computing such a requirement is the determination of the fasting catabolism. When a resting animal is required to fast, it derives the energy for its vital processes by catabolizing its own body tissues. It is reasonable to believe that under such conditions the body will expend the minimum of energy possible in order to spare its tissues. This is the assumption underlying the use of fasting catabolism in calculating maintenance requirements.

The energy metabolized by a fasting animal appears as heat that may be measured either in a calorimeter or by methods of indirect calorimetry (Chapter 25). To obtain a basic value for this expenditure of energy, influences that might increase heat production must be kept at a minimum. The heat production of an animal under these conditions is called *basal metabolism*.

Basal metabolism defined Basal metabolism then represents the energy expended by an animal that is completely relaxed and at rest in a reclining, comfortable position, in a temperature within the zone of thermal neutrality, and after digestion and absorption of the last food ingested have ceased. The energy used under these conditions is only that required to run the automatic life processes, and to maintain the normal tone of the tissues.

With the human these conditions are relatively easy to meet. Basal conditions occur 12–15 hours after feeding. The energy metabolized for a given individual under these conditions is reproducible to within 5%, and hence is, for practical purposes, a biological constant. However with many domestic animals, basal conditions are not easily met, and they may not represent the most practical "base" for figuring nutritive energy requirements. For example, it may be argued that basal conditions normally never occur with farm animals. Basal conditions involve complete rest. Animals in calorimeters move about in getting up and lying down, and such movements require energy. In the case of ruminants in calorimeters, correction is made for this activity, and records are expressed on a 12-hour standing, 12-hour lying day. With cattle, standing increases basal requirements by 25%.

A postabsorptive state is reached by humans without hardship, but in many other animals this is not so, because digestion and assimilation proceed for a much longer period following the intake of food. Most data show that with cattle 30–70 hours lapse between a feeding and cessation of its absorption. Animals cannot fast for that long a time without manifesting conditions that increase basal metabolism.

Resting metabolism   Because of these difficulties, metabolism under "resting" instead of "basal" conditions has been proposed as a basis for computing energy requirements for all animals, including humans. If the conditions are defined in such a way that they yield reproducible values, *resting metabolism* should be as satisfactory a point of reference as basal metabolism. Resting metabolism, as defined by Brody,* differs from basal metabolism only in that the animals are not in a postabsorptive state. In practice, it is the metabolism measured at some fixed time after feeding (usually 4 hours).

Basal metabolism and body surface area   Because total heat production is related to body size, it is necessary to devise some unit of reference in which to express energy values if they are to be applicable to different animals.

---

*Dr. Samuel Brody was chairman of the Committee on Growth and Energy Metabolism at the College of Agriculture, University of Missouri, Columbia, Mo., that constituted the research committee for a cooperative, long-time study of bioenergetics. From time to time Brody and his coworkers published in *Missouri Research Bulletins* the results of specific researches, and at the completion of the broader project an integrated report under Brody's authorship, titled *Bioenergetics and Growth*, was published in 1945 as a 1,000-page volume by Reinhold Publishing Corp. To its date of publication this volume is the most complete compilation of the scientific data on this subject, and today it is an invaluable source of fundamental information. Many of the data and equations referred to or used in this and the succeeding two chapters have been taken from, or are based on concepts obtained from, Brody's report.

From observation investigators have long known that the heat produced by small animals is greater per unit of body weight than that produced by larger animals. Perhaps this is because the surface area of smaller animals is greater in proportion to body weight than that of large animals. Because of the relatively larger surface area, heat loss is greater, and hence in homeotherms, heat production (i.e., basal metabolism) must be greater. M. Rubner is responsible for the concept that basal metabolism is directly proportional to body surface. Data from various sources on various animals support a constant value of 1,000 kcal per square meter of body area as the heat produced by resting animals. Some of these data, as given by H. H. Dukes, are listed in Table 28.1.

Table 28.1
Heat produced by resting animals of various species as a function of body weight and body surface area

| Species | Weight (kg) | Heat produced in 24 hours (kcals) | |
		per kg weight	per sq meter of surface
Horse	441	11.3	948
Pig	128	19.1	1,078
Human	64.3	32.1	1,042
Dog	15.2	51.5	1,037
Goose	3.5	66.7	969
Fowl	2.0	71.0	943

SOURCE OF DATA: Dukes, H. H., *The Physiology of Domestic Animals* (5th ed.), Comstock Publishing Associates, Ithaca, New York (1942).

Measurement of surface area   There is a serious objection to the use of surface area as a unit of reference in basal or in resting metabolism because of the practical problem of measuring body surface. The surface area of an animal is usually estimated from its weight, with or without additional measurements such as height or girth. An early formula for calculating body surface area was proposed in 1879 by K. Meeh.[*] It was expressed as:

$$S = kW^{.66}$$

where S is in square decimeters and W is in kilograms. This is based on the formula for the area of a cube in relation to its volume:

---

[*]Meeh, K., cited by Armsby, *The Nutrition of Farm Animals*, Macmillan, New York (1917):259.

$$V = (\text{height})^3$$
$$S = 6(\text{height})^2$$

Therefore

$$S = 6(V)^{2/3}$$
$$= kV^{.66}$$

For a given substance, volume is proportional to weight. Therefore

$$S = kW^{.66}$$

In Meeh's formula the value of k was a constant within a species, but was different for different species, and represented the relative weight of each unit of volume. For example:

Species	k
Human	12.3
Child	10.3
Dog	11.2
Calf	10.5
Pig	8.7
Rat	9.1

The body surface area of a 70-kilogram man would be calculated:

$$S = 12.3 \times 70^{.6666}$$
$$= 12.3 \times \text{antilog} (\log 70 \times .6666)$$
$$= 12.3 \times \text{antilog} (1.84510 \times .6666)$$
$$= 12.3 \times 16.98 = 209 \text{ dcm}^2$$
$$= 2.1 \text{ m}^2$$

Meeh's value for a k of 12.3 for humans is now known to be too high, but for many years it was the standard. Eventually scientists decided to obtain a more accurate equation, if possible, and in 1916 an electrical engineer named D. DuBois undertook the task of measuring the surface area of a human.[*] His procedure was novel. A subject was dressed in a tightly fitted suit of underwear (a section of the underwear fitting over his head and neck) and thin socks and cotton gloves. Strips of Manila paper were pasted on this groundwork until a flexible but inelastic mold of the body was completed. This was then marked out in different regions of the body according to the

---

[*]DuBois, D., and DuBois, E. F., *Arch. Internal Med.* **17**

bony landmarks, and the whole covering was removed by means of curved bandage scissors. The mold of each region of the body was then given a coat of paraffin and was cut into pieces small enough that they would lie flat. The pieces were put in a large printing frame which was placed over sheets of weighed photographic paper, and prints were made by exposure to the sun. The portions of unexposed photographic paper, that had been under the pieces of the mold, were cut and weighed. Since the weight of a square inch of the paper was a constant and known, the total area of the mold could be calculated from the total weight of the pieces. The method appears to have been accurate; when it was applied to a large bowling ball the results differed by only 0.13% from the surface area as calculated from the average diameter.

DuBois measured the surface area of five subjects of widely differing shapes, and from the results he worked out the following formula by which to calculate surface area in square centimeters.

$$\text{Surface (cm}^2) = k \times W_{\text{kg}}^{.425} \times H_{\text{cm}}^{.725}$$

where $k = 71.84$, W_{kg} is weight in kilograms, and H_{cm} is height in centimeters.

It is interesting to examine this equation in the light of the Meeh formula. For a given individual we can write height in terms of weight because

$$H = \sqrt[3]{V}$$
$$= k\sqrt[3]{W}$$
$$= kW^{.33}$$

Substituting in the DuBois formula we write

$$S = k_1 W^{.425} \times k_2 W^{(.33 \times .725)}$$
$$= k_1 k_2 \times W^{.425 + (.33 \times .725)}$$
$$= kW^{.66}$$

which is the Meeh formula. According to present data the value for k should be 10.7 instead of 12.3 as used in the original equation.

The DuBois equation then is the Meeh formula, modified or expanded to utilize both height and weight in the estimate of surface area, thereby achieving some adjustment for differences in stature.

Many other formulae have been proposed for calculating body surface area, but not all workers subscribe to the idea of using surface area as an index of basal metabolism. J. A. Harris and F. G. Benedict* did not believe that basal metabolism is necessarily related to body surface, and they proposed a for-

---

*Harris, J. A., and Benedict, F. G., *Carnegie Institute of Washington Publication 279* (1919).

mula which provides the best statistical fit of the basal metabolism data to height, weight, and age. For adult males (human) they proposed

$$\text{kcal per day} = 66.473 + 13.752\,W_{kg} + 5.003\,H_{cm} - 6.755\,A_{yr}$$

In 1932 M. Kleiber* made a critical statistical study of basal metabolism data reported from many sources. His findings supported Harris and Benedict's rejection of Rubner's "Surface Law" that basal metabolism of all animals is close to 1,000 kcal per 24 hours per square meter of body surface. The discrepancies from the Surface Law as found by Kleiber are illustrated in a table condensed from Kleiber's original report (Table 28.2).

These data clearly show that there is a tendency for larger animals to have higher values, and smaller animals to have lower values, than the expected 1000 kcal per square meter of body surface area. For each increase of 1 kilogram of body weight there is an increase of 0.125% in the heat of basal metabolism per square meter of surface. Some, and perhaps a large part, of this discrepancy lies in the calculation of the body surface. There appear to be nearly as many formulae as investigators, and values for surface area calculated by different formulae on the same individual may differ appreciably.

Nevertheless, it is evident that basal metabolism is more closely related to calculated surface area of the body than to the first power of its live weight. Measured by the same criteria, the coefficient of variation of the values for heat produced per unit of weight is more than twice that found using surface. This is a statistical way of saying that when weight to the first power is used to describe size, there is a greater tendency for heavier animals to have smaller values, and lighter animals to have larger values, than when surface area is used.

Metabolism related to a power of body weight   However, basal metabolism appears to be quite closely related to a fractional power of body weight. The standard deviation drops, not only for nonruminants but also for all other groups, to as low as 6%–8%. The power of body weight most closely related to basal metabolism is 0.75 for all groups, or 0.73 if ruminants are excluded. If this relation between basal metabolism and some power of body weight were a constant, plotting logarithms of basal metabolism against logarithms of the body weight should give a straight line, the slope of which would be the power of body weight to which the basal metabolism is most closely related. Statistically

$$\text{kcal} = W^n$$

$$\text{Log kcal} = n \times \log W$$

---

*Kleiber, M., *Hilgardia, Cal. Agr. Expt. Sta.* **6**(1932), no. 11.

Table 28.2
Relation between 24-hour basal metabolism and the weight of an animal or its calculated body surface

Animal	Average weight (kg)	Kilocalories 24 hr B.M.	Body surface (m²)	Calories heat produced per unit of				Formula for calculating body surface
				$W^{.66}$	$W^{.73}$	$W^{.8}$	W^1	
Steer	342	6255	1465	128	89	59	18	$0.1081 \times W^{5/8}$
Man	64	1632	926	102	78	59	26	$71.84 \times W^{.425} \times L^{.725}$
Sheep	46	1220	1163	105	75	57	27	$0.124 \times W^{.561}$
Dog	16	525	776	85	71	59	34	$0.112 \times W^{2/3}$
Hen	2	106	676	68	65	62	54	$5.86 \times W^{.5} \times L^{.6}$
Rat	0.23	26	600	69	75	84	113	$0.1136 \times W^{2/3}$
All groups, average:*			914 ± 34%†	90 ± 24%	75 ± 8%	65 ± 22%	54 ± 80%	
Groups except ruminants, average:*			730 ± 16%	78 ± 17%	73 ± 6%	70 ± 19%	71 ± 62%	

*From Kleiber's complete table.
†Coefficient of variation between species.

From such a plot Kleiber obtained a value of 0.75 for the slope of the regression (i.e., for the value of n in the equation above). It is not possible, however, to determine the best-fitting power of weight relating kilocalories of basal metabolism to body size within one species, except for dogs and horses, which have a large enough range in weights to adequately fix the regression.

Brody summarized the case for the use of a power of weight rather than surface area as a reference base in metabolism as follows:

> We do not see the logic involved in computing surface area from body weight, and then relating heat production to the computed area. Why not relate heat production to the body weight directly? Obviously, if surface area is computed as KW^n and if heat loss is proportional to surface, it is also proportional to the W^n. If W^n is or can be the same for all animals, the one method is as correct as another and the choice should lie with the one which is best defined—and by all odds—this is the weight.[*]

The Kleiber formula for caloric needs of adult humans   Kleiber examined data published by Harris and Benedict for human subjects and found by statistical studies that there is a decrease in basal metabolism per yearly increase in age amounting to about .4% of the basal metabolism at age 30 years. Basal metabolism is also affected by body build; however, height alone is not a satisfactory index of body shape. If both weight and height could be used in some generalized way to obtain an index to which basal metabolism is related, the problem would be solved. Kleiber argued that because weight is proportional to volume, the cube root of weight is proportional to one of its linear dimensions:

$$W = kV$$

and

$$V = L^3$$

therefore

$$W = kL^3$$

or

$$W^{.33} = kL$$

Hence, the ratio of height to $W^{.33}$ is an index of stature which is independent of size. As an example, let us compare two persons as follows:

---

[*]Brody, S., Comfort, J. E., Mathews, J. S., *Missouri Agricultural Experiment Station Research Bulletin No. 115* (1928).

	A	B
Weight	216 lb	125 lb
Height	73 in.	60.5 in.
Specific stature	$\dfrac{73}{\sqrt[3]{216}}$	$\dfrac{60.5}{\sqrt[3]{125}}$
	$= 12.1$	$= 12.1$

Thus, both of these persons have the same stature or body build.

Insofar as body build is concerned, Kleiber found Benedict's data indicated that for each unit increase in specific stature the basal metabolism (BM) per $W^{.75}$ increases 1% in man and 1.8% in woman. From these data he formulated an equation for basal metabolism:

$$\text{kcal} = c \times W^n [1 + \alpha (A - a) + \sigma (s - S)]$$

where

c = coefficient for sex or species: 71.2 for man; 65.8 for woman

W = body weight in kilograms

n = exponent .75

α = coefficient of age: .4%

A = standard age: 30 years if c = 71.2

a = actual age

σ = coefficient of build: 1% of BM at age 30 for man; 1.8% of BM at age 30 for woman

S = standard specific stature: 43.4 for man; 42.1 for woman

s = actual specific stature

The Kleiber formulae for normal basal metabolism are:

Male: $\text{kcal} = 71.2\, W^{.75} [1 + .004(30 - a) + .01(s - 43.3)]$

Female: $\text{kcal} = 65.8\, W^{.75} [1 + .004(30 - a) + .018(s - 42.1)]$

The following example illustrates the use of these formulae.

Given a male adult 35 years old, weighing 65 kg, and standing 165 cm in height,

$$\text{kcal} = 71.2 \times 65^{.75} \left[1 + .004(30 - 35) + .01\left(\frac{165}{\sqrt[3]{65}} - 43.4 \right) \right]$$

Specific stature $= \dfrac{165}{4.02} = 41$; and $65^{.75} = 22.9$, whence

$$kcal = 71.2 \times 22.9[1 + (-.02) + (-.024)]$$
$$= 71.2 \times 22.9(.956)$$
$$= 1558$$

The basal metabolism calculated without correction for age and stature is 1,630 kcal (71.2 × 22.9), and the correction itself amounts to −4.4% of this, or 72 kcal.

The Kleiber formulae were tested by comparing the basal metabolism values calculated from them with values of experimentally determined basal metabolism. The standard deviations of the difference between the calculated and experimentally determined values were:

Sex	Formula	SD of difference
Male	As given	±6.16%
	Without correction	±7.72%
Female	As given	±7.94%
	Without correction	±11.80%

Metabolic size   Nutritionists now generally agree that basal metabolism is proportional to a fractional power of body weight, but they are not in agreement as to what power should be used in specific cases. We shall therefore summarize the more important findings on which the values adopted in this book are based.

As far back as 1932 Kleiber* examined basal metabolism data from ten different species of adult mammals and found the best power of their kilogram weight, n, to be 0.739; in the same year Brody and R.C. Procter,† and in 1934 Brody and U. S. Ashworth,† proposed 0.734 as the value of n. The Conference on Energy Metabolism‡ sponsored by the Committee on Animal Nutrition of the U.S. National Research Council and held at Pennsylvania State College in 1935 endorsed the figure of 0.73, and in 1945 Brody suggested $(W^{kg})^{.75}$ be taken as the measure of "metabolic size" to which basal metabolism is proportional. In 1947 Kleiber** reported on his analysis of the data of 26 species, which did not include the ten species analyzed in the data published previously (1932). In this 1947 study he found n to be 0.756.

---

*Kleiber, M., *Hilgardia, Cal. Agr. Expt. Sta.*6 (1932).

†Brody, S., *Bioenergetics and Growth*, Reinhold Publishing Corp., New York (1945): Chapters 13 and 14.

‡NRC (U.S.), *Conference on Energy Metabolism*, U.S. National Research Council (1935).

Kleiber, M. *Physiol. Rev.* **27 (1947):511.

The experimental evidence about the power to which body weight (in kilograms) must be raised to best describe metabolic size indicates that it lies somewhere between 0.734 and 0.756, and the standard deviations applicable are of the order of 7%. It is therefore useless to argue about the relative validity of any value within this range. Biologically, one is as good as another. The logical choice can justifiably be made on the basis of simplicity of computation; and this choice is obviously 0.75, which power of a number can be computed by simple arithmetic whereas all others within this range require the use of logarithms.

For example, for a 65-kilogram man,

$$65^{.75} = 65^{3/4} = \sqrt[4]{65^3}$$
$$= \sqrt[4]{274,625}$$
$$= \sqrt{524.5}$$
$$= 22.8$$

$$65^{.74} = \text{antilog } (\log 65 \times 0.74)$$
$$= \text{antilog } (1.8129 \times 0.74) = \text{antilog } 1.341546$$
$$= 21.95$$

$$65^{.76} = \text{antilog } (1.8129 \times 0.76) = \text{antilog } 1.377804$$
$$= 23.85$$

Once metabolic size, W^n, is calculated, the kilocalories expended at basal metabolism per unit of metabolic size are found by dividing the experimentally measured heat loss at basal conditions by the value W^n. In studies of 36 groups of adult mammals, the 24-hour fasting heat production (measured in a calorimeter as heat loss) was found to be 69 ± 1.2 kilocalories per unit of metabolic size.[*]

Consequently, for all practical purposes in nutrition, the 24-hour basal metabolism of all adult mammals can be taken as

$$70(W_{kg}^{.75}) \text{ kcal}$$

Comparable individuals within and between species may deviate from this value by as much as 7%. This variation is not greater than is "normal" for other biological measurements, and therefore the value can be considered a biological constant.

To many, the use of a power of weight to express size is a needless complication. Why not relate nutrient needs directly to weight? The important reason is perhaps not at once evident, because to describe the energy needs of

---

[*]Kleiber, M., *Physiol. Rev.* **27**(1947):511.

Mr. Jones who is of average weight (65 kilograms), and at average work, and shown by experiment to need let us say 3,200 kcal to maintain his weight, it is immaterial whether we express this requirement as:

$$\text{Daily kcal for Mr. Jones} = 3{,}200 \text{ kcal}$$
$$\text{kcal per kilogram weight: } 3200 \div 65 = 49(W^{1.0}) \text{ kcal}$$
$$\text{kcal per unit metabolic size: } 3200 \div (65^{.75}) = 140(W^{.75}) \text{ kcal}$$

But if we must adjust this allowance to fit Mr. Smith who weighs 80 kg and also to fit Miss Black who weighs only 50 kg, both of whom do work comparable to that done by Mr. Jones, we find the "requirements" as follows:

Kilocaloric "requirements" computed from $(W^{1.0})$ *vs.* $(W^{.75})$

	49 $(W^{1.0})$	140$(W^{.75})$	Difference
Mr. Jones (65 kg)	3200	3200	0
Mr. Smith (80 kg)	3920	3750	17 kcal in excess
Miss Black (50 kg)	2400	2620	220 kcal in deficit

Compared to the biologically correct relationship between size and caloric requirement, allowances based directly on weight are *too meager* for the lighter person and needlessly excessive for the heavier person. The more the individual deviates from average size, the greater the discrepancy (see Figure 28.1).

A caloric excess may or may not be of practical importance to the individual in everyday living, though it obviously does not help the person who is attempting to curtail gains in weight. However, in allocating foods to large groups, as in rationing, it is important to avoid either unnecessary excesses or unrecognized deficiencies.

The maintenance energy requirement

Having derived a way of calculating basal metabolism kilocalories [i.e., $70(W_{kg}{}^{.75})$], we can now derive equations for calculating the amount of dietary energy needed to supply them. The maintenance energy requirement is the amount of energy required to maintain the "idle" body in energy equilibrium. Under fasting conditions it would be represented by the basal metabolism value. For maintenance under normal conditions, the basal value must be increased because the energy necessarily expended for activity is in excess of the basal value.

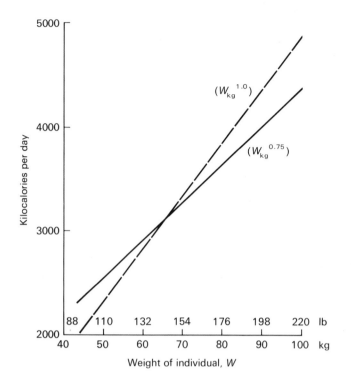

Figure 28.1
Daily energy requirement computed on the basis of $W_{kg}^{1.0}$ or $W_{kg}^{.75}$.

From the data on the metabolism of species varying in size from that of elephants to mice, Brody found that basal metabolism kilocalories represent about 75% of the kilocalories of dietary energy needs for the maintenance of idle adult, monogastric, nonherbivorous species if the values are expressed as metabolizable kilocalories. For cattle and sheep, basal metabolism kilocalories are about 50% of the energy needed for maintenance if this is expressed as pounds of total digestible nutrients (TDN) carrying 4 kcal per gram or 1,816 kcal per pound (evidence indicates that TDN carries about 2,000 kcal per pound.*

*Crampton, E. W., Lloyd, L. E., and MacKay, V. G., *J. Animal Sci.* **16** (1957):541; Swift, R. W., *J. Animal Sci.* **16** (1957):753.

Based on these findings, the maintenance requirements of humans, pigs, and rats can be computed as follows:

$$\text{Metabolize kcal} = 1.33 \times 70(W^{.75})$$
$$= 93(W^{.75})$$

and those of cattle and sheep

$$\text{TDN}_{lb} = \frac{2 \times 70(W^{.75})}{4 \times 454}$$
$$= .078(W^{.75})$$

To express maintenance energy for the human, pig, or rat as digestible kilocalories it is reasonable to consider that urinary losses raise the requirement by 7% over metabolizable kilocalories:

$$\text{Digestible kcal} = 1.40 \times 70(W^{.75})$$
$$= 98(W^{.75})$$

Direct calculation of the kilocalories for "activity of idleness" (human)

J. B. Orr and I. Leitch of the Rowett Research Institute, Aberdeen, Scotland, approached the problem of the maintenance energy need of humans from a different viewpoint.* They assembled data for caloric requirements according to certain categories of activity at maintenance living. Values for two typical cases are shown in Table 28.3.

*Orr, J. B., and Leitch, I., *Nutrition Abstr. and Rev.* 7, no. 3 (1938).

Table 28.3
Typical energy expenditure of adult humans at maintenance living

Activity	Case I		Case II	
	Hours	*Kilocalories*	*Hours*	*Kilocalories*
Basal		1,700		1,700
Dressing	1	33	1	33
Sitting	7	105	5	75
Walking	2	230	2	230
"Gardening"	—	—	3	320
Standing	4	80	3	60
Total		2,148		2,418

SOURCE: Orr, J. B., and Leitch, I., *Nutrition Abstr. and Rev.* 7, no. 3 (1938).

Leitch said the average, adult human, 24-hour "maintenance" need is 2,200 kcal of metabolizable energy, and in her data the basal metabolism accounts for $1700 \times 100/2200 = 77\%$ of it. This means that the maintenance "activity energy" plus specific dynamic action is 23% of the total, and that to meet a given basal requirement the total maintenance energy allowance of metabolizable energy will have to be $100/77 = 1.30$ times the basal metabolism. By comparison, Brody gave a value of 1.33 as the general figure for all species.

Waste heat—specific dynamic action (SDA)   Limited data suggest that at maintenance about 10% of metabolizable energy is waste heat—that is, the specific dynamic action of energy metabolism. The exact percentage depends, of course, on the base on which it is calculated. It seems logical to express SDA as a percentage of some unit of energy other than basal

---

Box 28.1   Samuel Brody and bioenergetics

Samuel Brody (1890–1956) was a biochemist, physicist, dairy husbandry specialist, and master of bioenergetics. He conceived that the problems of bioenergetics (energy transformations in living things) were generalized by the first and second laws of thermodynamics. Few researchers were working in this field when Brody entered it, and few joined him in it during his active years.

Born in Lithuania, Samuel Brody immigrated to Canada at the age of sixteen. He worked there as a miner, peddler, and commercial fisherman before moving to New Hampshire to join an older brother. Having taught himself to read and write English, Brody was eventually admitted to the University of California at Davis where he was attracted by T. B. Robertson's theories on the dynamics of growth. There he received his undergraduate degree in biochemistry in 1917 and the M.A. degree in 1919.

Brody accepted a position on the staff of the Department of Dairy Husbandry at the University of Missouri in 1920; he remained associated with this institution for the remaining thirty-six years of his life. During a sabbatical leave from Missouri, he obtained his Ph.D. degree from the University of Chicago in 1928, under the direction of A. J. Carlson. In 1930 and 1931, Brody studied in five European universities on a Guggenheim Foundation fellowship.

Sixty-six Agricultural Experiment Station bulletins dealing with the growth and development of domestic and laboratory animals were issued from Missouri under Samuel Brody's coauthorship. During the ten years prior to his death, he published thirty-nine bulletins in the field of environmental physiology and shelter engineering.

metabolism, because under basal conditions there can be no SDA. Maintenance energy is the minimal practical level computable for all adults, and it is therefore logical to use the number of metabolizable kilocalories needed for maintenance as the base to express SDA, and to add to production rations an SDA allowance appropriate to the production anticipated.

Based on the Orr and Leitch figures, Table 28.4 shows how the metabolizable energy required for maintenance is utilized by an adult human of about 70 kg.

However, to compute dietary needs for maintenance it is necessary to relate the fractions of metabolizable energy that are used for various purposes to basal metabolism, which is the only measurable value. Table 28.4 can be rearranged as in Table 28.5 to show the kilocalories necessary as metabolizable energy to provide 1 kcal of basal metabolism.

The Orr and Leitch value of 1.30 is based on limited data; consequently,

In addition to his great output of Experiment Station bulletins, Brody was the author or coauthor of ninety-two journal articles between 1921 and 1957, dealing variously with growth, milk secretion, energy metabolism, thyroid function, ageing, environmental influences on dairy cattle performance, as well as with the philosophical aspects of population control and the world food supply. His writings also dealt with specific dynamic effect, net energy and feeding standards, the efficiency of animals and humans as transformers of energy, basal metabolic rate, and the energy cost of work.

Perhaps Samuel Brody's most famous work was his book *Bioenergetics and Growth* published in 1945. This volume consisted of 1,023 pages, carried more than 2,000 references, and provided more than 500 illustrations and some 113 tables of data. Probably the most useful feature of the book is the detailed accounts of methods of measuring heat production and of establishing production norms for such measurements. Brody discovered that the basal metabolism of all species varies not with surface area directly but with a power of body weight ($W^{.73}$), this measure representing "metabolically effective" body weight. In his investigation of bioenergetics, he extended his "efficiency calculations" to apply to practical agriculture, especially the production of milk and eggs.

Brody was constructively critical of the work of his students, and had a remarkable sense of humor, a philosophical mind, and little regard for material things. His scientific ambition was the driving force of his life and he left himself little time for anything other than his work. His death at the age of sixty-six was the result of a coronary occlusion.

For further information, see *J. Nutr.* **70**(1960):3.

Table 28.4
Partition of metabolizable kilocalories required
for maintenance living in a 70-kilogram adult human

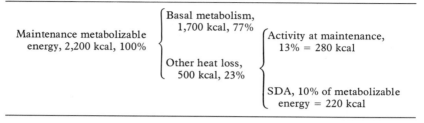

Table 28.5
Metabolizable kilocalories for maintenance relative to 1 kcal of basal metabolism

Maintenance metabolizable energy, 1.30 kcal
- Activity at maintenance, 0.17 kcal
- Heat loss, 1.13 kcal
  - Basal metabolism, 1.00 kcal
  - SDA, 0.13 kcal

Brody's finding that basal metabolism represents 75% of the maintenance metabolizable energy requirement, or that the maintenance metabolizable energy requirement is 100/75 = 1.33 times the basal metabolism, seems a more reliable value to accept at the present.

Maintenance allowances for humans proposed by the FAO Committee on Calorie Requirements   The Canadian Dietary Standard of 1948* was the first human standard to be based on the concept that body weight is a more satisfactory basis for estimating nutrient and energy requirements than age. It is interesting that the Food and Agriculture Organization (FAO) of the United Nations, in its bulletin *Calorie Requirements*,† and the Food and Nutrition Board of the U.S. National Research Council in the 1953 revision of its bulletin *Recommended Dietary Allowances*, also adopted weight rather than age as the basis for computing dietary requirements. (Feeding standards for animals other than humans have always used weight as a basis for determining ration needs.)

Canadian Bulletin on Nutrition **2**, no. 1 (1950).

†*Calorie Requirements*, FAO Nutrition Studies, No. 5 (1950).

In 1957 the revised FAO bulletin contained the following statement:

> The resting energy expenditure is represented . . . by basal metabolism. It may be estimated with reasonable accuracy from the body weight by an expression of the form: basal metabolism $= aW^n$, where a is a constant determined by age, sex, and the units employed, W is the nude weight and the exponent is about 0.73. If it is considered that resting energy expenditure should include seated as well as supine rest, the same equation holds but the constant a is somewhat larger. . . . The energy expenditure in the seated position is simply a multiple of that in the supine position, the multiplier being of the order of 1.3. . . . The energy expenditure associated with the ingestion of food is generally called the Specific Dynamic Action. It is subject to some modification by type of diet, but with ordinary mixed diets it is perhaps slightly less than 10% of the energy value of the total food metabolized and can therefore be taken as about 10% of the total energy expenditure when the individual is in caloric balance.[*]

This statement can be expressed algebraically as follows:

$$\text{Kilocalories for maintenance} = \left[1.3 \times 71(W_{kg}{}^{.73})\right] \times 1.11$$

In this equation a is given a value of 71 for the reference man (i.e., 91/1.3 = 70.7; see following subsection).

It is worth noting that the values proposed by the FAO committee were not arrived at by the same methods that form the basis of the Brody formula. Because of the fundamental significance of the energy requirement in determining dietary requirements for specific nutrients, we will examine in some detail the evolution of the FAO equation for computing the maintenance energy needs of adult humans.

The reference man The FAO committees (1950 and 1957) and the joint FAO/WHO[†] Ad Hoc Expert Committee (1973) established caloric standards on the basis of a reference man, described by the joint committee as being between 20 and 39 years of age, weighing 65 kg, and working 8 hours daily in an occupation involving moderate activity. He is assumed to require an average of 3,000 kcal daily to maintain a constant weight. This allowance is in accordance with most dietary survey data.

Maintenance energy needs The rate of *energy expenditure for maintenance* can be thought of as comprising two parts: basal metabolism and, in humans, the activities associated with sedentary living. Basal metabolism requires about 1.1 kcal per minute in the "reference man," and the mean expenditure

---

[*]*Calorie Requirements*, FAO Nutrition Studies, No. 15 (1957).

[†]*WHO* = World Health Organization of the United Nations.

for such sedentary activities as sitting, dressing, standing, and walking amounts to about 1.6 kcal per minute.

Because a man at maintenance living spends 8 hours lying down (sleeping or resting) and 16 hours at sedentary activity, we can calculate maintenance energy expenditure for a 65-kilogram man as follows:

$$\text{BM:} \quad 8 \text{ hr} \times 60 \times 1.1 = \quad 528 \text{ kcal}$$

$$\text{Sedentary pursuits:} \quad 16 \text{ hr} \times 60 \times 1.6 = 1{,}536 \text{ kcal}$$

$$\text{Total 24-hr maintenance} = 2{,}064 \text{ kcal}$$

To express these data as an equation of the Brody–Kleiber type we calculate, for a 65-kilogram man, the kilocalories per unit metabolizable body size by solving the equation

$$2{,}064 \text{ kcal} = a(65_{\text{kg}}{}^{.75})$$

$$a = \frac{2{,}064}{22.9}$$

$$= 90.1$$

Thus,

$$\text{Total 24-hr maintenance} = 90.1(W_{\text{kg}}{}^{.75}) \text{ kcal}$$

The energy expenditure of a typical 65-kilogram man living at a sedentary or essentially "idle" level of activity is approximately 1.33 times basal metabolism.

Brody and Kleiber each have produced evidence (see p. 406) that basal metabolism is the same for many homeotherms per unit of metabolic size and is numerically expressed as

$$\text{Kilocalories of BM per 24 hr} = 70(W_{\text{kg}}{}^{.75})$$

This basal figure must be increased by about 1.33 times to describe numerically the intake of metabolizable energy necessary to meet the energy expenditure at maintenance living. The increment multiple will be somewhat greater than 1.33 if the answer is to be in digestible or gross dietary kilocalories. Table 28.6 gives an idea of the multiples of the basal metabolism used to express the average, adult, 24-hour maintenance requirement for dietary energy in various species.

Generalized formula for computing adult maintenance energy needs From the figures in Table 28.6, it is possible to derive a generalized standard for the maintenance energy requirements of adult animals:

Table 28.6
Multiples of basal metabolism to compute daily energy requirements for adult maintenance in various species

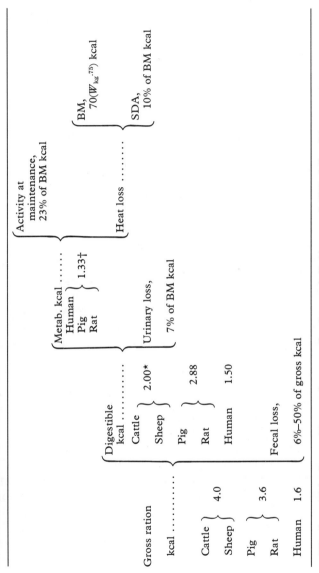

*The figure 1.7 is often used here on the assumption that metabolizable energy is 80% of digestible energy.
†Example: Metabolizable kcal for human maintenance = $1.33 \times 70(W_{kg}^{.75})$.

$$X = abW^n$$

where X is the energy requirement in kilocalories, a is the activity factor representing the increase in requirement for maintenance over basal conditions, b is the regression of basal kilocalories in W^n. Numerical values for a, b, and n are

a = 1.3 metabolizable kilocalories ⎫
⎬ carnivora and omnivora
    1.4 digestible kilocalories ⎭

  = 1.7–2.0 digestible energy as TDN} herbivora

b = 70 kcal

n = 0.75

Maintenance energy requirements for women   It is debatable whether there is any real difference in the maintenance energy requirements traceable to sex *per se*. Basal metabolism correlates fundamentally with the actively metabolizing mass of the body. If women carry appreciably more adipose tissue than men, we might expect (for individuals of the same weight) women to have a slightly lower basal metabolic rate. However, using data from the 1973 FAO/WHO bulletin on *Energy and Protein Requirements* we can show that the differences between sexes are largely due to differences in size.

	Reference man	*Reference woman*	*Difference*
8 hr bed rest at basal rate (kcal)	518	432	20%
Wt of subject (kg)	65	55	18%

About a quarter of the maintenance requirement in excess of that required for basal metabolism is utilized to cover activity, a large part of which consists of moving the body itself. Because average women weigh less than average men, the energy cost of their daily activity as individuals may be less than that of men. However, for individuals of equal weight it is illogical to expect muscle to differ in efficiency because of sex. R. Passmore and J. V. G. A. Durnin state that "energy expenditure was closely correlated with body weight, but not significantly with height, age, race, or sex."[*]

Consequently, it is unlikely that there are significant differences attributable to sex in maintenance energy needs per unit of metabolic size. The same

---

[*]Passmore, R., and Durnin, J. V. G. A., *Physiol. Rev.* **35** (1955):801.

equation can therefore be used to compute the maintenance requirement of adults of either sex:

$$\text{Total 24-hr maintenance} = 1.33 \times 70(W_{kg}{}^{.75}) \text{ kcal}$$
$$= 93(W_{kg}{}^{.75}) \text{ kcal}$$

The simplest way of presenting the data for humans of differing weights is in the form of a graph in which kilocalories are plotted against body weights, as is done in Figure 28.2. In this graph the weight range is a little greater than plus or minus twice the standard deviation of the weights of male adults of North America, and so includes over 95% of the population.

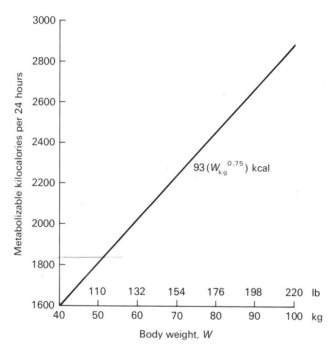

Figure 28.2
Metabolizable energy required by human adults at maintenance living: kcal = $93(W_{kg}{}^{.75})$.

Energy requirements for work   The greatest obstacle to establishing accurate dietary standards is the exact determination of the energy requirement for work: it is difficult to assess the average intensity of muscular effort necessary to execute the variety of tasks performed in an 8-hour day. During a single work shift, humans not only may engage in a variety of jobs, each requiring widely different energy expenditure, but they are also prone to eat with no conscious regard to actual needs. Appetite is usually a guide to energy needs when needs are high, but, unfortunately, not when they are relatively small.

Because the intensity of work during an extended period (such as an 8-hour work day) cannot be accurately expressed by ranking occupations according to whether they demand light, moderate, or heavy work, accurate statements

---

Box 28.2   Obesity: a problem of energy balance?

Obesity is a very real human problem of our time. It has been defined as an excessive accumulation of adipose tissue containing stored fat in the form of triglyceride. The changes in energy balance that occur when caloric intake exceeds caloric expenditure invariably cause obesity. This type of imbalance may result from an overconsumption of energy, an underexpenditure of energy, or more frequently from a combination of both. The quantity of food consumed as well as its quality and the frequency with which it is eaten may result in excessive energy intake. A predisposition to sedentary living habits will result in an underexpenditure of energy.

However, obesity is not always a cut-and-dried problem of simple energy imbalance. It is becoming increasingly recognized that a host of other factors may play a role in creating such imbalances. These include social, economic, biochemical, genetic, neural, and psychological factors, which exert interacting effects. The question of the regulation of food (energy) intake is complex, and numerous theories have been suggested about how the central nervous system receives signals that initiate the consumption of food. A 1975 report by T. B. Van Itallie suggests that eating may be controlled by satiety to a greater extent than by hunger.

The matter of childhood obesity is of particular interest. Excessive weight gain during infancy is related to greater incidence of obesity during later childhood, and this in turn tends to persist into the adult years. Obesity can be classified as hypertrophic or hyperplastic; one theory on what differentiates the two types postulates that hypertrophic obesity, associated with late onset, is

of energy requirements for work depend on the measurement of oxygen consumption over timed periods of activity at different intensities of muscular effort. Using a caloric equivalent for oxygen of 4.92 kcal per liter, Durnin and Passmore* determined the energy requirement for different forms of physical activity. Representative values are shown in Table 28.7.

The rates of energy expenditure given in Table 28.7 represent total energy expenditure, including the basal metabolism per minute *plus* the specific dynamic action (SDA) component *plus* the actual activity.

Because the increase in energy required for a particular activity is normally met through increasing the usual dietary intake, the SDA component re-

---

*Durnin, J. V. G. A., and Passmore, R., *Energy, Work and Leisure*, Heinemann Educational Books, London (1967).

---

caused primarily by an increased *size* of fat cell, whereas hyperplastic obesity, associated with early onset, has the added dimension of an increased *number* of fat cells. It has been reported that adipose tissue develops through stages of hyperplasia first, followed by hypertrophy. Because it appears to be more difficult to lose excess fat if obesity is of the hyperplastic form, it is important to determine the critical period of life during which the total number of fat cells becomes established in order to provide a rational basis for dietary control measures. In the human, this critical period is as yet unknown but appears to be anywhere from the last trimester of pregnancy to the first three years of life and perhaps even into adolescence.

Obesity can be prevented and, as with other diseases, prevention is definitely better than treatment. The discovery of means of identifying at an early stage the periods during which fat cells multiply and fat depots develop at an abnormal rate, together with steps to alter the development of this tissue before hypercellularity occurs, offers the best hope for the prevention of obesity in both children and adults.

The most sensible approach to the treatment of obesity is to restrict the dietary intake of high-energy foods and to accompany this with increased physical activity. Much less satisfactory are such techniques as therapeutic starvation, jejunoileal bypass surgery, various reducing dietary regimens, and the use of such hormones as human chorionic gonadotropin (HCG), thyroxine and triiodothyronine, human growth hormone, and progesterone.

For further information, see *Dairy Council Digest* **46**, no. 4 (1975).

Table 28.7
Rate of energy expenditure in relation to intensity of muscular work

Intensity of work	Rate for reference man (kcal/min)
Very light work (e.g., drafting)	1.5–2.3
Light work (e.g., carpentry)	2.9–5.0
Moderate work (e.g., pushing wheelbarrow)	5.0–7.1
Heavy work (e.g., splitting wood)	8.6–9.1
Very heavy work (e.g., boxing)	9.0–14.4
Basal metabolism*	1.1

SOURCE: Durnin, J. V. G. A., and Passmore, R., *Energy, Work and Leisure,* Heinemann Educational Books, London (1967).
*The energy expenditure at basal metabolism for a 65-kg man can be calculated as follows:

$$\text{Basal metabolism} = 70(W_{kg}^{.75})$$
$$= 70(65^{.75})$$
$$= 1{,}603 \text{ kcal}$$

$$1{,}603/1{,}440 \text{ min in 24 hr} = 1.1 \text{ kcal/min.}$$

mains a constant fraction of the energy requirement. Hence, for practical purposes, SDA can be considered an integral part of the increased requirement associated with that activity.

On this basis, carpentry (using a mean value of 3.9 kcal/min) would require an activity expenditure of 3.9 − 1.1 = 2.8 kcal per minute, and boxing (using a mean value of 12.0 kcal/min) would necessitate an activity expenditure of 12.0 − 1.1 = 10.9 kcal per minute.

The report of the second FAO Committee on Calorie Requirements (1957) contained formulae for relating energy requirements to body weight; the subsequent report (1973) acknowledged that the implied accuracy of these formulae was greater than justified. Therefore, the 1973 report simply related energy requirements to body weight and tabulated them for men and women within four different categories of activity: slightly active, moderately active, very active, and exceptionally active.

Energy requirement for pregnancy

During pregnancy energy expenditure increases as a consequence of increased body weight, growth of the fetus and associated tissues, and the 20% increase in basal metabolism that occurs in the last trimester. However, not until the last third of gestation is there any appreciable increase in an animal's energy demand. During this period a 20% increase in basal metabolic rate, based on the increased weight, would result in:[*]

$$\text{Basal, nonpregnancy:}\quad 70(55_{kg}{}^{.75}) = 1{,}413 \text{ kcal/day}$$

$$\text{Basal, last trimester:}\quad 1.2 \times 70(65_{kg}{}^{.75}) = 1{,}924 \text{ kcal/day}$$

$$\text{Increased need, last trimester} = \quad 511 \text{ kcal/day}$$

Coincidental with advancing pregnancy, the mother's physical activity may be curtailed, and, under these conditions, her total caloric intake should be adjusted downward according to the decline in activity. This decrease in caloric intake may be large enough to obviate any increase in total intake.

Energy requirement for lactation

The energy requirement for lactation depends on the quantity of mik produced, its energy value, and the efficiency of conversion of metabolizable dietary energy to milk energy.

Brody and R. C. Procter studied the energy cost of milk production in cattle, using the method of partial regression.[†] They assumed that digestible energy (total digestible nutrients) is partitioned between milk production (x_1), body maintenance (x_2), and body weight gain (x_3) as expressed in the equation

$$\text{TDN consumed} = b_1(x_1 - \bar{x}_1) + b_2(x_2 - \bar{x}_2) + b_3(x_3 - \bar{x}_3)$$

From data contained in 243 yearly lactation records they derived the following partial regression values.

$$\text{TDN} = 0.305\,x_1 + 0.053\,x_2 + 2.1\,x_3$$

This says that for each pound of milk produced, 0.305 pound of TDN is required. If we accept the assumption that there are 4 kcal per gram of TDN, we calculate $454 \times 4 \times 0.305 = 553$ kcal required for each pound of milk. Cow's milk of 4% butterfat contains 340 kcal per pound; therefore, the efficiency of TDN energy in producing cow's milk is

$$100(340/553) = 61\%$$

---

[*]See also Chapter 27.

[†]Brody, S., *Bioenergetics and Growth*, Reinhold Publishing Corp., New York (1945):840.

The FAO/WHO committee has proposed that 80% efficiency be used in calculating the energy needs for human lactation. The committee assumes women produce daily an average of 850 milliliters of milk containing about 600 kcal. To produce 600 kcal of milk energy daily with an efficiency of 80% would require 750 kcal daily of metabolizable dietary energy in addition to the energy required to fulfil other needs (e.g., maintenance and activity).

It would be legitimate to estimate that each nursing woman has a daily "lactation" requirement of $(750 \times 100)/850 = 88$ (or about 90) kcal per 100 ml of milk produced.

Energy requirements of children and adolescents

The energy requirements for children and adolescents found in dietary standards originate almost exclusively from diet surveys whereas those for young animals found in feeding standards are primarily the results of feeding trial data. None of the data rests on any fundamental metabolic basis, because none is known. With humans the caloric intake of growing individuals has been recorded and classified according to age and sex, weight, and height. From these data "normal" growth curves have been plotted. From such growth curves (cumulative time–weight–age curves) a value for expected size at some specified age, and/or the expected daily gain, can be computed. The caloric intakes that will result in these normal weights or weight increases are taken as the energy requirement for individuals of that age–size category.

The caloric needs of young children and adolescents, as well as of growing animals, are usually expressed in relation to age, sex, and weight attained. Compared to the requirements of the adult of the species, on the basis of relative weight, the needs of young individuals are invariably higher; this is because of the admittedly higher "normal" activity level among young animals and their requirement for energy to fuel the growth that is still taking place.

For adolescents 16–19 years of age, whose weights may well be the same as those of adults, the daily energy needs are only slightly higher than those of the adults. Again this is because adolescents are slightly more active than adults.

Energy requirements of the elderly

The FAO/WHO committee (1973) pointed out that "the energy expenditure of adults may alter with age because of (a) changes in body weight or body composition, (b) a decrease in the basal metabolic rate, (c) a decline in physi-

cal activity, and (d) an increased prevalence of diseases and disabilities."*
Consequently, the committee recommended that energy requirements be decreased by 5% for each decade between the ages of 40 and 59 years, and by 10% from 60 to 69 years, and by another 10% beyond age 70.

---

*FAO/WHO, *Energy and Protein Requirements*, WHO Technical Report Series No. 522, World Health Organization, Geneva; or FAO Nutrition Meeting Report Series No. 52, Food and Agriculture Organization of the United Nations, Rome (1973).

Suggested readings

Bureau of Nutritional Sciences, Health Protection Branch. *Dietary Standard for Canada.* Department of National Health and Welfare, Ottawa (1975).

Consolazio, C. F., and Johnson, H. L. "Measurement of Energy Costs in Humans," *Federation Proceedings* **30**(1971):1444.

Durnin, J. V. G. A., and Passmore, R. *Energy, Work and Leisure.* Heinemann Educational Books, London (1967).

Food and Agriculture Organization/World Health Organization. *Energy and Protein Requirements.* WHO Technical Report Series No. 522, World Health Organization, Geneva, or FAO Nutrition Meeting Report Series No. 52, Food and Agriculture Organization of the United Nations, Rome (1973).

Garrow, J. S. *Energy Balance and Obesity in Man.* American Elsevier, New York (1974).

National Academy of Sciences–National Research Council. *Recommended Dietary Allowances* (8th ed.). National Academy of Sciences, Washington, D.C. (1974).

Chapter 29
Protein requirements of the body

Protein requirements for adult maintenance

Analogous to fasting energy metabolism is nitrogen catabolism, for which there is a minimal amount associated with the maintenance of the vital body processes. It is measured by the minimal urinary nitrogen excreted on a nitrogen-free, energy-adequate diet. The direct determination of "endogenous" urinary nitrogen, however, offers at least two problems. First, edible nitrogen-free diets are difficult to prepare. Second, because of its ability to utilize deposit protein, the body must endure a relatively long nitrogen-free feeding period before it attains a constant minimum of nitrogen excretion, and animals refuse nitrogen-free diets after a short period.

Endogenous urinary nitrogen and basal metabolism Both endogenous nitrogen metabolism and basal metabolism are related to body weight, and it follows that they are related to each other. This is to be expected, because each represents minimal catabolism compatible with life. The first work showing the relationship was done by E. F. Terroine. When he included endogenous urinary plus metabolic fecal nitrogen in his calculation he found that for many species 2.4 mg of nitrogen are excreted for each kilocalorie of basal metabolism. He also found the excretion to be independent of factors not related to basal metabolic rate.*

D. B. Smuts, using endogenous urinary nitrogen only, confirmed Terroine's finding that the ratio is constant from species to species, but obtained a value of 2 mg of nitrogen excretion per kilocalorie of basal metabolism.†

After examining statistically a large body of data, Brody derived two equations that appear to be applicable to all species:‡

$$\text{Kilocalories of BM} = 70.5(W_{kg}{}^{.73})$$

$$\text{Milligrams of endogenous N} = 146(W_{kg}{}^{.72})$$

The ratio between Brody's values for basal kilocalories and milligrams of endogenous urinary nitrogen is

$$\frac{146(W^{.72})}{70.5(W^{.73})} = 2.1 \text{ mg N/kcal of BM}$$

Thus, endogenous nitrogen may be estimated from data on basal metabolism.

Determining protein requirement from metabolic size   It is possible to calculate minimal nitrogen losses of adults at maintenance living:

1. Endogenous urinary nitrogen is sometimes calculated as

$$\text{Milligrams of N} = 140(W_{kg}{}^{.75})**$$

2. Metabolic fecal nitrogen, on the basis of Brody's and other data, is taken as being equal to a constant fraction of endogenous urinary nitrogen that quantitatively amounts to

    40% for carnivores and omnivores
    60% for nonruminant herbivores
    80% for ruminant herbivores

Therefore, the digestible protein of 100% biological value (BV) required daily to replace the sum of the endogenous urinary and metabolic fecal nitrogen losses would be

Carnivores and omnivores: 1.4 times endogenous urinary nitrogen

Nonruminant herbivores: 1.6 times endogenous urinary nitrogen

Ruminant herbivores: 1.8 times endogenous urinary nitrogen

---

*Terroine, E. F., *Arch. Internal Physiol.* **29**(1927):121.
†Smuts, D. B., *J. Nutr.* **9**(1935):403.
‡Brody, S., *Mo. Agri. Sta. Bull. No. 220* (1934).
**The error of about 1% from the original $146(W^{.72})$ is disregarded.

In practice Brody used a value of 50% BV for the protein of a mixed diet. With such rations the amount of digestible diet protein necessary to replace the endogenous urinary nitrogen loss would be twice the endogenous loss. The daily digestible nitrogen requirement for adult maintenance can therefore be expressed as

$$\text{Daily digestible nitrogen (mg)} = m \times q \times 140(W_{kg}^{.75})$$

where the value for m are 1.40 for humans, pigs and rats; 1.60 for horses; 1.80 for cattle and sheep; and the value for q is 2 for all species.

The requirement value is converted to protein by the conventional factor, 6.25, and to grams by dividing by 1,000. Thus, for humans or pigs:

$$\text{Digestible crude protein (g)} = \frac{1.4 \times 2 \times 140(W_{kg}^{.75}) \times 6.25}{1000}$$

$$= \frac{17.5 \times 140(W_{kg}^{.75})}{1000}$$

$$= 2.45(W_{kg}^{.75})$$

To obtain a value for dietary crude protein, it is necessary to assume a digestibility coefficient. For humans, 92% is often used:

$$\text{Dietary crude protein (g)} = \frac{2.45(W_{kg}^{.75})}{0.92} = 2.66(W_{kg}^{.75})$$

The relation between the nutritional "fractions" of dietary protein required for adult maintenance according to Brody's proposal can be shown in chart form in a manner similar to that used to show the partition of energy (see Table 29.1).

Physical activity   Table 29.1 does not provide for any protein for physical activity or work. Maintenance need is merely the amount of protein required to replace endogenous urinary loss plus metabolic fecal loss, adjusted to an assumed 50% biological value of the dietary protein. This is in accordance with the generally accepted evidence that muscular activity *per se* does not increase nitrogen catabolism (we shall mention this again in a later paragraph).

Thus, we can estimate, according to the Brody scheme, the probably daily digestible crude protein requirement (DCP) for a 65-kilogram man:

Table 29.1
Nutritional partition of dietary crude protein (at maintenance living)

Total crude protein (g),
(N × 6.25)

Metabolizable protein

Dig. crude protein (g),
$$\frac{m \times q \times 140(W^{.75}) \times 6.25}{1000}$$

- New tissue or other production
- Repair; end. nitrogen (mg) $= 140(W_{kg}^{.75})$

Loss from deamination
(50% of dig. crude protein)

Loss in dig. and met. nitrogen
Met. nitrogen $= 40\%$ of end. nitrogen for carnivores and omnivores
Met. nitrogen $= 60\%$ of end. nitrogen for nonruminant herbivores
Met. nitrogen $= 80\%$ of end. nitrogen for ruminants

$$DCP \text{ (g)} = \frac{1.4 \times 2 \times 140(65^{.75}) \times 6.25}{1000}$$

$$= 2.45(22.9)$$

$$= 56$$

If we assume a loss in digestion of 8% (an average applicable to most humans), we have 56/.92 = 61 g protein per day for a 65-kilogram adult man at maintenance living. In terms of body weight this is 0.94 g per kilogram of weight.

It now becomes clear that the generalized formula for maintenance energy requirements (Chapter 28)

$$X = abW^n$$

can also be used for calculating protein requirements (keeping in mind that a is now the product of the increase needed to cover the loss from imperfect biological value q, plus that to replace metabolic fecal loss m; and that b is milligrams of endogenous urinary nitrogen).

Determining protein requirement by nitrogen balance   The nitrogen balance method of estimating maintenance protein requirements has been the principal method used in arriving at values applied to human diets. I. Leitch and J. Duckworth conducted one of the early studies in which nitrogen equilibrium was the criterion of adequacy.*

To determine the maintenance protein requirements of an adult man, they made use of correlation and regression. Their procedure consisted of grouping all nitrogen balance tests according to whether the results showed a positive or a negative balance. They argued that although with intakes above minimum the balance in any given test may be either positive or negative, there must be:

1. A level of intake below which balances are always negative.

2. Another level of intake above which balances are always positive.

These two points of reference can be located by fitting regression lines separately to the data for trials that gave negative balances and to the data for trials that gave positive balances. Statistically, the procedure is merely plotting, for the two sets of data, intake against corresponding nitrogen output on typical mixed diets. Regression lines are then fitted to the two groups of data by the method of least squares. The values obtained by Leitch and Duckworth yielded the following equations, shown in graph form in Figure 29.1:

---

*Leitch, I., and Duckworth, J., *Nutrition Abstr. and Revs.* 7(1937):257.

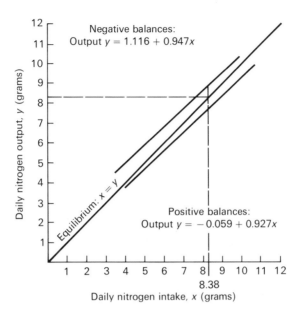

Figure 29.1
Leitch-Duckworth method of finding probable protein
requirements of adult man by correlation and regression
analysis of nitrogen balance.

$$\text{Positive balances:} \quad y = -0.059 + 0.927x$$

$$\text{Negative balances:} \quad y = 1.116 + 0.947x$$

$$\text{For equilibrium, of course:} \quad y = x$$

The level of intake at which the chances of positive or negative balance are
equal is the one of most significance, and it is indicated by the point at which
the regression line for the negative balances and that for the positive balances
are equidistant from the line of equilibrium (i.e., where $y = x$).

In the Leitch–Duckworth study, the point in question corresponded to
8.39 g of nitrogen, which is equivalent to 52.4 g of protein, and this, they
believed, represents approximately the average daily protein requirement for
equilibrium over a long period of time. It is interesting to compare the value
obtained by this method with values proposed by various other groups as the
protein requirement of adult humans (Table 29.2). Some of these have been
stated as the minimum necessary to attain nitrogen equilibrium, whereas
others are more liberal amounts that include a margin of safety in excess of
the minimum needed.

Table 29.2
Average daily protein intake recommended for adult human
as proposed by different authorities

Authority	Year	Protein (g/day)	Body weight (kg)	Grams protein per day per kg body wt
A. Minimum intake				
Bricker et al.	1945	25	65	0.38
Hegsted et al.	1946	27	70	0.38
Rose	1949	25	65	0.38
Leverton	1954	20	65	0.31
FAO/WHO	1973	22	65	0.34
B. Desirable intake				
Sherman et al.	1920	44	70	0.63
Leitch and Duckworth	1937	52	65	0.80
FAO/WHO	1973	53	65	0.82
NAS–NRC (U.S.)	1974	56	70	0.80
Canadian Dietary Standard	1975	56	70	0.80

The important things to note in Table 29.2 are the general agreement on the "minimum" figure, and the extent of the margin above this that different workers recommend for practical feeding.

The figures in Table 29.2 also suggest that nutritionists now agree on the amount of protein that should be included in the diet of adult humans. It seems fairly safe to conclude that intakes of less than about 25 g of protein per day will not maintain nitrogen equilibrium in an average-sized man (65 kg); but above this level, almost any intake up to 0.8 g per kilogram body weight would be desirable.

However, the wide variation in the biological value of different sources of protein raises some doubt that protein intakes of between 25 g and 50 g per day will consistently result in nitrogen equilibrium.

Therefore, on the basis of experimental and epidemiological observations, it would appear that to meet their maintenance needs for nitrogen, adult humans require close to 0.80 g of dietary protein per kilogram of body weight. This amounts to about 55 g of protein per day for a 65-kilogram man and about 45 g of protein per day for a 55-kilogram woman.

We can now compare this value of 55 g of protein per day for the "reference" man with that obtained using the Brody formula (p. 426).

$$\text{Adult protein requirement for maintenance (Brody)} = \frac{1.4 \times 2 \times 140(W_{kg}^{.75}) \times 6.25}{1000 \times 0.92}$$

$$= 61 \text{ g per day}$$

The difference between the values results primarily from different assumptions about the biological value of the protein ingested, which is 50% in the Brody formula.

In feeding farm animals, the determination of minimal values commensurate with nutritional adequacy is an economic necessity; with laboratory animals, such values are of experimental interest; but in human dietetics they are of little or no significance except in emergencies where the variety and/or amount of food are limited, or in the armed forces or institutions where the makeup of rations is not a matter of individual free choice. Thus it is not surprising that the most abundant and reliable data on protein needs are found in figures for species other than humans. When it becomes necessary to define human needs, it is not only possible, but also scientifically obligatory to make full use of the comparative data from all species. Any relevant figures that do not conform to the common pattern should be considered suspect and subject to critical reexamination.

Adjustment for imperfect biological value   The effect of an imperfect assortment of amino acids in the dietary protein is a demand for an increase in total protein intake sufficient to provide adequate intake of the amino acids that, because of their suboptimal concentration, limit the usefulness of the protein component of the ration. But increasing protein intake results in a "wastage" of the increasingly larger surplus of other amino acids. This reduced utilization is, by definition, expressed quantitatively in percentage figures of less than 100. For example, Brody postulated that the average dietary protein mixture has an effective biological value of about 50%.

To solve the problem of meeting the protein needs of a population group whose customary source of dietary protein has a low biological value, nutritionists have basically two choices. They can recommend an average intake of more than 55 g per day of the available protein of low biological value, which would result in wastage of the amino acids already present in sufficient amounts; or they can recommend that a daily intake of 55 g of protein be maintained, but that the biological value of the dietary protein be improved. The latter could be achieved either by introducing into the diet protein of high biological value such as milk, eggs, or fish, *or* by making use of protein sources, which themselves may not be of high biological value, but which contain amino acid assortments that are complementary to those in the customary protein source. An example of complementary supplementation would be the introduction of legumes into a basically cereal diet.

Practical level of protein intake   The Leitch and Duckworth method of dealing with published nitrogen balance data appears to produce results that can be taken as a reliable indication of what a practical or normal intake of protein should be. About 0.8 g per day per kilogram for a 65-kilogram adult is one value that has gained wide acceptance.

This value can serve as a basis for computing the desirable intakes for adults weighing in the range of 40 kg–100 kg. Sex does not affect the amount of protein required for maintenance.

The equation on page 428 makes it possible to compute values adjusted for both the weight of the individual and the biological value of the dietary protein. Representative data are presented graphically in Figure 29.2.

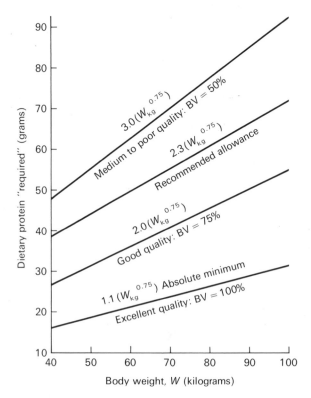

Figure 29.2
Daily protein requirements according to the size of individual and the quality of protein consumed.

Protein requirements for pregnancy and lactation   Chapter 27 discussed the extra protein required during pregnancy to meet the needs associated with not only growth of the fetus but also the increase in size of the uterus and mammary glands and the expansion of blood volume to serve these tissues. The FAO/WHO Expert Committee on Energy and Protein Requirements* suggested that the additional requirement for protein, of a quality equivalent to egg or milk, ranges from 1 g per day during the first quarter of pregnancy to 9 g per day in the last quarter. If we assume that biological value of the protein of the average North American diet is about 80% that of egg or milk, the increase in protein intake recommended during the last quarter of pregnancy is 11.25 g per day. The extra energy recommended for the same period is 350 kcal. Under normal conditions this additional energy would be met by increased consumption of the regular diet. In North America, protein supplies about 14%–16% of the kilocalories in the average diet.† Thus increased consumption of the regular diet to meet the additional 350 kcal of energy daily also will provide an additional 12 g–14 g of protein daily, which is adequate to meet the increase in intake recommended for pregnancy by the FAO/WHO committee.

Feeding standard recommendations for pregnant farm animals parallel those for pregnant women. No change is recommended in the percentage of protein in the sow's ration during pregnancy. The feeding of dairy cows during pregnancy is usually complicated by the concurrent milk production from the previous reproduction–lactation cycle. Increases in food needs for pregnancy are partly balanced by declining needs for the now declining milk yield. Furthermore, the increased calories and protein recommended for the last third to last quarter of the lactation are not made because of any demands of the current pregnancy. The committee responsible for the NAS–NRC (U.S.) 1971 Nutrient Requirements of Dairy Cattle states, "Liberal feeding during the last 2 or 3 months of gestation insures proper fetal development and adequate body condition of the cow for maximal milk production after parturition." No mention is made anywhere in this bulletin of any increased allowance because of pregnancy.

It would seem therefore that little if any change need be made in the "normal" percentage of protein in the diet to meet reproductive needs. The need for extra protein is met by the increased intake of the customary diet necessitated by the augmented requirement for energy.

Meeting the protein needs for lactation with any species of mammal is a matter of replacing the protein lost from the body in the milk secreted. With cattle the efficiency of the use of dietary protein for milk synthesis is of the

---

Energy and Protein Requirements, WHO Technical Report Series No. 522, World Health Organization, Geneva (1973).

†Beaton, G. H., and Swiss, L. D. *Am. J. Clin. Nutr.* 27 (1974):485.

order of 75%.* For each unit weight of milk protein, an estimated 1.33 units of dietary protein must be consumed.

Whatever degree of efficiency is applicable, the dietary protein necessary to meet the needs of lactation can be calculated as

$$\text{Units dietary protein} = c(\text{units milk} \times \% \text{ protein of milk})$$

where c is a constant for species and is the factor representing the increase in dietary protein needed to produce one unit protein in the milk. The following equations can be used to compute the amount of protein to be added to the daily maintenance allowance in order to meet the total daily requirement for this nutrient.

For cattle:

$$\begin{aligned}\text{Extra protein (kg)} &= 1.33(\text{kg milk} \times 0.033)\\ &= 0.044 \text{ kg per kg milk}\end{aligned}$$

For humans:

$$\begin{aligned}\text{Extra protein (g)} &= 1.33(850 \text{ g milk/day} \times 0.012)\\ &= 13.5 \text{ g/day}\end{aligned}$$

In computing the makeup of the ration or diet for lactation it must be remembered that there is also an increased energy requirement, and that this is usually met by increases in intake of the regular diet. In the average North American diet, approximately 15% of the calories is supplied by protein.† The increased energy for lactation required by most women is estimated as 550 kcal per day, from which we calculate that $(550 \times 15\%)/4 = 21$ g of extra protein (more than enough to meet the extra requirements of lactation) will come from the increase in the regular food intake to meet energy needs.

The extra protein required for each unit of milk produced by dairy cattle is negligible, providing the additional energy requirement of lactation is met by an increased intake of the regular components of the ration.

From these considerations of the protein requirements for work, pregnancy, and lactation the following conclusions can be drawn. The relation of extra protein needed to extra calories needed is about the same, quantitatively, as that in the normal maintenance rations of animals (including the human). Rather than any change in the protein-to-energy ratio, what is required is more total ration. Indeed, this is in accordance not only with biological reasoning but also with accepted and demonstrably successful feeding practice. We shall see in the next chapter that this applies, in general, to most of the nutrients normally included in the rations or diets of adults.

---

*Maynard, L. A., *Proceedings of Princeton Conference on Human Protein Requirement* (1955):129.
†Beaton, G. H., and Swiss, L. D. *Am. J. Clin. Nutr.* 27(1974):485.

Juveniles

Like the values used to represent energy needs, those for the protein requirements of growing individuals are based on amounts that appear to permit "normal" growth. Commonly accepted levels for children range from about 2.2 g down to 1.2 g per day per kilogram body weight. The ratios of protein to the probably energy requirement according to age and weight are shown in Table 29.3.

The values in Table 29.3 for the recommended grams of protein per individual per kilogram weight, and for kilocalories of metabolizable energy per day are taken from the report of the Joint FAO/WHO Expert Committee on Energy and Protein Requirements (1973); these values represent levels of intake that permit normal growth in children up to the late teens. The average body weights for the various age categories are, of course, approximate, and in practice actual weights should be used to compute specific dietary allowances.

According to these data, during the growing period there is a progressive increase in the number of grams of protein and kilocalories of metabolizable energy required per day, but if these values are expressed relative to body size, there is a progressive decrease in the protein and energy required. However, the percentage of metabolizable kilocalories from protein remains relatively constant with increasing age and body weight.

There is no satisfactory way of deriving separately the maintenance, growth, and activity components of the dietary requirements of growing subjects, although it is generally conceded that work or activity *per se* does not increase the requirement for protein.

Growing farm animals

Feeding standard data giving the requirements for growing livestock are, in the main, averages or summaries of figures from feeding trials that have been designed to establish the optimal level in the diet of energy, or of some specific nutrient, using daily gains in live weight as the principal criterion of the performance of the test animals. Usually, optimum can be defined as maximum, though in some cases, as with young dairy animals, optimum may be something less than maximum because with full feeding appreciable but undesirable fattening can also take place.

By assembling and suitably grouping the data from a large number of such feeding tests, so-called normal growth curves have been prepared for most species and breeds of farm animals. These curves become the yardsticks of acceptable rates of growth for the young of each stock. In employing the curves, agriculturalists define optimal intake as that which promotes live

Table 29.3
Protein-to-calorie ratios for juveniles

Age (years)	Body weight (kg)	Protein per day (score 70)* (g)	Protein per kg body wt (g)	Metabolizable kcals per day	Metabolizable kcals per kg wt	% Metabolizable kcals from protein
Children						
1–3	13.4	23	1.7	1,360	101.5	6.8
4–6	20.2	29	1.4	1,830	90.6	6.3
7–9	28.1	35	1.2	2,190	77.9	6.4
Male adolescents						
10–12	36.9	43	1.2	2,600	70.5	6.6
13–15	51.3	53	1.0	2,900	56.5	7.3
16–19	62.9	54	0.9	3,070	48.8	7.0
Female adolescents						
10–12	38.0	41	1.1	2,350	61.8	7.0
13–15	49.9	45	0.9	2,490	49.9	7.2
16–19	54.4	43	0.8	2,310	42.5	7.4

SOURCE: Compiled using data from FAO/WHO, *Energy and Protein Requirements*, World Health Organization Technical Report Series No. 522, Geneva, or Food and Agricultural Organization Nutrition Meeting Report Series No. 52, Rome (1973).
*Score 70 is an estimate of the quality of the protein usually consumed relative to that of egg or milk (which have a score of 100).

weight gains matching those indicated by the appropriate normal growth curve.

If the weight data shown in feeding standards for successive ages or attained weights of growing animals are plotted, it is possible to reproduce approximately the normal growth curve for that species or breed. If, in addition, the age or attained weight points of the graph are converted to a scale representing some least common denominator for several types, such as "percentage of adult weight attained," and if the nutrients are expressed as a percentage of the digestible energy required, it is possible to compare directly the nutrients required for the growth of these groups. H. R. Guilbert and J. K. Loosli have made such a study of seven kinds of mammalian farm livestock, including five species and two types within two of these species, and have stated:

> The data [for protein] for horses, dairy cattle, beef cattle, sheep, and swine are sufficiently similar to suggest that they may well be identical. The hypothesis is advanced, therefore, that the ratio of required protein to available energy is the same for various species at physiologically equivalent growth stages. The ratio changes, however, with alterations in the composition of growth increments with advancing age.*

Table 29.4 gives some figures computed from the data presented by Guilbert and Loosli.

Table 29.4
Protein requirements of growing farm animals with advancing maturity

	Percentage of mature weight attained					
Nutrient	*10*	*20*	*30*	*40*	*50*	*60*
Total digestible nutrients (TDN)	100	100	100	100	100	100
Dig. protein as % of TDN	19	15	13	11.5	10.5	10
Dig. kcal per gram TDN	440	440	440	440	440	440
Dig. kcal per gram dig. protein	23	29	34	38	42	44
Grams protein per 1,000 dig. kcal	43	34	30	27	24	23

A separate statement of the daily protein requirement of young farm animals is usually found in feeding standards, but in practice the more useful information is (1) the necessary percentage of protein in the ration (or in the meal portion of the ration of herbivores) which this represents, or (2) the

---

*Guilbert, H. R., and Loosli, J. K. *J. Animal Sci.* **10** (1951):22.

percentage of the digestible energy which should be protein. The latter appears to be the same for different species and breeds of animals, but because of differences in the digestibility of typical rations the corresponding concentration of digestible protein in the feed as fed may differ, especially between the rations of herbivores and those of nonherbivores.

For example, provision of 100 weight units of total digestible nutrients in typical rations requires for growing cattle about 160 weight units of feed, and for pigs about 133 weight units. Thus, 15% of TDN as *digestible protein* becomes 9.3% of the air dry feed of growing cattle, but 11.2% in that of pigs; comparable total crude protein percentages would be about 13% and 14%, respectively.

Suggested readings

Blaxter, K. L. "Protein Metabolism and Requirements in Pregnancy and Lactation." In *Mammalian Protein Metabolism*, Vol. II. Edited by H. N. Munro and J. B. Allison. Academic Press, New York and London (1969):173.

Bureau of Nutritional Sciences, Health Protection Branch. *Dietary Standard for Canada*. Department of National Health and Welfare, Ottawa (1975).

Food and Agricultural Organization/World Health Organization. *Energy and Protein Requirements*. WHO Technical Report Series No. 522, World Health Organization, Geneva, or FAO Nutrition Meeting Report Series No. 52, Food and Agricultural Organization of the United Nations, Rome (1973).

National Academy of Sciences–National Research Council. *Maternal Nutrition and the Course of Pregnancy*. National Academy of Sciences, Washington, D.C. (1973).

National Academy of Sciences–National Research Council. *Recommended Dietary Allowances* (8th ed.). National Academy of Sciences, Washington, D.C. (1974).

Chapter 30
Dietary and feeding standards

It is not within the scope of this book to dwell upon the specific quantities of each of the nutrients believed to be necessary components of an adequate diet or ration. Rather, it is our intention to deal with dietary and feeding standards in a general way by discussing their origin and purpose, and by examining how they should be used in practice.

According to common definition, a human dietary or farm animal feeding standard is a tabulation of the amount of energy and the quantity of each nutrient (for which there are data) believed by the author(s) of the standard to be needed daily by groups of individuals to maintain nutritional health; to permit normal growth, reproduction, synthesis of some product; and/or to perform work.

Historical development of standards

Until recently people have had few feeding guides for themselves beyond instinct and folklore. However, for their flocks and herds they have systematically observed and recorded the effects on performance of the kinds and amounts of feed offered. It is not surprising, therefore, to find that feeding standards for domestic animals appeared long before dietary standards for the human family evolved.

The first feeding standard for farm animals was proposed in 1859 by Grouven, and it included the total quantity of *protein, carbohydrate,* and *ether extract* found in feeds as determined by chemical analysis. It was based on the total rather than the digestible portion of these ration entities.

In 1864 E. Wolf published the first feeding standard based on the digestible nutrients in feeds. It gave the amounts believed to be actually needed to meet the physiological needs of the animal. W. O. Atwater in 1874 called attention in the United States to the need for animal feeding standards, and in 1880 H. P. Armsby published his *Manual of Cattle Feeding.*

Thus the beginning of "scientific" animal feeding in North America dates from 1880 and, fittingly enough, in 1917 Dr. Armsby, then Director of the Institute of Nutrition, Pennsylvania State College, was made Chairman of the United States National Academy of Sciences (NAS) Subcommittee on Protein Metabolism in Animal Feeding. In that same year, Armsby's textbook, *The Nutrition of Farm Animals,* appeared.

Two years after Armsby's Subcommittee on Protein Metabolism was organized, a Committee on Food and Nutrition was created in the new Division of Biology and Agriculture of the National Research Council (NRC), with Dr. J. R. Murlin of Rochester University as chairman. The activities of this Committee on Food and Nutrition were assigned to two subcommittees: the Subcommittee on Human Nutrition and the Subcommittee on Animal Nutrition; Armsby served as chairman of the latter.

In 1927 the NAS–NRC Committee on Food and Nutrition was discharged, and in 1928 the Subcommittee on Animal Nutrition became a full-fledged committee of the NAS–NRC Division of Biology and Agriculture with Dr. Paul E. Howe of the USDA Bureau of Animal Industry as chairman. The original Subcommittee on Human Nutrition became the NAS–NRC Food and Nutrition Board, with a Subcommittee on Dietary Allowances. Since 1940 one of the major activities of each of these committees has been the development of nutrient requirement standards for humans, and for domestic and laboratory animals. Each committee has also sponsored the preparation of extensive tables of the energy and nutrient composition of *human* foods and *animal* feedstuffs, as necessary adjuncts to the preparation of diets and rations meeting the requirements set out in feeding standards.

The Food and Nutrition Board published its first issue of *Recommended Dietary Allowances* in 1941, and revised it in 1943, 1945, 1948, 1953, 1958, 1964, 1968, and 1974.

The Committee on Animal Nutrition began publishing the *Recommended Nutrient Allowances for Farm Animals* in 1944, with separate reports for each of the major classes of farm livestock and for poultry. In 1953 this committee decided that all future reports would be designated as *Nutrient Requirements* for each of the species. These reports are revised periodically, and at present there are reports available on the nutrient requirements of

Dairy cattle   Rabbits
Beef cattle   Poultry
Sheep   Dogs
Swine   Laboratory animals
Horses   Mink and foxes
Trout, salmon, and catfish

Philosophy and purpose of human dietary and livestock feeding standards

Both human dietary standards and livestock feeding standards serve as a basis for the formulation of food rules or rules-of-thumb for feeding. Indeed it is in these abbreviated forms that standards actually serve the general public or livestock feeder as guides to both the selection of proper foods or feed, and the determination of adequate diet or ration allowances.

Feeding standards for livestock are important determinants of the formulation of rations for farm animals and poultry, and the rationale for their existence is thus primarily economic. Nutritional well-being in livestock is likely to be related either to the rate of growth of young animals destined within a few weeks or at most a few months to become human food, or to the milk- or egg-producing capacity of adults for periods of up to 10 years. Efficiency of food conversion in these functions is intimately dependent on the nutrient balances of the rations. Because the efficient conversion of feedstuffs into eggs, milk, and meat is almost as important to a nation as it is to individual livestock producers, governments have traditionally sponsored the continuous review, expansion, and revision of livestock and poultry feeding standards.

The intakes recommended in livestock feeding standards represent actual requirements derived directly from experimental data on amounts found to be adequate for normal growth, health, and productivity. In fact, the Committee on Animal Nutrition of the National Research Council (U.S.) decided in 1953 to change their designation from "recommended nutrient allowances" to "nutrient requirements." Inherent in this decision was the abandonment of their earlier policy of including "margins of safety." Thus all revisions of the NRC publications setting forth "nutrient requirements for livestock and poultry" since 1953 have been based on *average levels* found necessary to achieve normal health, growth, and productivity. Changes in these "nutrient requirements" are made only as new experimental findings become available.

On the other hand, human dietary standards are primarily intended to serve as goals in planning food supplies for *population groups* and as guides for the interpretation of food consumption records of *groups of people*. It is important to note that the daily nutrient intakes contained in human dietary standards are *recommended intakes considered, in the opinion of the committee, as adequate for the maintenance of health of nearly all persons for whom the standard is intended.* Thus human dietary standards are designed to meet the physiological needs of practically all persons in a population and, with the exception of recommendations for energy intake, exceed average requirements by amounts judged necessary to meet the needs of those individuals in any population group who in fact have particularly high requirements. Although dietary standards stipulate allowances that are in general higher than average requirements, it should be kept in mind that these requisite allowances are lower than the amounts of various nutrients that may be needed under pathological conditions or in rehabilitation following depletion.

Because human health is a major concern of all nations, it is not surprising to find that virtually all dietary standards are sponsored by governments or international agencies.

Box 30.1   Lord Boyd Orr and world food problems

John Boyd Orr (1880–1971), born in Ayrshire, Scotland, lived a long and productive life, and is remembered as a true humanitarian whose consuming passion was the nutritional well-being of the human race.

His university years resulted in degrees in Arts, Science, and Medicine between the years 1903 and 1914. His better-known honors include the following: Nobel Peace Laureate, Chancellor of Glasgow University, first Director-General of the Food and Agricultural Organization of the United Nations, first Director of the Rowett Research Institute, originator and elder statesman of the World Food Council, and first President of the British Nutrition Society. John Boyd Orr was knighted in 1935.

At the age of sixty-nine, he resigned his position as Director-General of the FAO and his peerage to become Lord Boyd Orr of Brechin. At this time, like Malthus centuries before him, he was most concerned with the impact of an ever-expanding world population whose rate of growth was outpacing the increase in world food resources. He warned that unless immediate and concerted action was taken to bring the world's food production into balance with its increasing population, world famine would eventually result.

As a physician and scientist, John Boyd Orr's concerns with the nutritional problems of both humans and domestic animals were borne out by the nature of his own and his colleagues' research efforts during his tenure as Director of the Rowett Research Institute in Aberdeen. This research included studies on min-

Traditionally, the purpose of dietary standards has been to:

1. Assess the adequacy of diets of population groups and of national food supplies.

2. Provide basic information for establishing national production and consumption policies, and for planning programs to achieve adequate and equitable distribution of food supplies.

3. Assist in the planning of diets for population groups.

4. Provide reference information for the epidemiological study of nutritional deficiencies.

More recently, the purpose of dietary standards has been extended to include such functions as appropriate guidelines for the development of new products, nutritional labeling, and the regulation of nutritional quality in food products.

---

erals, vitamins, milk, meat, and wool, as well as on the relationship of nutrition to immunity.

More relevant to this chapter, however, was Boyd Orr's involvement in dietary surveys in the United Kingdom. The first of the larger dietary surveys with which he was associated examined 607 families in 7 cities and towns in Scotland. He also initiated the large-scale Carnegie U.K. Dietary Survey. This and an earlier demonstration (supported by the Empire Marketing Board) of the value of milk for school children were of great benefit to the dairy industry and to school children in the U.K. The application of newer knowledge of nutrition to such dietary surveys led Boyd Orr to publish his classic report on *Food, Health and Income.*

During World War II, Boyd Orr organized a national food policy based on nutritional needs, giving priority to the protective foods required to maintain the health of women and children. Sir David Cuthbertson described the outcome of that program as follows:

> The result was that we emerged as a nation from the war in better nutritional state than when we entered it. The poor had more and better-balanced food; the wealthy had no surfeit and consequently were in better health.

Obviously, Lord Boyd Orr knew the value of dietary standards and how to apply them under very practical conditions.

For further information, see *J. Nutr.* **105**(1975):519.

A human dietary standard—practical application

An example of a human dietary standard, Table 30.1 reproduces daily dietary allowances recommended by the Food and Nutrition Board of the National Academy of Sciences–National Research Council in 1974.

Examination of this table reveals that recommended daily dietary allowances are provided for energy, protein, three fat-soluble vitamins, seven water-soluble vitamins, and six minerals. In addition, the standard distinguishes two age and weight groups of infants, three age and weight groups of children, male and female adolescents (11–14 years), four categories of adulthood according to age and weight for both sexes, and finally, pregnant and lactating females.

Except for the recommended allowances for pregnancy and lactation, all values given for adults are for maintenance living at the particular stage of development indicated and at a level of activity classified as light. If activity or work is carried out at a level that can be classified as moderate or heavy (e.g., at a level that expends more than 2.5 kcal per minute), additional allowances for energy must be made according to the actual energy expenditure of the activity being undertaken (see Table 28.7).

Although it was emphasized earlier that human dietary standards can be applied to populations or groups of people with greater validity than to individuals, we will illustrate the potential use of the data in Table 30.1 by showing how it can be applied to an 8-month-old infant weighing 10 kilograms; a 13-year-old boy weighing 42 kilograms; and a 24-year-old woman weighing 58 kilograms and nursing a baby.

The infant falls, of course, in the 0.5–1.0-year age group, and hence his or her recommended daily allowance for

1. energy is 10 kg × 108 = 1080 kcal;

2. protein is 10 kg × 2.0 = 20 g.

All other nutrients can be read directly from the table.

The adolescent boy falls in the age group of 11–14 years (males) and his weight is close enough to the average (44 kg) that no further adjustments are required. Hence his recommended daily allowance for energy, protein, and all other nutrients can be read directly from the table.

The nursing woman falls in the age group of 23–50 years (females) and her weight is identical to the average given for this group. Her recommended daily allowance for

1. energy is 2000 kcal + 500 kcal = 2500 kcal;

2. protein is 46 g + 20 g = 66 g;

3. niacin is 13 mg + 4 mg = 17 mg;

4. riboflavin is 1.2 mg + 0.5 mg = 1.7 mg;

5. thiamin is 1.0 mg + 0.3 mg = 1.3 mg.

All other nutrients can be read directly from the table.

If this infant, this boy, and this woman all had requirements that were in fact higher than the averages for individuals in their categories, then the specific daily allowances shown above would be quite applicable. However, if their actual requirements were average or lower than average for their categories, the specific daily allowances recommended would exceed their actual needs.

Thus the normal application of human dietary standards results in a certain degree of overnutrition. However, in dealing with humans, nutritionists have opted to sacrifice efficiency in favor of adequately nourishing the upper extremes of each population category. Conversely, in the philosophy guiding the feeding of domestic animals, efficiency is the crucial consideration.

A livestock feeding standard—practical application

The NAS–NRC (U.S.) 1973 publication, *Nutrient Requirements of Swine*, will serve as our example of a livestock feeding standard. The daily nutrient requirements specified by the NRC Subcommittee on Swine Nutrition for growing pigs and for breeding stock are reproduced in Tables 30.2 and 30.3.

The tables list daily requirements for: digestible energy, metabolizable energy, and crude protein; four inorganic nutrients (with sodium and chlorine given simply as salt for breeding swine); ten vitamins for growing swine and eight for breeding stock (with vitamin A requirements being stated as both β-carotene and vitamin A for both classes); and the ten amino acids essential for swine. Requirements for these nutrients are given for five weight classifications (from 5 kg to 100 kg liveweight) for growing swine (Table 30.2) and for six categories of breeding stock (Table 30.3). However, daily nutrient requirements for bred gilts and sows are identical. The tables also specify the intakes of corn-based diets that will meet the requirements set out in these tables.

Feeding standards for livestock are statements of the average nutrient requirements of groups of animals. Because livestock feeding standards are used extensively in formulating rations, the standards also give the nutrient requirements of swine on the basis of amount per kilogram of diet. Examples of the amounts per kilogram of each nutrient that must be provided in a corn-based diet in order to meet the daily requirements of growing and breeding stock are presented in Tables 30.4 and 30.5. It will be noted that the same weight groups are used in Table 30.4 as in Table 30.2, but that only three diets are outlined in Table 30.5 to provide the daily nutrient requirements for

Table 30.1
Example of a human dietary standard—Recommended Daily Dietary Allowances

	Age (years)	Weight (kg)	Weight (lbs)	Height (cm)	Height (in)	Energy (kcal)*	Protein (g)	Water-Soluble Vitamins Ascorbic Acid (mg)	Folacin† (µg)	Niacin†† (mg)	Riboflavin (mg)	Thiamin (mg)	Vitamin B_6 (mg)	Vitamin B_{12} (µg)
Infants	0.0–0.5	6	14	60	24	kg × 117	kg × 2.2	35	50	5	0.4	0.3	0.3	0.3
	0.5–1.0	9	20	71	28	kg × 108	kg × 2.0	35	50	8	0.6	0.5	0.4	0.3
Children	1–3	13	28	86	34	1,300	23	40	100	9	0.8	0.7	0.6	1.0
	4–6	20	44	110	44	1,800	30	40	200	12	1.1	0.9	0.9	1.5
	7–10	30	66	135	54	2,400	36	40	300	16	1.2	1.2	1.2	2.0
Males	11–14	44	97	158	63	2,800	44	45	400	18	1.5	1.4	1.6	3.0
	15–18	61	134	172	69	3,000	54	45	400	20	1.8	1.5	2.0	3.0
	19–22	67	147	172	69	3,000	54	45	400	20	1.8	1.5	2.0	3.0
	23–50	70	154	172	69	2,700	56	45	400	18	1.6	1.4	2.0	3.0
	51+	70	154	172	69	2,400	56	45	400	16	1.5	1.2	2.0	3.0
Females	11–14	44	97	155	62	2,400	44	45	400	16	1.3	1.2	1.6	3.0
	15–18	54	119	162	65	2,100	48	45	400	14	1.4	1.1	2.0	3.0
	19–22	58	128	162	65	2,100	46	45	400	14	1.4	1.1	2.0	3.0
	23–50	58	128	162	65	2,000	46	45	400	13	1.2	1.0	2.0	3.0
	51+	58	128	162	65	1,800	46	45	400	12	1.1	1.0	2.0	3.0
Pregnant						+300	+30	60	800	+2	+0.3	+0.3	2.5	4.0
Lactating						+500	+20	80	600	+4	+0.5	+0.3	2.5	4.0

		Fat-Soluble Vitamins				Minerals					
Age (years)	Vitamin A Activity (RE)§	(IU)	Vitamin D (IU)	Vitamin E Activity (IU)‡‡	Calcium (mg)	Phosphorus (mg)	Iodine (µg)	Iron (mg)	Magnesium (mg)	Zinc (mg)
Infants										
0.0–0.5	120‡	1,400	400	4	360	240	35	10	60	3
0.5–1.0	400	2,000	400	5	540	400	45	15	70	5
Children										
1–3	400	2,000	400	7	800	800	60	15	150	10
4–6	500	2,500	400	9	800	800	80	10	200	10
7–10	700	3,300	400	10	800	800	110	10	250	10
Males										
11–14	1,000	5,000	400	12	1,200	1,200	130	18	350	15
15–18	1,000	5,000	400	15	1,200	1,200	150	18	400	15
19–22	1,000	5,000	400	15	800	800	140	10	350	15
23–50	1,000	5,000		15	800	800	130	10	350	15
51+	1,000	5,000		15	800	800	110	10	350	15
Females										
11–14	800	4,000	400	12	1,200	1,200	115	18	300	15
15–18	800	4,000	400	12	1,200	1,200	115	18	300	15
19–22	800	4,000	400	12	800	800	100	18	300	15
23–50	800	4,000		12	800	800	100	18	300	15
51+	800	4,000		12	800	800	80	10	300	15
Pregnant	1,000	5,000	400	15	1,200	1,200	125	18+**	450	20
Lactating	1,200	6,000	400	15	1,200	1,200	150	18	450	25

SOURCE: Reproduced with permission of the National Academy of Sciences from NAS–NRC (U.S.), *Recommended Dietary Allowances* (8th ed.), National Academy of Sciences–National Research Council, Washington, D.C. (1974).

NOTE: The allowances are intended to provide for individual variations among most normal persons as they live in the United States under usual environmental stresses. Diets should be based on a variety of common foods in order to provide other nutrients for which human requirements have been less well defined.

*Kilojoules (kJ) = 4.2 × kcal.

†The folacin allowances refer to dietary sources as determined by *Lactobacillus casei* assay. Pure forms of folacin may be effective in doses less than one-fourth of the recommended dietary allowance.

††Although allowances are expressed as niacin, it is recognized that on the average 1 mg of niacin is derived from each 60 mg of dietary tryptophan.

§Retinol equivalents.

‡Assumed to be all as retinol in milk during the first six months of life. As retinol equivalents, three-fourths are as retinol and one-fourth as β-carotene when calculated from international units. As retinol equivalents, α-tocopherol and 20 percent other tocopherols.

‡‡Total vitamin E activity, estimated to be 80 percent as α-tocopherol and 20 percent other tocopherols.

**This increased requirement cannot be met by ordinary diets; therefore, the use of supplemental iron is recommended.

[447]

Table 30.2
Example of a livestock feeding standard—Daily Nutrient Requirements of Growing Swine

Liveweight (kg):	5–10	10–20	20–35	35–60	60–100
Feed Intake (air-dry) (g):	600	1,250	1,700	2,500	3,500
Nutrients	*Requirements*				
Energy and protein*					
Digestible energy (kcal)	2,100	4,370	5,610	8,250	11,550
Metabolizable energy (kcal)	2,020	4,200	5,390	7,920	11,090
Crude protein (g)	132	225	272	350	455
Inorganic nutrients (g)					
Calcium	4.8	8.1	11.0	12.5	17.5
Phosphorus	3.6	6.3	8.5	10.0	14.0
Sodium	——	1.3	1.7	——	——
Chlorine	——	1.6	2.2	——	——
Vitamins					
Beta-carotene† (mg)	2.6	4.4	4.4	6.5	9.1
Vitamin A (IU)	1,300	2,200	2,200	3,250	4,550
Vitamin D (IU)	132	250	340	312	437
Vitamin E (mg)	6.6	13.8	18.7	27.5	38.5
Thiamin (mg)	0.8	1.4	1.9	2.8	3.9
Riboflavin (mg)	1.8	3.8	4.4	5.5	7.7
Niacin‡ (mg)	13.2	22.5	23.8	25.0	35.0
Pantothenic acid (mg)	7.8	13.8	18.7	27.5	38.5
Vitamin B_6 (mg)	0.9	1.9	1.9	——	——
Choline (mg)	660	1,125	——	——	——
Vitamin B_{12} (μg)	13.2	18.8	18.7	27.5	38.5
Amino acids (g)					
Arginine	1.6	2.8	3.4	4.4	5.7
Histidine	1.5	2.5	3.1	3.9	5.1
Isoleucine	4.1	7.0	8.5	10.9	14.2
Leucine	5.0	8.4	10.2	13.1	17.1
Lysine	5.8	9.8	11.9	15.3	19.9
Methionine + cystine§	4.1	7.0	8.5	10.9	14.2
Phenylalanine + tyrosine††	4.1	7.0	8.5	10.9	14.2
Threonine	3.7	6.3	7.6	9.8	12.8
Tryptophan	1.1	1.8	2.2	2.8	3.7
Valine	4.1	7.0	8.5	10.9	14.2

Source: Reproduced with permission of the National Academy of Sciences from NAS–NRC (U.S.), *Nutrient Requirements of Swine* (7th ed.), National Academy of Sciences–National Research Council, Washington, D.C. (1973).

*These suggested energy levels are derived from corn-based diets. When barley or medium- or low-energy grains are fed, these energy levels will not be met. Formulations based on barley or similar grains are satisfactory for pigs weighing 20–100 kg, but feed conversion will normally be reduced with the lower-energy diets.

These are approximate protein levels required to meet the essential amino acid needs. If cereal grains other than corn are used, an increase of 1 or 2 percent of protein may be required.

†Carotene and vitamin A values are based on 1 mg of beta-carotene equaling 500 IU of biologically active vitamin A. Vitamin A requirements can be met by carotene or vitamin A or both.

‡It is assumed that all the niacin in the cereal grains and their by-products is in a bound form and thus is largely unavailable.

§Methionine can fulfill the total requirements; cystine can meet at least 50 percent of the total requirment.

††Phenylalanine can fulfill the total requirement; tyrosine can fulfill 30 pecent of the requirments.

[448]

Table 30.3
Example of a livestock feeding standard—Daily Nutrient Requirement of Breeding Swine

Nutrients	Bred Gilts	Bred Sows	Lactating Gilts	Lactating Sows	Young Boars	Adult Boars
Liveweight (kg):*	110–160	160–250	140–200	200–250	110–180	180–250
Feed Intake (air-dry)(g):	2,000	2,000	5,000	5,500	2,500	2,000
	Requirements					
Energy and protein						
Digestible energy (kcal)	6,600	6,600	16,500	18,150	8,250	6,600
Metabolizable energy (kcal)	6,340	6,340	15,840	17,420	7,920	6,340
Crude protein (g)	280	280	750	825	350	280
Inorganic nutrients (g)						
Calcium	15.0	15.0	37.5	41.2	18.8	15.0
Phosphorus	10.0	10.0	25.0	27.5	12.5	10.0
NaCl (salt)	10.0	10.0	25.0	27.5	12.5	10.0
Vitamins						
Beta-carotene (mg)	16.4	16.4	33.0	36.3	20.5	16.4
Vitamin A (IU)	8,200	8,200	16,500	18,150	10,250	8,200
Vitamin D (IU)	550	550	1,100	1,210	690	550
Vitamin E (mg)	22.0	22.0	55.0	60.5	27.5	22.0
Thiamin (mg)	3.0	3.0	5.0	5.5	3.8	3.0
Riboflavin (mg)	8.0	8.0	17.5	19.3	10.0	8.0
Niacin (mg)	44.0	44.0	87.5	96.3	55.0	44.0
Pantothenic acid (mg)	33.0	33.0	65.0	71.5	41.3	33.0
Vitamin B_{12} (μg)	28.0	28.0	55.0	60.5	35.0	28.0
Amino acids (g)						
Arginine	—	—	17.0	18.7		
Histidine	4.0	4.0	13.0	14.3		
Isoleucine	7.4	7.4	33.5	36.9		
Leucine	13.2	13.2	46.4	51.0		
Lysine	8.4	8.4	30.0	33.0	†	‡
Methionine + cystine	5.6	5.6	18.0	19.8		
Phenylalanine + tyrosine	10.4	10.4	46.9	51.6		
Threonine	6.8	6.8	25.5	28.1		
Tryptophan	1.4	1.4	6.5	7.2		
Valine	9.2	9.2	34.0	37.4		

SOURCE: Reproduced with permission of the National Academy of Sciences from NAS–NRC (U.S.), *Nutrient Requirements of Swine* (7th ed.), National Academy of Sciences–National Research Council, Washington, D.C. (1973).
*Expected daily gain for bred gilts is 0.35 kg–0.45 kg; for bred sows, 0.15 kg–0.30 kg; and for young boars, 0.25 kg–0.45 kg.
†Data unavailable; intakes 25 percent greater than those of bred gilts are suggested as adequate.
‡Data unavailable; intakes equal to those of bred sows are suggested as adequate.

Table 30.4
Example of a livestock feeding standard—Nutrient Requirements of Growing Swine expressed as amounts per unit of diet

Liveweight (kg):	5–10	10–20	20–35	35–60	60–100
Daily Gain (kg):	*0.30*	*0.50*	*0.60*	*0.75*	*0.90*
Nutrients	*Requirements*				
Energy and protein					
Digestible energy* (kcal)	3,500	3,500	3,300	3,300	3,300
Metabolizable energy* (kcal)	3,360	3,360	3,170	3,170	3,170
Crude protein† (%)	22	18	16	14	13
Inorganic nutrients (%)					
Calcium	0.80	0.65	0.65	0.50	0.50
Phosphorus	0.60	0.50	0.50	0.40	0.40
Sodium	——	0.10	0.10	——	——
Chlorine	——	0.13	0.13	——	——
Vitamins					
Beta-carotene (mg)	4.4	3.5	2.6	2.6	2.6
Vitamin A (IU)	2,200	1,750	1,300	1,300	1,300
Vitamin D (IU)	220	200	200	125	125
Vitamin E (mg)	11	11	11	11	11
Thiamin (mg)	1.3	1.1	1.1	1.1	1.1
Riboflavin (mg)	3.0	3.0	2.6	2.2	2.2
Niacin‡ (mg)	22.0	18.0	14.0	10.0	10.0
Pantothenic acid (mg)	13.0	11.0	11.0	11.0	11.0
Vitamin B_6 (mg)	1.5	1.5	1.1	——	——
Choline (mg)	1,100	900	——	——	——
Vitamin B_{12} (μg)	22	15	11	11	11
Amino acids (%)					
Arginine	0.28	0.23	0.20	0.18	0.16
Histidine	0.25	0.20	0.18	0.16	0.15
Isoleucine	0.69	0.56	0.50	0.44	0.41
Leucine	0.83	0.68	0.60	0.52	0.48
Lysine	0.96	0.79	0.70	0.61	0.57
Methionine + cystine§	0.69	0.56	0.50	0.44	0.41
Phenylalanine + tyrosine††	0.69	0.56	0.50	0.44	0.41
Threonine	0.62	0.51	0.45	0.39	0.37
Tryptophan	0.18	0.15	0.13	0.11	0.11
Valine	0.69	0.56	0.50	0.44	0.41

SOURCE: Reproduced with permission of the National Academy of Sciences from NAS–NRC (U.S.), *Nutrient Requirements of Swine* (7th ed.), National Academy of Sciences–National Research Council, Washington, D.C. (1973).

*These suggested energy levels are derived from corn-based diets. When barley or medium- or low-energy grains are fed, these energy levels will not be met. Formulations based on barley or similar grains are satisfactory for pigs weighing 20 kg–100 kg, but feed conversion will normally be reduced with the lower-energy diets.

†Approximate protein levels required to meet the essential amino acid needs. If cereal grains other than corn are used, an increase of 1 or 2 percent of protein may be required.

‡It is assumed that all the niacin in the cereal grains and their by-products is in a bound form and thus is largely unavailable.

§Methionine can fulfill the total requirement; cystine can meet at least 50 percent of the total requirement.

††Phenylalanine can fulfill the total requirement; tyrosine can fulfill 30 percent of the total requirement.

Table 30.5
Example of a livestock feeding standard—Nutrient Requirements of Breeding Swine
expressed as amounts per unit of diet

	Bred Gilts and Sows	Lactating Gilts and Sows	Young and Adult Boars
Liveweight (kg):	110–250	140–250	110–250
Nutrients	Requirements		
Energy and protein			
Digestible energy (kcal)	3,300	3,300	3,300
Metabolizable energy (kcal)	3,170	3,170	3,170
Crude protein (%)	14	15	14
Inorganic nutrients (%)			
Calcium	0.75	0.75	0.75
Phosphorus	0.50	0.50	0.50
NaCl (salt)	0.5	0.5	0.5
Vitamins			
Beta-carotene (mg)	8.2	6.6	8.2
Vitamin A (IU)	4,100	3,300	4,100
Vitamin D (IU)	275	220	275
Vitamin E (mg)	11.0	11.0	11.0
Thiamin (mg)	1.5	1.0	1.5
Riboflavin (mg)	4.0	3.5	4.0
Niacin (mg)	22.0	17.5	22.0
Pantothenic acid (mg)	16.5	13.0	16.5
Vitamin B_{12} (μg)	14.0	11.0	14.0
Amino acids (%)			
Arginine	—	0.34	
Histidine	0.20 [*]	0.26	
Isoleucine	0.37	0.67	
Leucine	0.66 [*]	0.99	
Lysine	0.42	0.60	
Methionine + cystine	0.28	0.36	[†] [‡]
Phenylalanine + tyrosine	0.52 [*]	1.00	
Threonine	0.34	0.51	
Tryptophan	0.07	0.13	
Valine	0.46	0.68	

SOURCE: Reproduced with permission of the National Academy of Sciences from NAS–NRC (U.S.), *Nutrient Requirements of Swine* (7th ed.), National Academy of Sciences–National Research Council, Washington, D.C. (1973).
[*]This level is adequate; the minimum requirement has not been established.
[†]All suggested requirements for lactation are based on the requirement for maintenance + amino acids produced in milk by sows fed 5 kg–5.5 kg of feed per day from which amino acids are 80 percent available.
[‡]No data available; it is suggested that the requirements will not exceed that of bred gilts and sows.

the six classes of breeding stock given in Table 30.3. The fact that only three diets are needed for breeding stock stems from the fact that the levels of all nutrients relative to energy are the same for bred gilts and sows, for lactating gilts and sows, and for young and adult boars.

Let us consider specific examples of how a feed manufacturer would use this information in the formulation of swine rations. Suppose that a farmer required feed for 100 weanling pigs, 35 days of age; 100 growing pigs averaging 75 kg liveweight; and 20 lactating sows.

Pigs weaned at 35 days of age would usually fall in the 10 kg–20 kg group of growing swine. Pigs of this weight gain an average of 0.50 kg daily (Table 30.4) and consume an average of 1,250 g of feed per day (Table 30.2). The amount of a corn-based diet needed for these 100 weanling pigs is 2,500 kg:

$$(10 \div 0.5) \times 1.25 \times 100 = 2500 \text{ kg}$$

The feed manufacturer would simply formulate 2,500 kg of diet containing the levels of nutrients listed for 10 kg–20 kg swine in Table 30.4. This amount of feed would be sufficient to carry this group of pigs into the next weight category of 20 kg–35 kg.

Growing pigs weighing 75 kg consume approximately 3.5 kg per day of a corn-based diet. Thus approximately 5,000 kg of diet would be needed to supply the feed requirements for this group of pigs for two weeks:

$$3.5 \times 100 \times 14 = 4900 \text{ kg}$$

In this case the feed manufacturer would formulate 5,000 kg of diet containing the levels of nutrients specified for 60 kg–100 kg swine in Table 30.4.

Twenty lactating sows would require 2,300 kg of a corn-based diet over a two-week period:

$$5.5 \times 20 \times 14 = 2310 \text{ kg}$$

The feed manufacturer would simply formulate 2,300 kg of feed according to the requirements listed for lactating gilts and sows in Table 30.5.

The diets for the weanling pigs, the 75-kg growing pigs, and the lactating sows are formulated to meet the average requirements for swine in each of these categories. Thus one would expect the diet to exceed the requirements of some pigs in each group while being under the requirements for others. However the diets should provide optimal efficiency for each *group* of swine.

If the feed manufacturer were to use a cereal other than corn—for example, barley—in the formulation of the diet for the 75-kg growing pigs, he would have to adjust the nutrient concentration in the diet on the basis of the lower energy content of barley. The rationale here is that pigs tend to eat quantities of feed that will meet their energy requirements. Because barley provides about 3,100 kcal of digestible energy per kilogram compared to approximately 3,600 kcal for corn, the feed manufacturer would reduce the *concentration* of other nutrients, except protein, by about 15 percent because the pigs will now be consuming more total feed.

The protein level in the diet, on the other hand, would probably have to be increased slightly to meet the requirements for the essential amino acids. Barley would contribute a greater proportion of the total protein than corn in a diet formulated to contain 13% protein. The protein in cereals is of a lower quality than that of most protein concentrates, such as soybean meal, and therefore more than 13% protein may be required to meet the requirements for the essential amino acids.

Most of the work in feed formulation is now done by linear programming. The nutritionist simply specifies the minimal levels of nutrients that must be provided per kilogram of diet, the ingredients available for making up the diet, the nutrient composition of these ingredients, and any restrictions that might apply to any particular ingredient (such as maximal allowable level), and the computer formulates a diet.

Limitations of human dietary standards

It has already been pointed out that human dietary standards are primarily intended to serve as goals in planning food supplies for population groups and as guides for interpreting the food consumption records of groups of people. For this reason, the data found in most human dietary standards represent not specific nutrient requirements, but rather "recommended dietary allowances." In most cases, the latter are arrived at by first determining average nutrient *requirements* from the literature, and then, to each of these, adding an arbitrary amount to cover the upper extreme of the population group.

Recommended dietary allowances, except those for energy, are therefore estimated to exceed the actual requirements of most individuals in a population. Hence, in order to adequately nourish that segment of a population group whose requirements are higher than average, the majority of individuals within the group will receive nutrients well in excess of their actual needs. This aspect of human dietary standards appears to be wasteful and inefficient; however, because we are dealing with humans and not with animals, there seems to be no good alternative to this approach at present.

Some nutritionists have criticized the recommended dietary allowance figures in dietary standards because they give no indication of the *magnitude of the safety margin included.* In other words, some nutrition researchers or teachers would like to see recommended dietary allowance figures fractionated into their two components—i.e., actual average requirement *plus* the

Box 30.2   Nutrient fortification of foods

The practice of fortifying foods with specific nutrients, sometimes called enrichment, dates back to the nineteenth century when the French chemist J. B. Boussingault recommended the addition of iodine to table salt as a prevention against goiter in South America. However, the general adoption of this practice in the United States began during World War II. Prior to 1936, only the addition of vitamin D to milk and of iodine to table salt had been approved by the Committee on Foods of the American Medical Association. The Food and Nutrition Board (then the Committee on Food and Nutrition) of the National Research Council at its first meeting in November 1940 endorsed a program calling for the addition of thiamin, riboflavin, niacin, and iron to flour. As a result of this recommendation, a standard of identity for enriched flour for the U.S. became effective on January 1, 1942. Since that time many fortification programs have been adopted not only in the U.S. but throughout the world.

Regulatory agencies, such as the Food and Drug Administration in the U.S. or the Health Protection Branch in Canada, have taken a cautious approach to the enrichment of foods. With time, however, the criteria for the enrichment of foods have been updated to correspond more closely with the needs of a technological society. Today the regulations permit or make mandatory the enrichment of foods if there is nutritional justification for such additions. Specific criteria used in establishing these regulations include: (1) evidence of an inadequate intake of a nutrient (thus iodine is added to table salt); (2) removal of a vitamin or mineral from a staple food in the course of its manufacture (thus the addition of thiamin, riboflavin, and niacin to white flour); and (3) replacement of a food normally considered an important source of the nutrient (thus vitamin A is added to margarine and ascorbic acid to fruit drinks). The best-known examples of fortification in the United States and Canada are the enrichment of white flour used in bakery products with thiamin, niacin, riboflavin, and iron; fruit beverages and noncitrus fruit drinks with L-ascorbic acid; table salt with iodine; milk, dairy products, and dairy substitutes (e.g., margarine) with vitamins A and D; and water with fluorine.

The question of nutrient fortification is still frequently debated in spite of the ample evidence that justifies fortification and despite the fact that no ill effects, except for the now-famous instance of excessive intake of vitamin D by infants, have been reported in the 50 or so years that fortification programs have been in effect. One of the principal deterrents to the fortification of foods has been the somewhat naive concept (even among some nutritionists and food scientists) that the world food supply was somehow arranged to meet the nutrient needs of humans and to tamper with the nutrient levels in foods is to contravene nature. Added to this deterrent has been the lack of distinction between nutrient fortification and the question of nonnutritive food additives.

arbitrary amount judged necessary to adequately nourish those individuals with higher-than-average needs.

In devising supplements to a diet that is inadequate, or imbalanced, or is intended for temporary use in disaster situations, the person responsible for defining such additions obviously needs some guide to the actual overall daily requirement of the group consuming the diet.

One obstacle to the widespread use of human dietary standards in the feeding of the normal human population is undoubtedly that they are not stated in "ready-to-use" terms; they require translation to make them fit a particular case. Thus people must have access to such derived feeding guides as *Canada's Food Guide* or the U.S. *Food for Fitness—A Daily Food Guide*,* which provide practical interpretations of dietary standards.

Unfortunately, human dietary standards seldom have any important *direct* bearing on what people buy or prepare to feed their families. Custom, habit, prejudice, erroneous beliefs, and finances all affect their choices so that it is only with difficulty that human beings can be induced to alter their dietary habits for nutritional reasons. Indeed it would hardly be worth the effort and cost of assembling a reliable, nutritionally sound dietary standard for human use if it had no purpose other than as an everyday guide to food selection.

Although recommended daily allowances for energy and the various nutrients are of little direct value to the general public as they appear in dietary standards, they are useful guides to practicing nutritionists and dietitians who recommend food policies, order food supplies, or assemble meals for population groups.

Limitations of livestock feeding standards

As mentioned previously, the NAS–NRC (U.S.) feeding standards for livestock are designated as "nutrition requirements." The recommendations contained in these publications are based principally on experimental data and represent the average intakes considered adequate for normal growth, health, reproduction, and production of groups of animals. Because livestock feeding standards are based on experimental evidence, they present information only for those nutrients for which quantitative data are available. The daily nutrient requirements for swine presented in Tables 30.2 and 30.3 summarize the entire recommendations of the Subcommittee on Swine Nutrition, with the exception of minimal information on trace minerals. Although feeding standards are intended as up-to-date guides which merit wide applications by producers and feed manufacturers, their use in practical feeding operations

---

*Hertzler, A. A., and Anderson, H. L., *J. Am. Diet. Assoc.* **64**(1974):19.

requires interpretation in terms of conditions prevailing at a particular instant.

For example, no safety factor has been intentionally added in drawing up current livestock feeding standards. Thus in applying these standards some margin of safety may have to be added to take care of particular stress conditions. The amount of nutrient to be added will vary with the nutrient and with the conditions that make the increased intake necessary. Relationships among nutrients also must be borne in mind when nutrient intakes are modified, because changing the level of one nutrient frequently alters the requirement for or availability of another.

In addition, economic considerations affect practical feeding operations. Although feeding standards give the average nutrient requirements found adequate for normal health and performance of a group of animals, modifications may be called for to generate the rate of weight gain or level of egg or milk production that is most economical in view of the prevailing cost of feed and the market price of the products being produced. These modifications may even take into account the effect of specific nutrient intake level on such characteristics as carcass quality or butterfat content of milk.

Feeding standards are only partial guides to the formulation of rations. They give no indication of the combination or combinations of feedstuffs that will supply the nutrient requirements specified. Although the NRC publications on the nutrient requirements of domestic animals give the approximate nutrient composition of feeds commonly used in rations for the species in question, there is no information on the availability of nutrients from the various feedstuffs. The nutrient requirements given in Tables 30.4 and 30.5 as a percentage or amount per kilogram of diet assume optimal availability of the nutrients. Nutritionists are aware that this situation does not always prevail. Factors such as palatability and the physical nature of the ration also influence the effectiveness of a ration. Finally, antibiotics and other drugs are frequently administered through the feed; thus nutritionists have the responsibility of adjusting nutrient intakes to compensate for known or suspected drug–nutrient interactions.

Livestock feeding standards are useful guides to ration formulation only when interpreted in terms of end use.

Interpretation of dietary or feeding standards

It must be stressed once more that dietary or feeding standards should be used primarily as guides applied to fulfilling the nutritional needs of normal and healthy members of specific population groups.

Regardless of the purposes for which they are intended (e.g., determining the recommended daily allowances of nutrients for a group of adolescent boys, or the nutrient requirements of a group of pregnant sows), or the function assigned to time (e.g., calculating a hospital's food budget, or computing feed costs in a beef cattle operation), it cannot be overemphasized that it is practically impossible for a lay person to interpret dietary or feeding standards intelligently or meaningfully.

We strongly recommend that a nutritionist be consulted in the interpretation of dietary or feeding standards. For example, to select the proper food or feed ingredients to make up a diet or ration for a particular purpose, a person must know: the composition of food or feed ingredients; the food habits and food preferences in the case of humans, as well as the effect of method of food preparation on nutrient content, availability, etc.; the palatability and cost of individual ingredients used to formulate livestock rations; what effects nutrients have on each other; how drugs and nutrients interact; etc., etc.

It is well recognized that most politicians, food or feed processors, physicians, social workers, or chemists do not possess this combination of knowledge. It is, however, the responsibility of nutritionists, whether they have been trained to function in the field of human or animal nutrition, to have such knowledge and to apply it in interpreting dietary or feeding standards.

Suggested readings

Beaton, G. H. "The Use of Nutritional Requirements and Allowances." In *Proceedings Western Hemisphere Nutrition Congress III*, edited by P. L. White. Futura, Mount Kisco, New York (1972):356.

Bureau of Nutritional Sciences, Health Protection Branch. *Dietary Standard for Canada*. Department of National Health and Welfare, Ottawa (1975).

Harper A. E. "Recommended Dietary Allowances: Are They What We Think They Are?" *Journal of the American Dietetic Association* **64**(1974):151.

National Academy of Sciences–National Research Council. *Recommended Dietary Allowances* (8th ed.). National Academy of Sciences, Washington, D.C. (1974).

National Academy of Sciences–National Research Council. *Nutrient Requirements of Domestic Animals. Beef Cattle* (1971); *Dairy Cattle* (1971); *Dogs* ((1972); *Horses* (1973); *Laboratory Animals* (1972); *Mink and Foxes* (1969); *Poultry* (1971); *Rabbits* (1966); *Sheep* (1968); *Swine* (19730; *Trout, Salmon and Catfish* (1973). Published by National Academy of Sciences, Washington, D.C.

Index

QP
141
.C77
24,556
24,1

CAMROSE LUTHERAN COLLEGE
Library

CKKD

DATE DUE
DATE DE RETOUR

	DEC 0 5 1985		
NOV 0 6 '80			
MAR 0 5 '8	APR 0 7 1998		
OCT 0 7 1991	MAR 1 9 1998		
DEC 8 1982	APR 1 2 2001		
NOV 9 1983	MAR 2 6 2001		
NOV 2 3 1983	MAR 0 1 2002		
DEC 9 1983	MAR 1 1 2002		
JAN 2 6 198			
MAR 2 0 1984			
NOV 1 8 1985			
APR 0 2 1987			
DEC 2 1987			
FEB 2 5 1994			
APR - 6 1994			
DEC 0 5 1994			
DEC 0 1 1994			
NOV 1 5 1995			
12/06/95			

LOWE-MARTIN No. 1137